28TH EUROPEAN STRABISMOLOGICAL ASSOCIATION MEETING

TRANSACTIONS

28th European Strabismological Association Meeting

TRANSACTIONS

BERGEN, NORWAY, JUNE 19-21, 2003

Edited by:

Jan-Tjeerd de Faber

The Rotterdam Eye Hospital

Rotterdam, The Netherlands

CRC Press

[redacted]

Published 2004 by CRC Press
Taylor & Francis Group
6000 Broken Sound Parkway NW, Suite 300
Boca Raton, FL 3487-2742

ISBN-13: 978-90-265-1965-9 (hbk)

Visit the Taylor & Francis Web site at
http://www.taylorandfrancis.com

and the CRC Press Web site at
http://www.crcpress.com

Transactions 28th Meeting European Strabismological Association, de Faber (ed.)
© 2004 European Strabismological Association, ISBN 90 265 1965 6

Table of Contents

Session 11: Varia

Posters

Transactions 28th Meeting European Strabismological Association, de Faber (ed.)
© 2004 European Strabismological Association, ISBN 90 265 1965 6

Preface

The 28th meeting of the European Strabismological Association took place in Bergen, Norway from June 19-21 2003 as a co-production and joint meeting with the Nordic Strabismologic Association. The organizing committee performed an excellent job with this memorable, well runned, joint meeting. Although the weather gods provided rain for the entire 3 days of the meeting, the sun did shine during the post congres tour and we enjoyed a sunny "Norway in a nutshell". A special compliment is earned by our local host and organizer Dr. Olav Haugen and his staff for the excellent social program.
I would like to express my gratitude to all the authors who delivered their transaction in time. I am grateful to the Council and Membership of the ESA for having me selected as the editor of the Transactions. I would like to thank my wife Cris for her invaluable secretarial assistance and moral support.

Jan-Tjeerd de Faber, editor
Rotterdam, July 2003

Transactions 28th Meeting European Strabismological Association, de Faber (ed.)

Executive Committee of the European Strabismological Association

Until June 16th 2003

M. SPIRITUS	BELGIUM	PRESIDENT
J.T. de FABER	THE NETHERLANDS	VICE-PRESIDENT
R. FROSINI	ITALY	VICE-PRESIDENT
A. PECHEREAU	FRANCE	VICE-PRESIDENT
V. HERZAU	GERMANY	SECRETARY/TREASURER
O.H. HAUGEN	NORWAY	COUNCILLOR
S.B. ÖZKAN	TURKEY	COUNCILLOR
G. KLAINGUTI	SWITZERLAND	COUNCILLOR
J.T. de FABER	THE NETHERLANDS	EDITOR

After June 16th 2003

M. SPIRITUS	BELGIUM	
S.B. ÖZKAN	TURKEY	VICE-PRESIDENT
J. LEE	UNITED KINGDOM	VICE-PRESIDENT
A. PECHEREAU	FRANCE	VICE-PRESIDENT
C. SCHIAVI	ITALY	SECRETARY/TREASURER
O.H. HAUGEN	NORWAY	COUNCILLOR
R. LIANO de GOMEZ	SPAIN	COUNCILLOR
H.D. SCHWORM	GERMANY	COUNCILLOR
J.T. de FABER	THE NETHERLANDS	EDITOR

Transactions 28th Meeting European Strabismological Association, de Faber (ed.)
© 2004 European Strabismological Association, ISBN 90 265 1965 6

ESA meeting organization 2003

Scientific Committee

J.P. Lee
A. Pechereau
L. Lindberg
O.H. Haugen

Local Organizer

O.H. Haugen

Transactions 28th Meeting European Strabismological Association, de Faber (ed.)
© 2004 European Strabismological Association, ISBN 90 265 1965 6

Obituary Professor Krystyna Michalina Krzystek-Walka

1924-2002

On 11th July 2002 professor Krystyna Krzystek-Walka PhD died in Cracow. Michalina Krzystek was born in 1924 in Cracow, Poland. She passed her maturation exams (in the Polish wartime underground education system) in Cracow in 1944. That same year she and her mother were arrested by the Gestapo and sent to Ravensbruck concentration camp. After liberation she was transported to Sweden, from where she returned to Poland in 1947 but continued to uphold contacts, both private and academic, with Sweden for the rest of her life.

Between 1947-1952 she studied medicine at the Medical Faculty of the Jagiellonian University in Cracow (later the Cracow Medical Academy). She commenced her clinical and academic career in 1951 at the Cracow Medical Academy's Clinic of Ophthalmology under professor Marian Wilczek. Here, from 1954-1958, she specialised in ophthalmology. She completed her doctorate studies in 1961 with the thesis "Investigations into darkness adaptation in glaucoma" and gained her PhD with the paper "Disorders in retinal correspondance in strabismus and their changes after therapy"; after which she was nominated decent at the Clinic of Ophthalmology. In 1977 she received her nomination as extraordinary professor, and in 1987 achieved the status of ordinary professor.

In 1959, while still working at the Cracow Clinic of Ophthalmology, she was responsible for organising the Department of Strabismus and Amblyopia Therapy at the Vojevodship Ophthalmic Hospital in Cracow-Witkowice. This department, founded and run by her until 2002 was to become Polands' largest centre for medical and surgical therapy of strabismus and other disorders of binocular function.

In the years 1967-1977 professor Krzystek was a senior consultant at the M.Wilczek Strabismus Rehabilitation Sanatorium in Sobotka near Wroclaw (Breslau), of which she was co-founder. For 20 years, from 1975, she was the national consultant for strabismus and paediatric ophthalmology in Poland. In 1965 she also founded the Cracow School for Orthoptists and it was due to her efforts that Orthoptists were officially recognised as qualified medical personnel.

Professor Krzystek founded the Department of Visual Pathophysiology and Neuroophthalmology at the Cracow Ophthalmology Clinic in 1980, of which she was head until 1996.

Professor Krystyna Krzystek was a member of numerous academic societies; she was a founder member and head of the strabismus section of the Polish Ophthalmological Society fromi 973-2001, long time member of the national board and secretary of the Cracow section of the Polish Ophthalmological Society. From 1967 she was a board member ofCosilium Europaeum Strabismi Studio Deditum (later the European Strabismological Association), of which she was secretary from 1970-1990, a board member of the International Strabismological Association, member of the American Association ofPediatric Ophthalmology and Strabismology (AAPOS),the French Ophthalmological Association, the Swedish Ophthalmological Association, the International Association for Orbital Disorders and the Sensory Commitee of the Medical Department of the Polish Academy of Sciences. Moreover she maintained working relationships with many European and American physicians who shared her interest in Strabismology and neuro-ophthalmology. In 1973 she was delegated by the World Health Organisation to Morocco as paediatric ophthalmology consultant. She helped organise the foundation of strabismus centres in Sweden between 1967 and 1987, cooperated with them academically and lectured annually at the Higher School for Orthoptists in Stockholm.

Professor Krzystkowa readily passed on her knowledge and experience- she organised dozens of courses in strabology for ophthalmologists, oversaw academic placements for 15 overseas postgraduate students , was head of specialisation for 23 Ophthalmological consultants, promoter for 11 doctorate and 2 PhD students and review board member for 29 doctorates and 8 PhD's. Her academic achievements include 145 papers, including 5 original textbooks pertaining to strabology. Most of her work regarded neuroophthalmology, disorders of ocular motility, paediatric strabismus, mono- and stereoptic vision following facial trauma, diagnosis and operative therapy of double vision disorders. She classified various forms of strabismus and her analysis of rare oculomotor disorders were based on hundreds of cases. She undertook experimental work in visual pathophysiology and retinal correspondance. She introduced, described and propagated new operative methods in strabismus, congenital nystagmus and other congenital disorders. She was a pioneer of the introduction of Botulin A toxin to strabismus therapy and introduced penalisation therapy in strabismus to Poland. Professor Krzystek was the recipient of many Polish and international awards and honours.

With the passing of professor Krystyna Krzystek we have lost an exceptional academic, teacher and lecturer to generations of ophthalmologists, one of the shining lights of Polish strabology and a remarkable physician. She will ever remain in the minds of her colleagues, pupils and the patients for whom she cared as a devoted, friendly and upstanding human being.

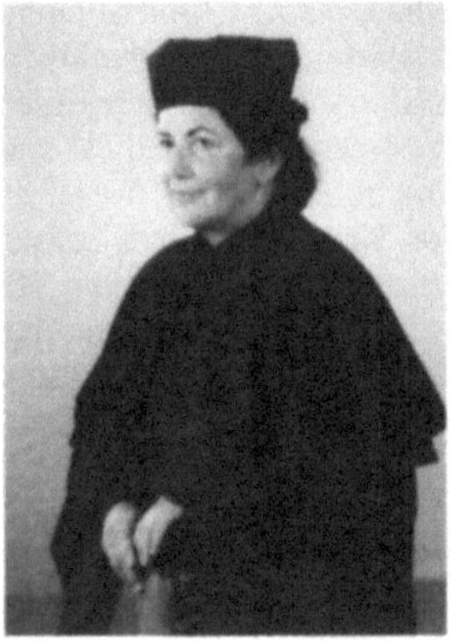

Professor Krystyna Krzystek-Walka

Transactions 28th Meeting European Strabismological Association, de Faber (ed.)
© 2004 European Strabismological Association, ISBN 90 265 1965 6

Obituary Professor Dr. med. Alfred Bangerter

April 22th, 1909 – March 23th, 2002

Only a few of the present members of the European Strabismological Association (ESA) had the opportunity to meet Professor Bangerter. Having retired from his position as head of the Eye Department of the St-Gallen Kantonspital in 1974, he no longer participated at any meetings after the ESA succeeded in 1981 to the Consilium Europaeum Strabismi Studio Deditum (CESSD).

There are at least two reasons, however, for his name to remain familiar to all strabismologists and orthoptists : firstly Bangerter foils, marketed by Ryser Opticians (St-Gallen) and used daily in strabismological and orthoptic practice; secondly, the excellent Bangerter hooks, used by many surgeons in eye muscle surgery.

Professor Bangerter was born in Biel (Switzerland) in 1909. His father was a surgeon and gynaecologist and his mother one of the first woman doctors in Switzerland. After his bilingual French/German schooling and completion of his medical studies in 1936 he specialized in ophthalmology at the Bern Medical School Eye Department under Professor Hans Goldmann (1936-1941). It was here that he opened, in 1941, the first visual training unit (Sehschule) in continental Europe. From 1942 to 1946 he was senior-resident, successively consultant and, in 1946, Privatdocent.

In this same year he was promoted to head of the Eye Department in St-Gallen, position that he retained until his retirement in 1974. In 1983 he opened a private practice that was extended to a day clinic in 1989, and worked there with a team of collaborators until his demise in 2002. He was elected Vice-President of the CESSD in 1962 and became an Honorary Member in 1976 [1].

His 28 years of intensive work as head of the Eye Department in St-Gallen were above all devoted to Strabismology and eye muscle and plastic surgery, areas in which he was a pioneer. In 1947 he created the first Pleoptic and Orthoptic School (POS, later OPOS). From 1954 on he organized courses for ophthalmologists on Pleoptics and Orthoptics and, from 1959, on surgery. He also organized amblyopia screening in the schools of eastern Switzerland, thus reducing the incidence of deep amblyopia from 2,6% as it was in 1951, to 0,3% in 1971. During this period he developed several apparatus for monocular and binocular training (localizer, centrophore, pleoptophore, separation trainer etc.). Among his publications the monograph on amblyopia management ("Amblyopiebehandlung") in 1953, published again in 1955, marked a milestone. He gave a lecture at the XVIII Concilium Ophthalmologicum Belgica in 1958 on "Orthoptische Behandlung des Begleitschielens. Pleoptik" and was invited to lecture in New York and Montreal in 1962.

What remains for present-day strabismology from his intense activity lasting over half a century ? He was, closely followed by his contemporary Curt Cüppers (1910-1995), one of the pioneers in functional reeducation of comitant strabismus, breaking off with abusive occlusion which was the current method of treatment. Even if the methods and instruments for monocular and binocular training developed by Bangerter, together with those of Cüppers, "did not hold (their) initial promise"[2] and were progressively abandoned in the nineteen sixties, the impetus provided by Bangerter and Cüppers in the prevention and treatment of amblyopia was decisive, and continues to govern our strabismological practice with, of course, updated methods. One of the instruments developed by Bangerter was, and is still, fundamental to ophthalmic practice, this the modification of the ophthalmoscope in order to recognize fixation behaviour. This tool, developed with Cüppers and in collaboration with the Oculus Cie, became the "visuscope". In addition, Bangerter foils remain in daily use.

Professor Bangerter was also a remarkable surgeon, especially in the fields of eye muscle and plastic surgery. The hooks he developed are, in my opinion, the most suitable ones, the most logical in shape and probably the best in size for microsurgery. He also developed a number of instruments for eyelid surgery.

As is normal, the evolution of medical knowledge, concepts and techniques lead to change in the field of reeducation as well as that of surgical muscle procedures. Professor Bangerter's work represents a milestone on the way to continuing progress. Some of his major contributions remain, and will surely continue to remain, topical.

André Roth (Genève)

1.- HELBLING-STEIDELE M. – *Prof. Dr. med. Alfred Bangerter: Leben und Werk. Ein Rückblick zum 90. Geburtstag.* Bodensee-Galerie Verlag - Fausel Druck, CH-9400 Rorschach, 1999.

2.- LANG J. – The history of european Strabismology. In: NOORDEN G.K. von: *The history of Strabismology.* J.P. Wayenborgh, B-8400 Oostende 3, 2002, pp.71-116.

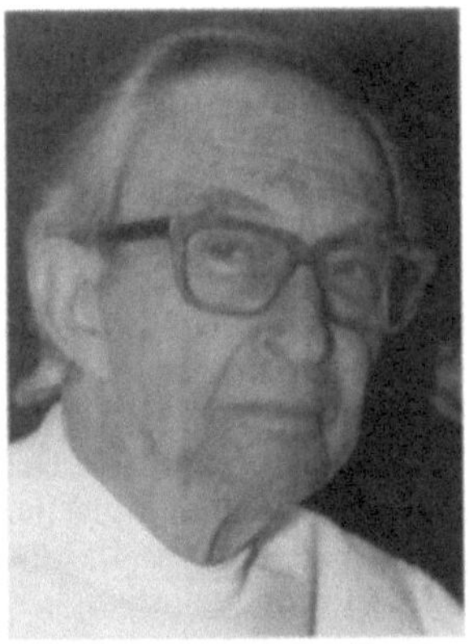

Professor Dr. med. Alfred Bangerter

Session 1
Screening

Transactions 28th Meeting European Strabismological Association, de Faber (ed.)
© 2004 European Strabismological Association, ISBN 90 265 1965 6

The Implementation of Primary Orthoptic Screening For 4-5yr old Children in Inner City Bradford

L. Mulley & A. Bruce
Bradford Hospitals NHS Trust, Bradford, West Yorkshire, UK

ABSTRACT: A review was undertaken of a new primary orthoptic school screening programme. It followed the latest recommendations of the UK National Screening Committee (Hall & Elliman 2002). An orthoptic assessment and auto refraction were carried out on 1936 children (93% uptake). The majority of children (15%) with refractive error only were referred via the local optometrist to the orthoptist for follow-up. Four percent were referred to the hospital eye service (HES) with ocular motility defects and/or gross amblyopia. Attendance via the optometrist was poor compared to the HES. The incidence of squint seemed to be normal but there was a higher than usually quoted incidence of refractive error. This may be linked to the ethnic make-up of Bradford's inner city population.

KEY WORDS: vision screening

1 Introduction

Following the recommendations from the Children's Sub-Group of the National Screening Committee UK an orthoptic primary vision screening programme was introduced into inner city Bradford where there was previously no orthoptic screening. An audit after the first 3 months helped change the referral criteria. This is a review of results after the audit so that all children were judged on the same protocol.

2 DESIGN

A retrospective review of results was made of the first year of the new screening programme.

3 METHOD

All children between the ages of 4 and 5 years of age in reception class in inner city Bradford schools were targeted. The orthoptist visited each school twice and performed an orthoptic assessment and autorefraction using the Welch-Allyn refractometer.
Orthoptic test regime:
- Uniocular visual acuity using Sonksen-Silver
- Cover test at 33cm and 6m
- Ocular movements
- Convergence
- Prism reflex test
- Stereoacuiy test

Criteria for referral: Any child with an ocular muscle anomaly and/or visual acuity < 6/36 was referred to the hospital eye service. Any child with visual acuity of <6/9 or 6/9 and suspected refractive error on autorefraction was referred to the orthoptist via their local optometrist. A letter was sent home in this instance requesting the parents to take the child to their local optometrist who would then complete the form and send the result on to the orthoptic department so that an orthoptic follow-up could be made at a community clinic.

4 RESULTS

In total 1936 children were screened resulting in a 93% uptake. The majority of children 1513 (78%) passed the assessment. Forty seven (3%) were found to be already attending either a local optometrist or the HES. Of these, 23 had refractive error only, 23 had ocular motility defects and 1 had optic nerve pallor. Seventy five (4%) were referred directly to the HES. Of these 54 had ocular moltility defects 20 had refractive error only and 1 had a family history of Stargart's Disease. Two hundred and ninety seven (15%) were referred initially to the local optometrist and then offered an orthoptic follow-up. The number of parents who failed to take their children to the optometrist after the initial letter and who needed a reminder was 186 (63%). Ultimately, only 57% of community referrals attended for follow-up. From the community referrals 35 (20%) were discharged after one orthoptic follow-up to the optometrist, 13 (8%) were discharged without glasses, 66 (39%) needed further review by the orthoptist because we were not happy with their level of vision and/or they needed occlusion, 47 (28%) failed to attend the orthoptic follow-up, 8 (5%) were referred on to the HES for further investigation and 1 had moved away.

The incidence of squint was 3.6% the majority of which (34) were intermittent exotropias.

5 DISCUSSION

This new programme aimed to implement the latest recommendations in the UK for vision screening. An audit of the existing health visitor screening in Bradford had highlighted a high false positive rate of referrals (80%). This information along with the new guidelines was used to make the case for a change in local current practice. A contract was set up with one of the primary care trusts in inner city Bradford which covers about half of Bradford's population to provide the school screening service. This involved meetings and road shows to educate schools, health visitors and school nurses of the change in practice since no active vision screening was to take place before the age of 4 years by any other agency in accordance with the recommendations. Electronic systems were set up to record the data so that it could be forwarded to school nurses and other appropriate child surveillance professionals. It was decided that the majority of referrals that were purely suspected as having refractive error could be managed by an optometrist and orthoptist. This relied on parents taking their children to a local optometrist and then attending a community orthoptic clinic in the inner city area thus relieving the HES of a number of referrals. The poor follow-up rate (57%) was disappointing and this pathway will be reviewed. We understand that a good screening regime takes into account the need for acceptable follow-up treatment patterns (Wilson & Junger1968). Attendance at the HES was almost 100%. It was felt that visual acuity of <6/36 in the absence of squint needed a fundus and media examination to rule out any pathology thus they were referred to the HES.

The initial audit of the service helped refine our pass/fail criteria especially the Welch-Allyn results. A LogMAR test is now used in place of the Sonksen-Silver visual acuity test.

The uptake was excellent (93%) since we had a captive audience in school.

The incidence of squint mirrors normal rates quoted in the literature (Oliver & Nawratzki 1971) but the referral rate of refractive error is significantly above what we expected. This may well be due to the ethnic make-up of the cohort screened which is predominantly Asian (Bradford

Council 1991-2001). Bradford's population is 25% Pakistani and inner city Bradford may well be higher than this.

6 CONCLUSIONS

We needed a high degree of administrative support to set up the service and there was a lot of initial work needed to educate the schools etc regarding the change in service.
The uptake was excellent but there is room for improvement in terms of follow-up treatment for the community referrals.
We have highlighted a higher than normal incidence of refractive error which needs further investigation in terms of ethnicity.

REFERENCES

Bradford Councils Population Forecasts 1991-2001.

Hall, D & Elliman, D 2002 National Screening Committee (Britain). Health for All Children 4th Edition Harlow Printing Ltd. 2002.

Oliver, M. & Nawratzki, I. Screening of pre-school children for ocular anomalies. II. Amblyopia. Prevalence and therapeutic results at different ages. *Br J Ophthalmol* 1971:55:467-71.

Wilson, JMG. & Junger, G. Principles and practice of screening for disease. *Public health papers No. 34 Geneva: WHO*, 1968

Transactions 28th Meeting European Strabismological Association, de Faber (ed.)
© 2004 European Strabismological Association, ISBN 90 265 1965 6

Vision screening in 3 year old children. Comparison between the Lea symbol chart and the HVOT (LM) chart.

G. Kvarnström, P. Jakobsson
Department of Ophthalmology, Linköping University Hospital, Sweden

G. Lennerstrand
Department of Ophthalmology, Karolinska Institute, Stockholm, Sweden

ABSTRACT: The aim of this prospective study was to compare visual screening at 3 years and at 4 years. At four Child Health Care Centres (CHCC) 478 children were tested at the age of 3. Of these children, 440 were tested again at the age of 4. Another group, consisting of 229 children, was examined at the age of 4 only. All children were tested with two different charts: The HVOT chart and the Lea LH symbol chart. The testability rate for 3 years was slightly more than 80% and for 4 years slightly more than 90%. The testing time was significantly longer at 3 years than at 4 years. Children who had been tested at 3 years had a significantly shorter time at 4 years than children who had not been tested previously. There was no statistical difference in the testability, mean testing time or visual acuity between the two charts.

KEYWORDS: screening, visual acuity, LH chart, HVOT chart, 3-year-olds, testability rate

1 INTRODUCTION

In Sweden screening has been generally in use since the mid 70-ies and in our earlier work we have shown that it is effective (Kvarnström et al. 1998). The attendance rate was more than 99%. The prevalence for deep amblyopia (visual acuity ≤0.3, 20/60) decreased from 2% to 0,2% with screening and treatment. Despite screening and treatment there are, however, a not insignificant number of children whose amblyopia is not cured. A reason for this could be the age of detection. The aim of this prospective study was therefore s to investigate if visual screening could be performed at age of 3 years instead of the regular 4 years.

Some reports have shown results that treatment of amblyopia gives better results the earlier treatment is initiated (Nordlöw & Joachimsson 1966). The treatment periods have been shown to be shorter for younger children (Lithander & Sjöstrand 1991). Visual acuity has been described as the best way to find amblyopia (Köhler & Stigmar 1973). The problem is to find a reliable visual chart for young children. We have compared the Anders Hedin's HVOT chart to Lea Hyvärinen's LH chart.

2 MATERIALS

In 1996 we started up a prospective study in Huddinge and Linköping with all 3 year old children (± 3 m) during one year, the study group (3y). A total of 478 children were included in this group. At the same time we let the 4 year old children (± 3 m, 229 children) on the regular examination at the Child Health Care Centres (CHCC) be tested with the same design as the study group. This group used as a control group (4y). One year later we tested the study group at 4 years again with the same design. This group is referred to as the follow-up group (3/4y) and consisted of 440 children.

Thirty-eight children dropped outs mostly because they moved from the area or the country. Only children or parents not familiar with the Swedish language were excluded and children who were already patients at the eye-department. Only a few did not want to participate.

3 METHODS

The children were tested with the HVOT chart and the LH chart. All children were tested with both methods, half of them with HVOT first and the other half with LH first. The HVOT (Hedin et al. 1980) chart has been in use since around 1980 in the Swedish screening system.The chart has the four letters HVOT in lines. The Lea symbol chart was introduced in 1980 by Lea Hyvärinen (Hyvärinen et al. 1980) but has not been commonly used in Sweden. This chart has also 4 different symbols in lines. All testing was performed at 3 meters. All children were occluded with a facial patch. The testing was performed by one orthoptist and 6 child nurses working regularly with screening. The children had a pointing chart in both methods but could also give a verbal response.The testability rate for the first session was calculated for each age and each method. The time was measured with a stopwatch and included the instruction time. All the children were tested and instructed individually. The average time per eye was calculated.

The maximum visual acuity was assessed for each child. When comparing the visual acuity between the two charts this was done for the first session. Four out of five optotypes in the LH-chart must be right and all except 2 optotypes in each line (lines 0.65, 0.8 and 1.0 have 12 optotypes) with the HVOT-chart. Children who did not pass the criteria (≥0.65 at 3 years and ≥0.8 at 4 years) were referred to the Eye Clinic. They were tested on three occasions before referring with approximately one month's interval. If the children needed a second examination, a copy of the two tests was given for practice at home before next visit. Children not cooperating well after 3 trials were also refereed.

4 RESULTS

4.1 *Testability*

The testability rate at the first examination was almost the same for both charts, as can be seen in Figure 1. There was no statistical difference between the methods at any age. There was, however, a statistically significant difference between ages in the ANOVA-test. The testability was approximately 10% better at the age of 4 and the t-test showed a significant difference ($p<0.002$) between 3y and 4y, and 3y and 3/4y but not between 3/4y and 4y. The most common problem was that the child refused to wear a patch. Children who were tested binocularly or with the parent's hand as an occluder were considered not testable. The testability rate increased at the second examination for the 3-year-olds and 60% of the children who could not be tested the first time, cooperated in the second session with at least one of the methods. This increased the testability rate at 3 years to 93%.

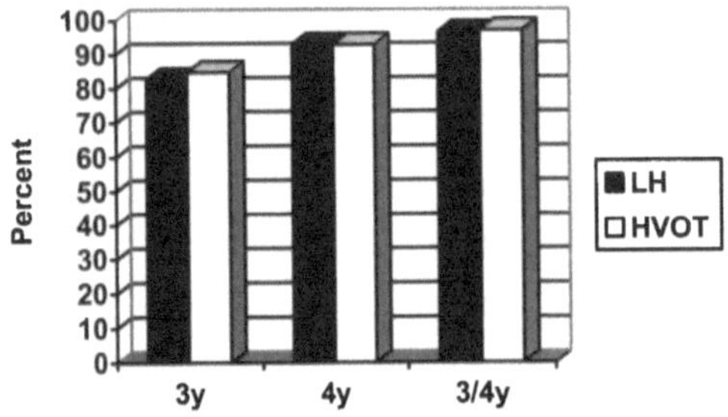

Figure 1. Testability rate with the two charts in the three age groups.

4.2 *Testing time*

The mean testing time for one eye in the first examination including instructions was 2:21 min (LH) and 2:28 min (HVOT) at 3 years, at 4 years 1:48 min (LH) and 1:50 min (HVOT) and for 3/4 years 1:21 min (LH) and 1:29 min (HVOT). This is shown in Figure 2. There was no statistical difference (ANOVA) in the time for examination between the two charts. A significant difference ($p<0.003$) between all different age groups was observed for both methods. The largest difference was between 3y (study group) and 3/4y (follow-up group). Children who had been tested at 3 years had a significantly shorter time (average 24 sec) at 4 years (3/4y) than children who had not been tested previously at 3 years (4y).

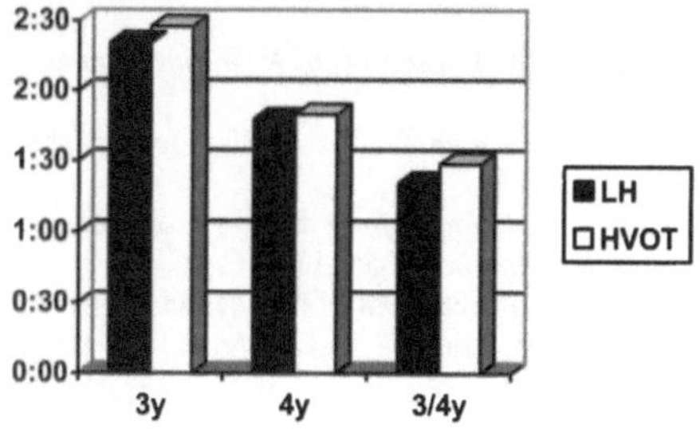

Figure 2. Mean testing time per eye in the three age groups.

4.3 *Visual acuity*

Since each child was tested with both methods it was possible to compare the visual acuity in each eye with both methods. This comparison was performed for the first examination. There was no statistical difference between the methods except at the age of 4 where the HVOT chart gave higher visual acuities than LH ($p=0.014$). The mean difference at this age was small however (0.01).

4.4 *Sensitivity*

Only one "missed" child was found at the age of 4. The boy had microtropia and should possibly have been detected at the age of 3. However, the boy was difficult to examine even after retesting and a third examination was intended but the parents preferred to wait until the age of 4 years. He achieved full visual acuity after treatment. No other false negative or missed cases were detected at the 4-year examination. The positive predictive value was 74%.

5 DISCUSSION

The testability rate in 3 years old children was more then 80% for both the LH and the HVOT chart, which is acceptable for a screening test. Testability rate is better at four years, especially for those who had also been tested at 3 years. The explanation for this is probably a training effect.

Hered and co-workers (Hered et al. 1997) have compared Leas symbol with one variant of the HVOT test and found that Leas Symbol chart had a better testability rate at 3 years than the HVOT chart. There are, however, some differences in procedure compared to our study. As far as we can understand their results are based upon the second test session in a selected group (777 children out of 1135). The children were instructed in a group before the examination.

The positive predictive value was 74% and is slightly better than our previous study (Kvarnström et al. 1998) for 4-year-olds (68.9%).

Our conclusion is that visual acuity can be tested in most children at three years. The testability rate at 3 years was about 80%, which permits mass screening. The mean testing time is half a minute longer at 3 years compared to 4 years, which is acceptable and the visual acuity can be tested equally well with both charts

REFERENCES

Hedin, A. & Nyman, K.G. & Derouet, B. 1980. A modified letter matching chart for testing young children's visual acuity. *J Ped Ophthalmol Strabismus* 17: 114-118.

Hered, R.W. & Murphy, S. & Clancy, M. 1997. Comparison of the HOTV and Lea symbols charts for preschool vision screening. *J Pediatr Ophthalmol Strabismus* 34: 24-28.

Hyvärinen, L. & Näsänen, R. & Laurinen, P. 1980. New visual acuity test for pre-school children. *Acta Ophthalmol (Copenh)* 58: 507-511.

Köhler, L. & Stigmar, G. 1973. Vision screening of four year old children. *Acta Paediatr Scand* 62: 17-27.

Kvarnström, G. & Jakobsson, P. & Lennerstrand, G. 1998. Screening for visual disorders in children, evaluation of the system in Sweden. *Acta Paediatr* 87: 1173-1179.

Lithander, J. & Sjöstrand, J. 1991. Anisometropic and strabismic amblyopia in the age group 2 years and above: a prospective study of the results of treatment. *Br J Ophthalmol* 75: 111-116..

Nordlöw, W. & Joachimsson, S. 1966. The incidence and results of treatment of reduced visual acuity due to refractive errors in four year old children in a Swedish population. *Acta Ophthalmol (Copenh)* 44: 152-165.

Transactions 28th Meeting European Strabismological Association, de Faber (ed.)

Vision screening program for 4 year old children

A. Yaman
Fellow, Department of Ophthalmology, Dokuz Eylül University, Izmir, Turkey

A T. Berk
Professor, Department of Ophthalmology, Dokuz Eylül University, Izmir, Turkey

M. Erbezci
Opthalmologist, Ozel Saglik Hastanesi Izmir, Turkey

G. Ergör
Asocc. Professor, Department of Public Health, Dokuz Eylül University, Izmir, Turkey

Aim: Our aim is to test the sensitivity and specificity of general practitioners in diagnosis of amblyopia and manifest strabismus and recommend a regular screening program in younger age such as 4-year-old in public health centers.
Methods: 1430 children were included in the study. Thirty general practitioners were trained about examination of children. Snellen E visual acuity test, Lang stereotest, Hirschberg test for manifest strabismus were performed by general practitioners in health centers. The children who were unable to pass 20/40 visual acuity, who had two line differences between eyes or who had manifest strabismus in initial examination and control subjects were referred to ophthalmologist.
Study design: Prospective double blind,
Results: One thousand seventy five of 1430 children (75.2%) were examined by general practitioners in health centers. 158 children were referred to ophthalmologist. 2.2% of children were pathologic referral. Amblyopia was diagnosed in 1.5% of them. The cause of amblyopia was refractive or anisometropia in 7 (43.75%), deprivation in 1(6.25%), strabismus in 8 (50%). The sensitivity of general practitioners was 95.8%, the specificity was 60%. False positive referral was 46.9%. The attendance rate at ophthalmologist was 57.6%. The socioeconomic status of the patients statistically determined the attendance to ophthalmologist.(p:0.029, chi-square: 2.5)
Conclusion: The Snellen visual acuity testing is practical and can be performed in public health centers by general practitioners. General practitoners could be used confidentaly in vision screening program. The socioeconomic status of subjects is a barier for attendance to ophthalmologist. Education of parents for importance of child's eye care is mandatory.

Keyword: Preschool vision screening, amblyopia,

Vision screening program for 4 year old children

Introduction: The early detection and treatment of amblyopia, strabismus and significant refractive errors are important to maximize a child's visual potential. The goal of all vision screening is to detect poor vision or risk factors that interfere with vision and normal visual potential at a young age during sensitive period for treatment.

Amblyopia is the commonest cause of defective vision in childhood with prevalence of 1% to 4%.(1) It develops durıng the sensitive period of visual maturation which continuous until about 8 years of age. Visual acuity assesment is currently the most effective screening test for amblyopia. Preschool vision screening has been obligated for many years as a part of several fedaral programs in many countries.. In Turkey; there are no laws, guidelines and for recommendations for preschool vision screening. Many children underwent a visual acuity assesment by elementary school teachers at 7 years old which was too late for the diagnosis and an effective treatment

Our aim was (1)to identify valid and efficient methods for vision screening of preschool children,(2)to standardize the general practitioner's eye examination for vision screening, (3) to demonstrate their sensitivity and specifity and (4)to recommend a cost-effective preschool vision screening guidelines and policies in Turkey

Method: Thirteen public health centers out of 39 which were in the area of same district health directorate were enrolled into study. The list of children who at the age of 4 years were obtained from records of public health center. 110 children selected randomly from each health center. 30 general practitoners were used in screening. Considerable variability in the educational backround of the general practitoners used in screening were standardized by a pediatric ophhalmologist (AT.B). The children were examined by general practitioner in public health center. A description of the screening procedure can be seen in table 1.

Visual acuity assesment with Snellen E acuity testing from 5 meters.
Stereo testing with Lang Stereotest
Ocular alignment using corneal light reflex(Hirshberg testing)

Table 1: tests performed during the screenig program in public health center

The criteria for referral for further examination at the ophthalmology clinic are shown in table 2. To find out the specifity and negative predictive value of general practitoners children who had normal eye examination were referred after each pathologic referrals.

Two lines of differences between two eyes
OR
Visual acuity under 20/40
OR
Presence of manifest deviation supported by negative lang stereotest

Table 2:The criteria for the referral of children fron health center to an ophthalmologist

Ophthalmologists performed a full ophthalmic and orthoptic examination in a blind fasion without knowing the general practitoner's diagnosis.The ophthalmologist's examination included snellen acuity testing with Snellen E chart, stereotest, detection of strabismus by cover test, cycloplegic refraction, ophthalmoscopy and slit-lamp examination. The presence of amblyopia among children was determined using Snellen acuity testing. Amblyopia was defined as a best corrected Snellen acuity of 20/40 or worse in either eye and/or interocular difference of two Snellen lines or more.

The examiners were masked to results of the screening. The findings at screening in public health center and on subsequent attendance to ophthalmologist were recorded on specially designed card. All data were stored and compared.

Results: Preschool vision screening was offered to 1430 children. 1089 children were attended to public health center. 14 subjects were excluded because of insufficient medical record. 1075 (75.2%) children were examined by general practitioners. 158 subjects were referred to ophthalmologist but only 91 subjects (57.6%) were able to examined by an ophthalmologist. 24

subjects (2.2%) had pathologies according referral criteria. The prevelance of amblyopia was 1.5 % in the study population.

The sensitivity of general practitioners was find out 95.8%. Their specifity was 60.0 %. The positive predictive value was 46.9%. Negative predictive value of general practitoners was 97.5 %. General practitoners referred 49 patients with suspicion of pathology which turned out to 23 after examination by an ophthalmologist and GPs referred 40 patients as normal eye examination, except one the remaining 39 were in accordance with ophthalmolgist's diagnosis. Twenty six patients found to be false positive referrals had failed screening for the following reasons: manifest deviation (13cases), poor cooperation (5 cases), reduced vision in one or both eye(8 cases). It was observed that 50% of the GPs referred the subjects with suspision of strabismus but their visual acuities and the stereotests were normal. There was an overdiagnosis of strabismus. The reasons of false positivity were summarized in table 3.

No:26	Practitioners	Ophthalmologist
13	Lang (+) VA 20/20 Esotropia (+)	12 strabismus (-) 1 foria (+)
5	Cooperation (-)	3 (+) 2(-), 1 MMR
8	Visual acuity (6) one eye (2) two eyes	1 strabismus Amblyogenic factors (-)

Table 3: The reasons of false positivity

Children with amblyopia:

Sixteen patients had amblyopia; 7 patients (43.75%) were refractive-anisometropic (straight eyed) amblyopia, 8 patients (50%) were strabismic(7) and strabismic-anisometropic amblyopia(1), one (6.25%) were ambliyopic because of deprivation.

In refractive anisometropic group; 6 children had astigmatism(>2 diopters), one had hyperopia (>4 diopters). Lang stereotest was positive in 6 of 7 patients. In the strabismic and strabismic-anisometric amblyopia group; 5 children had hyperopia (range + 3.75 to + 7.75 diopters), one had astigmatism (>2 diopters), 2 children were emmetropic. Lang stereo test was negative in 6 of 7 patients with strabismic ambliyopia.

Ametropia was diagnosed in 7 patients. All these patients had astigmatism (range 0.50 to 1.5 diopters).

We evaluated effectivitiy of Lang stereotest. It's sensitivity was 23.1 %. It's specivity was 95.5 %. Lang stereotest is good at detection of strabismic cases but misdiagnosed the detection of refractive amblyopia.

The effect of socioeconomic status on attendance were examined. The ratio of attendance to public health center was 75.2%. The ratio of attending ophthalmolgist was 57.8%. The drop outs level increased as socioeconomic status decreased and this was found statistically significant(P:0.029 chi square:2.5). The attendance rate according to socioeconomic status was shown in table 4.

Socioeconomic status	Refered	Examined	%
High	22	17	77.3
Medium	47	32	68.1
Low	89	42	47.2

Table 4: Attendance rate according to socioeconomic status

Conclusion:

The primary purpose of preschool vision screening is to detect amblyopia in order to initiate treatment before the visual system matures and becomes resistant to treatment. Children are a difficult group to test but all children should be examined for ambliyopia or it's risk factors.

Preschool vision screening conducted by general practitioners is effective in detecting children with visual defects. Our screening achieved a positive predictive value of 46.9%. Apperently, suspision of strabismus at screening accounted for the majority of false positive referrals. Comperable studies have reported positive predictive values ranging from 74% to 94%. (2-5)

Every effort should be made to ensure that vision screening is performed using appropriate testing conditions, instruments and techniques. The most effective screening test for detection of amblyopia was visual acuity assesment, as reported previously. (5). We observed that Snellen E acuity testing was a simple and acceptable method for preschool vision screening program. Lang stereotest faciliates the diagnosis of manifest deviations but without visual acuity test it is not a sensitive method for the detection of amblyopia. General practitoners could be used confidentaly for screening programs and there remains the task of training sufficient general practitioners to provide this service throughout Turkey.

In this study, the attendance rate of our screening program was 57.8 %. Most other studies have reported that similar attendance rates,varying from 57% to 75% (2,3,5-7). It seemed that socioeconomic status of the population is a barrier for the attendance of further eye care and treatment. So a recommendation of a screening program solely is not enough, the education of the parents for the importance of childs eye care is mandotory.

References:

Simons K. 1996. Preschool vision screening: rationale, methodology, and outcome. Surv Ophthalmol; 41:3-30.

Wormald RPL. 1991. Preschool vision screening in Cornwall: performance indicators of community orthoptist. Arch Dis Child. 66:917-20.

Jarvis SN, Tamhne RC, Thompson L, Francis PM, Anderson J, Colver AF.1990. Preschool vision screening . Arch Dis Child. 65:288-94.

Köhler L, Stigmar G. 1973. Vision screening of four-year-old children. Acta Paediatr Scand. 62:17-27.

Williamson TH, Andrews R, Dutton GN, Murray G, Graham N.1995. Assesment of inner city visual screening programme for preschool children. 79:1068-73.

Edwards RS, Whitelaw AJ, Abbott AG. 1989. Orthoptists as pre-school screeners. Br. Orthopt J.46:14-9.

Ingram RM, Holland WW. Walker C et al. 1986. Screenig for visual defects in preschool children. Br J Ophthalmol. 70:16-21.

Transactions 28th Meeting European Strabismological Association, de Faber (ed.)
© 2004 European Strabismological Association, ISBN 90 265 1965 6

With an eye on vision screening in the Netherlands

Rotterdam Amblyopia Screening Effectiveness Study (RAMSES) up to date

V.K. Lantau, CO
TOV Foundation (Early Detection of Visual Disorders), Amsterdam, The Netherlands

J.H. Groenewoud, MD, PhD
Department of Public Health, Erasmus MC, Rotterdam, The Netherlands
on behalf of the RAMSES steering committee (The Netherlands)

ABSTRACT: The purpose of the RAMSES study is to evaluate the effectiveness and the efficiency of amblyopia screening activities as they are actually performed in Rotterdam child health care, during a follow-up period of 8 years. 4637 children born between September 1996 and May 1997 in Rotterdam have been included in the study. Vision screening data are collected at 7 occasions or 'rounds'. In children aged 9-24 months, vision is tested with the VOV-method, in children aged 3-7 visual acuity is assessed. The data of the first 5 rounds (up to the age of 4) have now been analysed. Some preliminary results will be presented here. We found that compliance with screening decreases with age, and that only part of the referred children visit the ophthalmic centre for further assessment. Our conclusion is that referral procedures after a positive test result must be improved.

KEYWORDS: screening, visual disorders, amblyopia, refractive errors.

1 INTRODUCTION

Amblyopia is the most common cause of monocular visual impairment in both children and young-aged adults (Attebo et al. 1998). In the Netherlands, a nation-wide organised screening programme for eye disease and visual abnormalities in children has been carried out since 1989. In June 2002, a standardised protocol on vision screening was published on instigation of the Dutch Ministry of Health (van Velzen-Mol, 2002).

Up to the age of 3, the VOV-method – which means Early detection of Visual disorders - is used for vision screening. The components of this VOV-method are assessed at four occasions (when the children are 1-2, 3-4, 6-9 and 14-24 months of age, respectively). In the first 6 months special attention is given to the fixation, the outer aspects of the eyes, the pupillary light reflex, the red fundus reflex and the binocular movements. From around 6-9 months of age ocular alignment is observed, as well as the monocular pursuit movements. Especially the monocular movements are indicative of the visual acuity of the child (Lantau et al. 1999). Visual acuity (VA) is assessed from age 3: at the age of 3 a picture chart is used, at ages 4 and 5½ a Snellen chart.

At the age of 5½, visual acuity is assessed at school health centres; the earlier examinations are carried out in Child Health Care centres (CHC). More than 97% of Dutch children attend a CHC in their first year of life. Screening is executed by skilled personnel: the VOV-method is performed by physicians; VA assessment by both physicians and nurses, who are all trained and retrained by orthoptists.

There has been a lof of debate about amblyopia screening and treatment. In 1997, Snowdon and Stewart-Brown concluded in their York Report that the efficacy of prevention programmes is not well substantiated (Snowdon & Stewart Brown 1997). They suggested that a conclusive judgement in this matter can only be reached by a randomised controlled screening trial (RCT); in response a RCT of treatment of amblyopia was set up in Newcastle. When a screening programme already exists, like in the Netherlands, it is very difficult to organise a RCT for the evaluation of such a programme: withholding a standardised protocol from those who normally would have had the opportunity to participate, will lead to strong resistance.

Moreover, the conclusions of the 2002 ALSPAC (Avon longitudinal study of parents and children) study support the hypothesis that early treatment for amblyopia leads to better outcomes than later treatment; this finding may be a stimulus for research into feasible screening programmes (Williams et al. 2002).

In 1996 the Rotterdam AMblyopia Screening Effectiveness Study (RAMSES) was started as an observational (practise based) study in order to establish a management plan for the optimisation of screening and treatment of amblyopia.

2 METHODS

4637 children born between September 1996 and May 1997 in Rotterdam were included in the RAMSES study. So far, data on vision screening have been collected at 5 occasions (ages 9, 14 and 24 months; 36 months; 45 months). The results of the first 3 occasions or 'rounds' were previously published (Juttmann 2001). Preliminary data on the 4th and 5th rounds concern 3764 children who by May 2002 still lived in Rotterdam.

3 RESULTS

3.1 *Coverage*

The coverage of screening in the 5 screening rounds is shown in Figure 1.

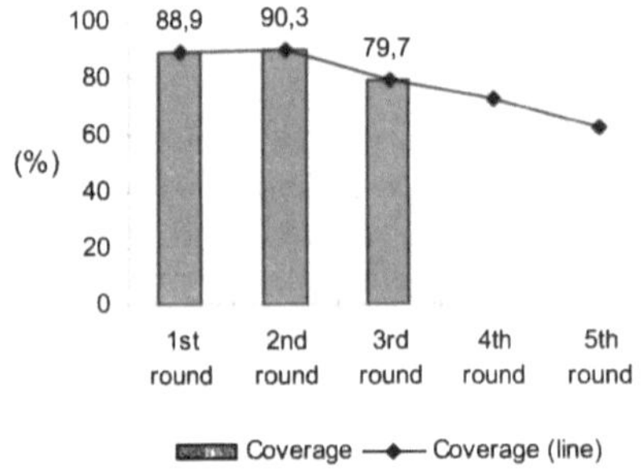

Figure 1. Coverage of vision screening in 5 rounds (up to the age of 4).

Attendance at the regular visits to the CHC turned out to be high in rounds 1, 2 and 3. Ninety-seven per cent of all children visited the CHC at least once up to the age of 24 months (first 3 rounds). Attendance at the 4th and 5th rounds showed a decrease.

3.2 *Referrals*

A total of 160 children (4% of the screened population) had at least one positive test after rounds 1, 2 and 3 (Juttmann 2001). After the 4th and 5th rounds, the number of children with at least one positive test had more than doubled (Figure 2).

All children with a positive test are to be referred to the general practitioner and subsequently to an ophthalmological centre for further diagnostic and possibly therapeutic procedures. Although the coverage of the screening programme itself is relatively high, referral procedures appear to be less efficient. Of children with a positive test in the first 3 rounds, 101 (63%)

visited an ophthalmological centre for diagnostic evaluation. Thus, one third of the children with a positive test after the 3rd round were not conclusively evaluated at an ophthalmological centre and may not profit from early treatment for amblyopia. After rounds 4 and 5, the number of referred children visiting an ophthalmological centre seems to be even smaller. The reasons for this non-compliance are unknown, but the rather small numbers may be due to parental non-compliance with referral (no visit to the general practitioner or the ophthalmological centre) or to doctor's delay (an unnecessary expectant attitude of general practitioners themselves). Poor follow-up may lead to missed or delayed detection of amblyopia cases. We believe that this part of the programme is eligible for improvement.

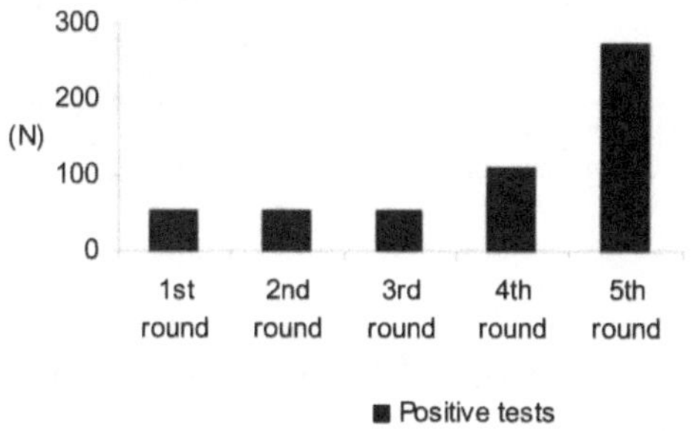

Figure 2. Children with a positive screening test (for the first time), absolute numbers.

3.3 *Ophthalmological evaluation*

For the first 3 rounds, the results of diagnostic evaluation at the ophthalmological centre and the entailing predictive values of a positive screening followed by an effective referral are presented in Table 1. We found that 64 (of 101) children after round 3 had some ophthalmological disorder. The PPV was 0.63 for any ophthalmological disorder and 0.42 for amblyopia. These results were published by Juttmann on behalf of the RAMSES steering group in 2001 (Juttmann 2001).

Preliminary analysis of the ophthalmological evaluation of children who were referred in screening rounds 4 and 5 shows that PPVs are comparable or even slightly better; however, data were not complete.

Table 1. Results of the evaluation at the ophthalmological centre and predictive value of a positive screening test followed by an effective referral (PPV) (from: Juttmann 2001).

Screening test		Evaluated by ophthalmologist (N)	Diagnosis		PPV	
			Visual disorder, not amblyopia	(Probably) amblyopia	All visual disorders	Amblyopia
VOV	9 months	41	*7*	15	*0.54*	0.37
	14 months	36	*9*	12	*0.58*	0.34
	24 months	24	*6*	15	*0.88*	0.62
Total		101	*22*	42	*0.63*	0.42

The PPV is a measure for the efficiency of the screening programme rather than for its effectiveness. It provides information about the number of screened individuals for whom the screening is not profitable but merely inconvenient and unnecessarily alarming (the false-positives).

Table 2. Literature data on positive cumulative incidence, number of false-positive test results, predictive value (PPV) and test sensitivity in child health care screening programmes for several disorders, per 1000 children (from: Juttman 2001).

		Incidence 0/00	False positives	PPV	Sensitivity
Phenylketonuria	Verkerk 1995	0.06	0.12	0.50	0.99
Congenital hypothyreodia	Verkerk 1996	0.29	1.7	0.17	0.98
Perceptive hearing impairments	van Leerdam 1998	2	70	0.024	0.86
Congenital heart malformations	Juttmann 1998	4	15	0.13	0.57
Idiopathic adolescent scoliosis	Yawn 1999	4	42	0.05	0.54
Developmental dysplasia of the hip	Boere-Boenekamp 1998	37	173	0.15	0.83
Amblyopia	present paper	20-40*	23	0.42**	not yet known

*Based on incidence estimations from the international literature.
**PPV of VOV-method calculated for amblyopia only and not for other ophthalmic disorders. PPV of VA assessment in rounds 4 and 5 is not yet known.

In comparison with published data on PPV and false positive rates of other screening programmes in CHC (Table 2), the VOV-method exhibits a quite favourable PPV, resulting in a relatively small number of false positives in spite of a relatively high incidence. Of course, screening for very rare disorders, such as PKU and CHT, causes very few false positives, even when the PPV is relatively low, as is the case in CHT screening,. Screening for other infrequent disorders, such as perceptive hearing impairments and idiopathic adolescent scoliosis, however, causes substantially more false positives than the VOV-method because of poor PPVs. Screening for developmental dysplasia of the hip, with an incidence similar to amblyopia, causes an eightfold increase in false positives compared with the VOV-method because of a less favourable PPV.

4 CONCLUSION

In the Netherlands, the predictive value of a positive test (VOV-method) is more favourable than of most other screening tests in child health care. Like vision screening using the VOV-method in the first three years of life, assessment of visual acuity at ages 3 and 4 may be effective in detecting visual and ocular disorders as well. The referral procedures after a positive test result must be improved.

Currently, we are collecting and analysing the data of round 6 (at age 5½). In 2004, when all children in the cohort have reached the age of 7, the prevalence and the severity of (still existing) amblyopia will be assessed by a team of independent orthoptists and ophthalmologists. These final results will be related to the compliance with the screening programme, the occurrence of a positive screening test, any diagnostic or therapeutic procedures, compliance with treatment and treatment outcomes. Results will also be compared with historical data on unscreened populations. In addition, we consider to follow the children up to the age of 9, if possible.

REFERENCES

Williams, C., Northstone, K., Harrad, R.A., Sparrow, J.M. & Harvey, I.; ALSPAC Study Team. 2002. Amblyopia treatment outcomes after screening before or at age 3 years: follow-up from randomised trial. *BMJ* 324(7353):1549.

Attebo, K., Mitchell, P., Cumming, R., Smith, W., Jolly, N. & Sparkes, R. 1998. Prevalence and causes of amblyopia in an adult population. *Ophthalmology* 105: 154-159.

Juttmann, R.; on behalf of the Rotterdam Amblyopia Screening Effectiveness Study (RAMSES) steering committee. 2001. The Rotterdam AMblyopia Screening Effectiveness Study (RAMSES):compliance and predictive value in the first 2 years. *Br J Ophthalmology* 85: 1332-1335.

Lantau, V.K., Juttmann, R.E., van der Maas. P.., de Faber, J.T.H.N., Simonsz, H., Hermans, J. & Paas, F. 1999. State of the Rotterdam Amblyopia Screening Evaluation Study (RAMSES). Orthoptics in Focus, pp.39-41. Transactions of the Ixth International Orthoptic Congress, June 21-24, 1999, Stockholm, Sweden.

Snowdon S.K., & Stewart-Brown, S.L. 1997. Preschool vision screening. *Health Technol Assess* 1(8): 1-83.

Van Velzen-Mol, H.W.M. (ed.). *JGZ-standaard Opsporing visuele stoornissen 0-19 jaar.* 2002 Houten/Diegem: Bohn Stafleu Van Loghum.

The Rotterdam Amblyopia Screening Effectiveness Study (RAMSES) steering committee consists of:
V.K. Lantau, CO, TOV Foundation (Early Detection of Visual Disorders), Amsterdam; H.J. de Koning, MD, PhD, Associate Professor, J.H. Groenewoud, MD, PhD & R.E. Juttmann, MD, PhD, Department of Public Health, Erasmus MC, University Medical Center Rotterdam; H.J. Simonsz, MD, PhD, Ophthalmic Department, Erasmus MC, University Medical Center Rotterdam; J.T.H.N. de Faber, MD, Rotterdam Eye Hospital; E. Hostmann, Rotterdam Homecare Foundation; W.C. Hoogeveen, MD, Rotterdam Municipal Health Department, all in the Netherlands.

Correspondence:
Kathleen Lantau, TOV Foundation, Velázquezstraat 5, 1077 NG Amsterdam, email: info@stichtingtov.nl.
Hanny Groenewoud, Department of Public Health, Erasmus MC, University Medical Center Rotterdam, PO Box 1738, 3000 DR Rotterdam, email: j.groenewoud@erasmusmc.nl.

Transactions 28th Meeting European Strabismological Association, de Faber (ed.)

New guidelines for screening of vision in children in Norway

T. Christoffersen
University Hospital of North Norway, Tromsø, Norway

J. Wirsching
Hospital of Vestfold, Tønsberg, Norway

ABSTRACT: In order to revise the guidelines for screening of vision in children, Norwegian health authorities established a multidisiplinary group in January 2001. The group was to review existing documentation and propose recommendations for visual screening in the primary health care. Large randomized controlled trials concerning this problem is lacking. However, there are a number of good clinical studies, especially from Sweden, evaluating screening and treatment for amblyopia. Also experts groups in different countries have considered the matter. Finally more than 30 years of systematic visual examinations in Norway were evaluated. Possible tests were considered according to the WHO criteria for screening. Red reflex examination at birth and at 6 weeks of age to detect congenital cataract and examination of visual acuity to detect amblyopia at 4 years of age are the only screening procedures recommended. What should be done in addition to screening is outlined, as are signs and symptoms of visual impairment.
KEYWORDS: Screening, children, vision, congenital cataract, amblyopia, strabismus.

1 INTRODUCTION

Since the late 1960-ies all children in Norway have been offered eye examinations. Almost all families, all over the country have brought their children to these examinations. In our scarcely populated country tests are performed by general practitioners and specially trained nurses, health visitors. Red reflex and inspection of the eyes are done in neonates. Eye motility and alignment are observed and visual development is assessed at short intervals until two years of age. Covertest for strabismus and visual acuity are examined between 4 and 5 years of age. In addition visual acuity are tested at different grades in school (Statens helsetilsyn 1998).

2 METHODS

Norwegian health authorities want guidelines for examination of vision to be evidence based and more standardized. A multidididiplinary group including orthoptist, optician, general practitioner, health visitor, low vision teacher, pediatrician, and two ophthalmologists has reviewed documentation and proposed new guidelines for examinations of vision in a primary health care setting.

3 RESULTS

Large randomized controlled trials concerning vision screening are generally lacking.

There are, however, a number of population based studies on amblyopia, and several non-controlled clinical studies evaluating screening and treatment for amblyopia (Campos 1995). In Sweden the frequency of amblyopia in screened populations nowadays is significantly lower compared to data from the same areas prior to screening (Kvarnström 2001, Lennerstrand

1996). We find this to be strong evidence in favor of screening and treatment for amblyopia. These studies are also of special interest since the Swedish health care system is similar to ours.

Evidence is strong in favor of early surgery for bilateral congenital cataract (Kugelberg 1992). A recent study from Sweden showed that treatment was initiated earlier in districts were red reflex examination was routine at birth compared to areas were it was postponed to the first visit in primary care (Magnusson 2002).

Early intervention in children with all kinds of visual impairment is important (Clarce 2000, Lanners 1999, Sameroff 2000).

Reviewing reports from expert groups in different countries, we found that the recommendations did not differ much (Snowdon 1997, Canadian Pediatric Society 1998, Hartmann 2001).

Evaluating the experience of more than 30 years of eye examinations in Norway, many of us felt that we had numerous cases were early treatment had been to the benefit of our patients. Unfortunately not very much data from our country has been published.

WHO has set up a number of criteria that should be fulfilled before a screening program is adapted (Wilson 1968). The health problem should be major, have a latent or early stage and its natural history must be understood. The test should be acceptable for the population and have high sensitivity and specificity. There must be consensus on whom to treat and how to treat. Finally there should be a positive cost-benefit balance concerning screening and treatment. Obviously many procedures will fail to fulfil these criteria.

4 RECOMMENDATIONS.

4.1 *Screening*

Two systematic screening procedures were recommended by the group.

Red reflex examination to detect cataract at birth by a pediatrician and at 6 weeks of age by a general practitioner.

Examination of visual acuity at 4 years of age to detect reduced visual acuity as a sign of amblyopia. Visual acuity can be tested using optotypes at an earlier age in many children. However, if it is to be done as screening a very high proportion of the children must be able to perform the test as specificity need to be high. We found the LEA chart suitable. It is a log MAR chart and it can easily be used with children from different ethnic backgrounds.

We do not recommend systematic screening for strabismus. In our experience manifest strabismus is often diagnosed early without screening. Besides evidence that the cover test or the light reflex test have sufficiently high sensitivity and specificity for screening in a primary health care setting is lacking, as it is concerning photorefraction. The stereotests are not good enough for screening (Ohlsson 2001). We do not recommend any screening above school age as we could not think of any serious condition with a latent stage affecting these age groups.

4.2 *Attention, observations and examinations*

All children are still to be seen for a number of reasons at short intervals from birth until late school years. Therefor attention should be paid to family history, birth history, psychomotor development and parental concern for the vision of the child. Symptoms and signs indicating a visual problem should be recognized and taken seriously. Health visitors and general practitioners must know how to examine children's eyes and vision. It should be easy to have children referred to a suitable specialist.

Children at high risk must be identified. The features of Cerebral Visual Impairment (Good 2001, Jacobson 2000) are emphasized in the report. Risk factors for visual impairment such as prematurity, hearing defects, mental retardation and others are outlined. Children with known high risk of visual problems, should be followed by specialists.

4.3 *Implementation*

Information, courses and training of all kinds of professionals involved in children with eye problems will be important for the implementation of new guidelines throughout the country.

REFERENCES

Campos C. 1995. Amblyopia. *Surv Ophthalmol* 40: 23-39.

Canadian Paediatric Society Clinical Practice Guideline. 1998. Vision screening in infants and children. *Paediatr Child Health* 3: 261-262.

Clarce A. 2000. *Early experience and the life path.* London: Jessica Kingsley Publishers.

Good W.V. et al. 2001. Recent advances in cortical visual impairment. *Dev Med Child Neurol* 43: 56-60.

Hartmann E.E. et al. 2001. Preschool vision screening: Summary of a task force report. *Ophthalmology* 108: 479-486.

Jacobson L.K. et al. 2000. Periventricular leucomalasia: An important cause of visual and ocular motility dysfunction in children. *Surv Ophthalmol* 45(1): 1-13.

Lanners J. et al. 1999. Early intervention for children with cerebral visual impairment: Preliminary results. *J Intellect Disabil Res* 43(1): 1-12.

Kugelberg U. 1992. Visual acuity following treatment of bilateral congenital cataracts. *Doc-Ophthalmol* 82(3): 211-215.

Kvarnström G. et al. 2001. Visual screening of Swedish children; an ophthalmological evaluation. *Acta Ophthalmol Scand* 79: 240-244.

Lennerstrand G. et al. 1996. Results of treatment of amblyopia with a screening program for early detection. *Acta Ophthalmol Scand* 74(suppl 219): 42-45.

Magnusson G. et al. 2002. Screening för kongenital katarakt sker bäst på BB – med kompletterande undersökning på BVC. *Läkartidningen* 99: 620-625.

Sameroff A.J. et al. 2000. Transactional regulation: The developmental ecology of early intervention. In Shonkoff J. & Meisels S.J. (eds), *Handbook of early childhood intervention*: 135-159. New York: Cambridge University Press.

Snowdon S.K. et al. 1997. Preschool vision screening: Results of a systematic review.*Report No 9.* York: NSH Centre for Review and Dissemination, University of York.

Statens helsetilsyn 1998. *Veileder for helsestasjons- og skolehelsetjenesten.* Oslo: Statens helsetilsyn.

Wilson J.M. et al. 1968. Principles and practice of screening for disease. Geneva: WHO.

Session 2
Amblyopia/Eye movements

Transactions 28th Meeting European Strabismological Association, de Faber (ed.)

The Relationship Between Stereopsis and Visual Acuity After Occlusion Therapy for Amblyopia

Se Youp Lee, M.D.
Department of Ophthalmology, Keimyung University, Dongsan Medical Center
Taegu, Korea

Sherwin J. Isenberg, M.D.
Department of Ophthalmology, Jules Stein Eye Institute, UCLA School of Medicine, Los Angeles, California,

ABSTRACT
Purpose: To investigate the relationship between visual acuity (VA) and stereoacuity after occlusion therapy in patients with various types of amblyopia.
Methods: 61 children with amblyopia caused by anisometropia with no strabismus (26 children), small angle (≤ 8PD) or intermittent strabismus (20), or both (15). All were treated with occlusion therapy. VA and near stereopsis using the Titmus test (Stereo Optical Inc, Chicago) were measured at each clinic visit.
Results: Mean age at initiation of therapy was 5.1 years (range 3.5 - 8) and mean follow-up 52.3 weeks (range 13 - 192). Mean duration of occlusion was 36 weeks (range 12 - 102). After occlusion treatment, mean VA of all children improved from 0.43 to 0.78 ($P < .0001$), while mean stereoacuity improved from 1167.4 seconds of arc to 101($P < .0001$). By the last visit, 85.2% (52/61) of patients demonstrated at least 2 lines improvement in VA. There was a significant linear relationship between VA and stereoacuity ($P < .001$). The 26 anisometropic patients without strabismus enjoyed a similar improvement in VA and stereopsis ($P < .0001$), as did the 35 with small angle or intermittent strabismus ($P < .0001$).
Conclusions: When employing occlusion therapy for amblyopia (due to anisometropia, small angle or intermittent strabismus, or a combination), as visual acuity improves, stereopsis generally also improves.

Keywords: Stereopsis, amblyopia, visual acuity

Amblyopia is a relatively prevalent developmental problem affecting about 5% of the population (Preslan,1996). It is the result of abnormal visual input during the critical phase of early development and generally affects one eye. The most effective way of treating amblyopia is by early detection, correction of any significant refractive error and abnormal ocular alignment, and occlusion or penalization of the dominant eye.

Occlusion of the good eye is the most widely accepted form of amblyopia treatment. It has been successful for over 250 years. In general, visual acuity (VA) will improve in patients with amblyopia after occlusion therapy if treatment is started before visual maturation. However, we are unaware of any previous study of the changes in stereoacuity as the VA of amblyopic eyes improve with occlusion therapy. The purpose of this study was to evaluate the relationship between VA and stereoacuity with occlusion therapy in amblyopes. A recently published clinical trial of amblyopic patients concluded that the visual acuity results at 6 months for those treated by occlusion or atropine were similar (PEDIG, 2002). If so, the major potential benefit for atropine treatment could possibly be better binocular vision or stereopsis since both eyes are always open during the treatment period. Our study was designed to investigate if stereopsis is improved with occlusion therapy.

MATERIALS AND METHODS

Patient Data

In this retrospective study, we reviewed the charts of 61 consecutive children (34 males) aged 3.5 to 8 years, who met our inclusion criteria. They presented between 1994 and 2001 at the Jules Stein Eye Institute of University of California Los Angeles and were diagnosed with amblyopia. Ages ranged from 3.5 to 8 years with a mean of 5.1 years. The groups did not significantly differ in mean age. Amblyopia was defined as a difference in vision of two lines or greater with the VA of the amblyopic eye less than 20/30 and were due to any combination of anisometropia, small angle strabismus (≤ 8 prism diopters, PD), and intermittent strabismus. Anisometropia was defined as a difference in either the sphere or cylinder of 1.5 D or greater (Weakly, 2001). Exclusion criteria were age over 8 years, previous eye surgery, inability to respond to stereopsis testing, and constant strabismus with best spectacle correction exceeding 8 PD.

Patients were divided into three groups by cause of amblyopia: anisometropia (Group I, N=26), strabismus (Group II, N=20) and both anisometropia and strabismus (Group III, N=15). Group II patients had intermittent strabismus or a manifest deviation less than 8 PD with glasses by simultaneous prism and cover test on an accommodative target. Group III patients had a small angle (within 8 PD of deviation angle) or intermittent strabismus combined with anisometropia.

All patients underwent a full initial ophthalmologic and orthoptic evaluation. All significant refractive errors were corrected based on cycloplegic refraction. Cycloplegic refractions were performed by instilling two drops of 1% cyclopentolate hydrochloride in each eye five minutes apart. At the first visit, refractive correction was given to anisometropic patients. Patients were instructed to wear their eyeglasses for 6 weeks after the first visit. If the VA had not improved by the second visit, part-time occlusion of the sound eye was initiated. Visual acuity was checked at each visit and expressed as a decimal. Monocular VA was measured using the Snellen letters or, if the child could not read letters, the Allen picture chart at 20 feet.

Stereopsis was quantitatively assessed with the Titmus test (Stereo Optical Inc, Chicago) with fly and graded circles. During the examination, the patients wore their regular spectacles underneath the polaroid lenses and the examiner used his index finger to guide fixation. The subject was enthusiastically asked to grab the wings of the fly and point to the circle that seemed to "jump" out of the book. When a mistake was made, the immediately preceding target was repeated. If a correct response was made on the preceding target, that target's disparity was used as the measurement. If that response was incorrect, further steps backward on the target series were made until the correct response was obtained. The last correct target identified was used as the child's stereopsis measurement.

Occlusion therapy consisted of part-time occlusion using adhesives patches. The number of hours per day of occlusion varied depending on the children's age, depth of amblyopia and other factors. The minimal initial patching schedule was 4 hours per day. If the VA did not improve, the number of hours of occlusion was generally increased. If the VA improved, hours of occlusion were reduced. Once the best possible VA in the amblyopic eye was obtained on two consecutive visits, the period of occlusion of the nonamblyopic eye was gradually reduced. No patients underwent occlusion after 9 years of age.

Statistical Analysis

For statistical analysis, patients with no measurable stereopsis were assigned to the worst measurable value of 3000 seconds as described previously (Weakly, 2001). The paired t test was used to test for change in VA and stereoacuity between the first and last visit of each patient. A *P* value of 0.05 or less was considered to be statistically significant. In order to include all subjects at all time periods, linear mixed regression models were used to test for an improvement over time for VA and stereoacuity and to evaluate the relationship between VA and stereoacuity after occlusion treatment.

RESULTS

The mean and standard deviation for follow-up time of all patients was 52.3 (± 26.4) weeks (range 13 - 192). Mean time interval from the previous visit to the next visit for all patients was as follows: Visit 1 to Visit 2: 7.0 (± 5.7) weeks, Visit 2 to Visit 3: 9.2 (± 7.3) weeks, Visit 3 to visit 4: 11.3 (± 8.7) weeks, Visit 4 to visit 5: 14.9 (± 11.6) weeks, and Visit 5 visit 6: 13.2 (± 7.1) weeks. The mean duration of patching for all patients was 36 (± 20.4) weeks (range 12 - 102). The mean duration of patching for Groups I, II, and III was 37.7 (± 15.3) weeks, 37.1 (± 24.2), and 31.7 (± 23.4) respectively.
The mean amount of anisometropia in Group I and III was 2.5 D (± 1.2) (range 1.5 - 5.5) in spherical power for anisomyopia and anisohypermetropia, and 1.8 D (± 0.6) (range 1.5 - 3.0) for anisoastigmatism. The mean deviation angle for all strabismic patients (N=35) was 6.2 PD (± 5.6), accommodative esotropic patients (N=27) 4.7 PD (± 2.9), intermittent strabismus patients (N=6) 15.6 PD (± 9.2), and for one exotropic and one nonaccomodative constant esotropic patient 5 PD.
Stereopsis was present in 48 patients (78.7%) before treatment. Mean stereoacuity improved from 555 to 55 sec in Group I (N = 23), 881 to 109 sec in Group II (N = 13), and 665 to 99 in Group III (N = 12). In 34 (70.8%) of them, it improved to 60 seconds of arc or better at last visit. Of the other 14 patients, 3 (beginning at 3000, 400, and 200 sec) improved to 80 sec, 5 (3 at 3000, 1 each at 400 and 200 sec) improved to 100 sec, and 1 each from 400 to 120, 3000 to 140, 400 to 200, and 3000 to 600 sec. Two patients with initial stereopsis of 100 and 400 sec did not improve. As a group, these 14 patients improved their mean stereopsis from 1464 to 164 sec at the last visit.
The 13 patients (21.3%) who gave a negative response on the Titmus test before occlusion therapy achieved a mean stereoacuity of 175 sec on the last visit. Seven patients (53.8%) achieved at least 100 seconds of arc stereoacuity. Of the other 6, 1 improved to 140, 2 to 200, and 3 to 400 sec. The mean stereopsis achieved on the final visit was 147 in Group I (N = 3), 214 in Group II (N = 7), and 99 sec in Group III (N = 3).
The mean corrected VA and stereoacuity for each group and all patients at first and last visit are listed in the table. At last visit, all three groups significantly improved VA and stereoacuity ($P < .05$). The anisometropic group (Group I) had the best stereoacuity outcome and subjects with both anisometropia and strabismus (Group III) had the best visual outcome, but there was no statistically significant difference among the groups in the final stereoacuity and VA. There was a significant improvement with time for both VA and stereoacuity in all patients and in each of the 3 subgroups ($P < .0001$).

Amblyopia Group	Initial Visual Acuity	Final Visual Acuity	Initial Stereopsis (sec arc)	Final Stereopsis (sec arc)
I	0.37	0.74	838	66
II	0.49	0.80	1622	146
II	0.47	0.81	1132	102
All	0.43	0.78	1167	101

At last visit, eighty-five percent of all patients achieved at least 2 lines improvement of corrected VA. Two patients each in the strabismic (Group II) and in the anisometropia and strabismus group (Group III) did not show improved corrected VA. The causes of treatment failure in these 4 patients were poor compliance with occlusion therapy in 3, and high hypermetropic anisometropia in one (amount: 5.5 D). There was a significant association between VA and stereoacuity for all patients and in subgroups with each follow-up ($P < .001$ for all exceptin group III, $P = .0027$).

DISCUSSION

While a number of case series of amblyopia after occlusion therapy have been reported in the literature, the relationship between changes in VA and stereoacuity after occlusion treatment in amblyopes has not been reported. In 1951, Burian stated that stereoacuity in a normal observer decreased approximately in the same ratio as does VA, but that VA can be normal without any stereopsis, or VA can be poor with good stereoacuity. However, Levy and Glick (1974) showed a linear relationship between stereoacuity and VA using the Titmus stereotest. In their study, they varied the VA in normal subjects in one eye only, while the fellow eye was maintained at 20/20. Goodwin and Romano (1985) stated that there is a statistically significant relationship between monoculary degraded vision and stereoacuity using experimental fogging with a spherical lens. Donzis and associates (1983) reported that when varying the binocular Snellen VA in normal subjects from 20/20 to 20/200, stereoacuity changed proportionally. Lavasik and Szymkiw (1985) found that induced anisometropia caused a non-linear loss of stereoacuity as measured by Titmus and Randot test. Sen (1982) showed that the improvement of VA in 49% of the patients who had anisohyperopic amblyopia without strabismus after part-time or full-time patching was accompanied by improved stereoacuity. However, he did not mention the relationship between VA and stereoacuity. In our results, there was a significant association between VA and stereoacuity for all patients and in subgroups with each follow-up ($P < .001$ for all except in group III, $P = .0027$). Thus, as VA improves with occlusion therapy, stereoacuity generally also improves significantly. Mitchel and associates (1983) found that occlusion therapy for amblyopia can produce significant improvements in stereoacuity. However, they did not mention the VA improvement and the relationship between stereopsis and VA.

One possible limitation of this study is the possibility of a learning effect producing improved stereopsis scores with repeated testing. Although possible, a few factors mitigate this alleged effect. The mean age of our patients at intake was 5.1 years. At this age, children can generally perform well on the Titmus test, especially with the encouragement we offer. Another consideration is that the children showed progressively better stereopsis scores on repeated visits. If there were a learning effect, one would expect that the maximum score to be achieved shortly after learning how to perform the test. The progressive improvement in stereopsis scored continued through as many as 6 visits. Thus, a learning effect probably does not account for the overall improved stereopsis found in this investigation. .

In conclusion,. in amblyopia due to anisometropia, small angle or intermittent strabismus, or a combination, as VA improves with occlusion therapy, stereoacuity generally also improves as well.

REFERENCES

Burian HM. 1951. Stereopsis. Doc Ophthalmol V-VI:169.

Ching FC, Parks MM, Friendly DS. 1986. Practical management of amblyopia. J Pediatr Ophthalmol Strabismus 23:12-16.

Cibis LM. 1969. Treatment of amblyopia. In: Becker B, Burde RM, eds. *Current Concepts in Ophthalmology 2*: 222. St Louis: Mosby.

Donzis PB, Rappazzo JA, Burde RM, Gordon M. 1983. Effect of binocular variations of Snellen's visual acuity on Titmus stereoacuity. Arch Ophthalmol 101:30-32.

Epelbaum M, Milleret C, Buisseret P, Dufier JL. 1993. The sensitive period for strabismic amblyopia. Ophthalmology 100:323-327.

Goodwin RT, Romano PE. 1985. Stereoacuity degradation by experimental and real monocular and binocular amblyopia. Invest Ophthalmol Vis Sci 26:917-923.

Hardman Lea SJ, Loades J, Rubinstein MP. 1989. The sensitive period for anisometropic amblyopia. Eye 37:83-90.

Kutschke PJ, Scott WE, Keech RV. 1991. Anisometropic amblyopia. Ophthalmology 98:258-263.

Lavasik JV, Szymkiw M. 1985. Effects of aniseikonia, anisometropia, accommodation, retinal illuminance, and pupil size on stereopsis. Invest Ophthalmol Vis Sci 26:741-750.

Levartovsky S, Gottesman N, Shimshoni M, Oliver M. 1992. Factors affecting long-term results of successfully treated amblyopia: Age at beginning of treating and age at cessation of monitoring. J Pediatr Ophthalmol Strabismus 29:219-223.

Levartovsky S, Oliver M, Gottesman N, Shimshoni M. 1995. Factors affecting long term results of successfully treated amblyopia: initial visual acuity and type of amblyopia. Br J Ophthalmol 79:225-228.

Levy NS, Glick EB. 1974. Stereoscopic perception and Snellen visual acuity. Am J Ophthalmol 78:722-4.

Malik SRK, Virdi PS, Goel BK. 1975. Follow-up results of occlusion and pleoptic treatment. Acta Ophthalmologica 53:620-625.

Mitchel DE, Howell ER, Keith CG. 1983. The effect of minimal occlusion therapy on binocular function in amblyopia. Invest Ophthalmol Vis Sci 24:778-781.

Preslan MW, Novak A. 1996. Baltimore vision screening project. Ophthalmology;103:105-109.

Sen DK. 1982. Results of treatment of anisohypermetropic amblyopia without strabismus. Br J Ophthalmol 66:680-684.

Sparrow JC, Flynn JT. 1979. Amblyopia: A long-term follow up. J Pediatr Ophthalmol Strabismus 14:333-336.

The Pediatric Eye Disease Investigator Group. 2002. A randomized trial of atropine vs. patching for treatment of moderate amblyopia in children. Arch Ophthalmol 120:268-278.

Weakley DR, Jr. 2001. The association between nonstrabismic anisometropia, amblyopia, and subnormal binocularity. Ophthalmology 108:163-171.

Transactions 28th Meeting European Strabismological Association, de Faber (ed.)
© 2004 European Strabismological Association, ISBN 90 265 1965 6

Citicoline treatment of amblyopia in elderly strabic children

A.Piantanida M.D.
Centro Lariano di Oftalmologia Pediatrica, Cernobbio (Como),Italy

ABSTRACT: Citicoline (Cytidine-5-diphosphocoline) is an endogenous substance intermediary for the synthesis of phosphatidilcholine.It is a fundamental phospholipid in the neuronal membrane and due to his role in the biosynthesis of structural phospholipids it increases the metabolism of cerebral structures and inhibits the degradation of phospholipids themselves. In the literature it has been referred that citicoline can ameliorate and improve the visual performance in amblyopic eyes "beyond the plastic period", due to its effects on noradrenaline and dopamine. We report the results of the treatment of 12 amblyopic children with citicoline. The age ranged from 7 to 12 years and all had strabismic amblyopia yet treated with occlusion therapy without success. All the children showed a visual improvement after one month from six months of follo-up and a decreasing of the V.A. reached from six to twelve months. According to the literature we stress the importance of citicoline in amblyopic patients "beyond the plastic period" with some cautions. KEYWORDS:Amblyopia, Occlusion ,Citicoline

Amblyopia is nowadays still a big ophthalmological problem expecially for those subjects that come to our observation after the "plastic period" (generally it is widely considered 6 or 7 years of age). Many articles have demonstrated a significative improvement in visual acuity after patchinng regimen even in children more than 8 years of age (Oliver 1986) and in previous presentations at the ESA meetings we have discussed about the importance in treating amblyopic elderly children.. (Piantanida A. 1999, 2001)
Now we want to point out the attention on this "quite new" treatment for amblyiopic subject and to discuss if this can ameliorate a situation that seems to have no Citicoline (Cytidine-5-diphosphocoline) is an endogenous substance intermediary for the synthesis of phosphatidiylcholine and a fundamental component of the neuronal membrane.
Citicoline increases the metabolism of cerebral tissues balancing the synthesis of phospholipids and inhibiting their degradation. It has been reported in several works of the literature about the citicoline role, that this substance has a neuroprotective effect in hypoxia and ischemia, increases the levels of different neurotransmitter like dopamine and noradrenaline, and in many articles it has been referred that citicoline enhances and improves the consciouness level in several brain disorders due to traumatic vascular or degenerative disease. (Boismare 1978, Serra 1981, Zappia 1985)
Citicoline stimulates the availability of different neurotransmitters like dopamine and for this reason it is used in Parkinson's disease. It is interesting to note that it has been reported the lack of side effects , even dose related , and a beneficial effect on vision: colours appear more saturated, letters seem more contrasted, in both normal and amblyopic subjects. (Gottlob 1992,Regan 1981)
It has been observed in glaucoma patients an improvement of cortical responses (VEP) and of retinal responses (PERG), and an amelioration of the index of neuronal conduction after citicoline treatment. (Parisi 1999)
According to these characteristics it has been proposed in some international papers the value of citicoline in the treatment of subjects with "poor vision due to amblyopia beyond the plastic period of the visual system". (Campos 1997)
possibility to be resolved.

MATERIALS AND METHODS

We considered 12 patients whose age ranged from 7 to 12 years (mean age 9 yrs); all the patients had strabismic amblyopia (microstrabismus). We decided to not consider anysometropic amblyopia since part of the improvement could have been due to the spontaneous amelioration of the visual acuity with full optical correction therapy.

All the patients were wearing a full optical correction and were already been treated with occlusion therapy in the past without improving their vision in 66.7% and a sligth amelioration in 33.3%. All had neglected patching for at least six months. All the patients underwent again a full ophthalmological examination, including cycloplegic refraction with cyclopentolate and an orthoptic examination: 8 of them were microesotrope (positive to Paliaga 8 diopters base-in test, Irvine 4 diopters base-out test ,absence of Lang stereotest), 4 of them were microexotrope and all did not alternate spontaneously and had an high suppression (tested with Bagolini red glasses and Worth test) .

About these subjects 8 (66,7%)were amblyopic due to a failure in patching regimen in the past caused by a lack of compliance (4 exotrope and 4 esotrope with high astigmatism). They refused to go on with patching due to a "slight improvement" in their vision and "the difficulties in doing ordinary activities at school and at home" so that they had interrupted spontaneously their occlusion from 6 months. (as referred from the parents).

Instead 4 (33,3%) underwent this therapy to ameliorate the result already reached with occlusion (4 esotrope with UHM).

All were treated with citicoline(500 mg i.m. daily for 15 days) and underwent a part time penalization therapy with Bangerter foils (0.4 three hours a day). The subjects were examinated after one months, three months , six months and one year. Linear visual acuity for Snellen charts was measured by means of a commercially available projector.V.A. of a patients was defined as that corresponding to the last complete line seen. V.A. was measured in at least four different session before starting the treatment, to establish no doubtfull baseline values.

RESULTS

All the children (100%) showed a visual improvement after one months from 6 months (confidence limits 95% : 73.54 - 100,00), and a decreasing from 6 months to the end of therapy in 33.3% (confidence limits 95% : 9.92 – 65.11) (Graphic 1)

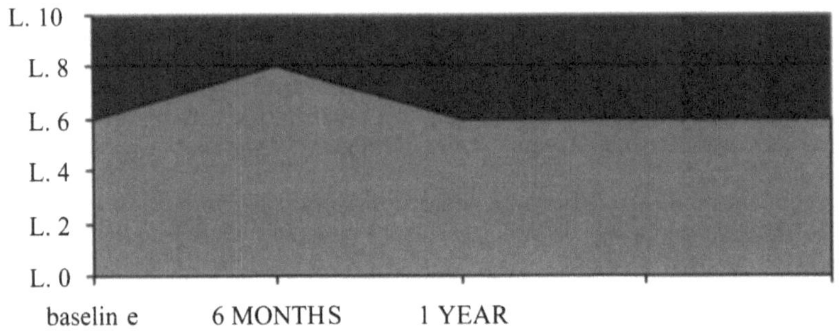

Graphic 1: Mean Visual Acuity durng follow-up measured in number of lines of Snellen as ordinal measures

The mean initial visual acuity was 0.6 (min 0.3, max 0.6) on the Snellen chart: among the exotrope children the initial V.A. was 0.3; among the esotropes the initial V.A. was 0.6. (Table 1)

TABLE 1: Mean baseline Visual Acuity : 0.6
(median statistically calculated as ordinal measures)

ET	XT	UHM+ET
0.6	0.3	0.6

The mean reached V.A. after 1 month was 0.8 (min 0.5, max 0.8) : the exotope children reached a visual acuity of 0.5, instead the esotrope ones 0.8 indipendently from the type of refraction and it lasted since the intermediate control after 6 months. (Table 2) No one of the subject referred for diplopia.

TABLE 2: Mean Visual Acuity after 6 months: 0.8
(median statistically calculated as ordinal measures)

ET	XT	UHM+ET
0.8	0.5	0.8

At the end of the follow-up after one year the mean visual acuity was 0.6 (min 0.5, max 0.8) (Table 3); all the patients but 4 manteined the V.A. reached: the 4 children who losted their improvement were all with an high astigmatic refraction.

TABLE 3: Mean Visual Acuity after 1 year : 0.6
(median statistically calculated as ordinal measures)

ET	XT	UHM+ET
0.6	0.5	0.8

DISCUSSION

There is a general agreement that amblyopia must be treated at an early age to achieve what we usaully say a "cured amblyopia" ; but in these last few years it has become more common to treat amblyopia in older people too, even if it is well known that the effect of the treatment is less beneficial. (Oliver 1986, Piantanida 1999, 2001)

Citicoline (Cytidine-5 diphosphocholine or CDP-choline) is a well known substance by the neurologists because it is commonly used to increase consciousness level in several brain disorders due to traumatic, vascular or degenerative causes. Citicoline has a dopaminergic action improving the availability of neurotransmitters and neuromodulators, and for this reason it is also used in Parkinson's disease patients. (Manaka 1971) Many studies have demonstrated the usefulness of citicoline treatment in improving general vision ameliorating retinal and cortical responses in glaucoma patients. (Gottlob 1992,Parisi 1999)

Recently it has been reported that the use of this treatment for strabismic and anisometropic amblyopia may improve the visual acuity of these patients irrespectively to the age. (Campos 1997)

In our study we want to point-out some consideration about compliance and citicoline treatment.

It is well known that antiamblyopia occlusion therapy relies on compliance and that usually it is imposssible *to cure* amblyopia beyond the plastic period, but it is also well known that it can be possible to ameliorate vision using patching regimen in "older age children" (8 years old or more). (Oliver 1986, Piantanida 1999, 2001) The big problem relies on compliance once more since elderly children usually refuse to wear patch for many reasons like psycological implications for and crowded activities of children at this age. The risk of non-compliance becomes also greater when the treatment period is prolonged. (Hussar 1975, Nucci 1992)

In our series we obtained good results in amelioration of visual acuity in accordance with the literature (2 lines on the Snellen charts after 6 months of follow-up) (Campos 1997, Porciatti 1998) We preffered, as suggested by others authors (Campos 1997),to make a part time occlusion that was well accepted by the patients and by the parents too, but we choose Bangerter's foils instead of total patching *to influence the less possible* the results of citicoline treatment and on the contrary to permit an alternation and consequently fixation of the amblyopic eye since all the children were non-alternating due to microstrabismus. In our opinion wearing a slight penalization for few hours a day (3 or 4 hours) can give us the possibility to reach the objective (fixation with the amblyopic eye) without influencing too much the daylife of our young patients and the amelioration of visual acuity with penalization therapy. (Lang 2000) For this reason it should be raccomandable to compare two groups of treated patients to see in a statistical way (Evidence Based Medicine) the significativity of this new therapy.(as reported in the literature)

Apparently surprisingly we could see an amelioration in 100% of the patients (confidence limits 95%: 73.54 – 100.00) that basically lasted for a long period (6 months) accordingly to the results of other authors, but in 33,3% of cases (confidence limits 95%: 9.92 – 65.11) we registered a worsening after one year and in 66.7% of the subjects (confidence limits 95%: 34.89 – 90.08) the Visual Acuity reached seemed stable (data not statistically significative since confidence limits overlap). The decreasing of visual acuity is statistically significant since the confidence limits don't overlap each other and it confirms the results reported in the literature where the electrophisiologic parameters and the retinal and visual pathway functions were similar to those observed before the start of the treatment after 6 months of washout. (Parisi 1999) According to E.Campos this work seems to justify that citicoline treatment in antiamblyopic therapy expecially in those cases where patching regimen was not possible. It is important to point-out that our results confirm the usefulness of a slight penalization therapy associated with citicoline since the combination of the two may enhance the results reached as reported in others reports.

As previously referred no one of the patients had diplopia during or after treatment even if the risk is higher in non alternating subject, since the suppression scotoma is weaker than in free alternator: we can say tha citicoline treatment seems to be apparently sure about diplopic vision since it improves general visual function stimulating the dopaminergic system, and we have to point-out that all our patients had microstrabismus, a condition where the suppression scotoma is well known to be high.

During the one year follow-up it was not obtained neither isoacuity nor free alternation stressing the demonstration of a practically impossibility "to cure amblyopia beyond the plastic period", but in our opinion this can't influence the possibility we have with this new therapy "to ameliorate visual acuity in elderly amblyopic children". (Porciatti 1998)

CONCLUSIONS

In conclusion it is clear that our results confirm the *efficacy* of this "quite new treatment" but not its complete *effectiveness*, although longer follow-ups should be needed. Efficacy defines the extent to wich a specific treatment produces a beneficial result under ideal conditions; effectiveness refers to the actual effect of a treatment in the real world of people (Paliaga 2003), and the effectiveness of our results is not so briliant . On these basis citicoline therapy points–out the possibility to manage amblyopia "beyond the plastic period". Statistical analysis and longer follow-up must be done to understand the real role of citicoline and the mechanism of cortical plasticity and methabolism that seem to be strictly related to visual function and amblyopia .

REFERENCES

- Boismare F.& Le Poncin M. et al 1978. Action of cytidinephosphocholine on functional and hemodynamic effects of cerebral ischemia in cats. *Pharmacology* 17,15-24.
- Campos E. & Bolzani R. et al 1997. Cytidin-5- diphosphocjoline enhances the effect of part-time occlusion in amblyopia. *Documenta Ophthalmologica* 93,247-263
- Gottlob I. & Charlier J. et al 1992. Visual acuities and scotomas after one week levodopa administration in human amblyopia. *Invest. Ophthalmol. Vis. Sci.* 33, 2722-2728
- Hussar D.A. 1975. Patient non-compliance. *J. Am. Pharm. Ass.* 15,183-190
- Lang J. 1999. An efficient treatment and new criteria for cure strabismic amblyopia: reading and Bangerter foils. *Binoc. Vis. and Strab.* 14(1), 9-10
- Manaka S. & Fuchinoue T. et al 1971. Mechanism of action of CDP-choline in Parkinsonism. *Brain and Nerve* 24,1051-1066
- Nucci P. & Alfarano R. et al 1992. Compliance in antiamblyopia occlusion therapy. *Acta Ophthalmologica* 70;128-131
- Oliver M. & Neumann R. et al 1986. Compliance and results of treatment for amblyopia in children more than 8 years old. *Am. J. Ophthalmol.* 102,340-345
- Paliaga G.P. 2003. *Ambliopia* Torino: Minerva Medica
- Parisi V. & Manni G. et al 1999. Cytidine-5-Diphosphocoline (Citicoline) improves retinal and cortical responses in patients with glaucoma. *Ophthalmology* 106(6), 1126-1134
- Piantanida A. & Vergani S. 1999. Successful occlusion therapy in compliant amblyopic elderly children. *Transaction 25th ESA* Meeting, Jerusalem, 41-45
- Piantanida A. 2001. Teen age visual acuity in treated amblyopic elderly children. *Transaction 27th ESA Meeting* Florence, 19-22
- Porciatti V. & Schiavi C. et al 1998. Cytidine-5-diphosphocholine improves visual acuity, contrast sensitivity and visually evoked potentials of amblyopic subjects. *Curr. Eye Research* 17,141-148
- Regan D. & Raymond J. Et al 1981. Contrast sensitivity, visual acuity and the discrimination of Snellen letters in multiple sclerosis. *Brain* 104, 330-350
- Serra L. & Aberghina M. et al 1981. Effect of CDP-choline on the biosynthesis of nucleic acids and proteins in brain regions during hypoxia. *Neurochem. Res.* 6, 607-618
- Zappia V. & Kennedy P. et al (Eds) 1985. *Novel Biochemical, pharmacological and clinical aspects of cytidinediphosphocholine.* New York: Elsevier

Transactions 28th Meeting European Strabismological Association, de Faber (ed.)
© 2004 European Strabismological Association, ISBN 90 265 1965 6

Contrast masking and spatial frequency properties of contour interaction in normals and amblyopes

O. Ehrt & R.F. Hess
Vision Research, McGill University, Montréal, Canada
Department of Ophthalmology, Ludwig Maximilians University, Muenchen, Germany (O. Ehrt)

ABSTRACT: We investigated some aspects of the cortical processes responsible for contour interaction, i.e. the detrimental effect of flanks on the discrimination of a central optotype. METHODS: Contrast thresholds for detection of the Landolt - C flanked by four high contrast bars and thresholds for discrimination of its orientation were measured for five normal subjects and five amblyopes. RESULTS: Detection thresholds for unfiltered stimuli did not change more than 30% when bars were brought in. Discrimination thresholds showed a much stronger threshold elevation for small stimuli and in amblyopia but not for large stimuli. Spatial frequency properties of contour interaction were unlike those of contrast masking. CONCLUSIONS: Low level contrast masking contributes to physiologic foveal contour interaction only for large stimuli whereas higher level processes seem to be involved in contour interaction for smaller stimuli and in amblyopia.

KEYWORDS: contour interaction, contrast threshold, spatial frequency, crowding, amblyopia

The detrimental effect of flanks on the discrimination of a central optotype is called contour interaction (Flom 1963). It is part of the crowding phenomenon and has clinical importance when we compare single optotype versus line acuity in amblyopes (Flom 1963) or the peripheral visual field (Bouma 1970, Toet 1992). In both conditions it is much stronger than in the normal fovea and contributes to the poor reading of amblyopes and patients with central scotomas (Leat 1999).

Little is knows about the cortical mechanisms underlying contour interaction. Previous work suggested a physical explanation of contour interaction but this has been refuted (Hess 2000). We set up a study to investigate the contribution of low level contrast masking and the spatial frequency properties of contour interaction in search for a better understanding of those mechanisms. Levi states that foveal contour interaction "is simple contrast masking" (2002). Others however claim that other mechanisms must be present (Chung 2001, Palomares 1999, Parkes 2001).

1 METHODS

1.1 *Equipment*

Landolt - Cs and four flanking bars (size 0.25° - 2°, thus 3 - 12-times the size at the acuity limit) were presented on a 10 cd/m² mid grey background of a calibrated monitor (Ehrt 2003). Contrast thresholds for detection of the Landolt - C and thresholds for discrimination of its orientation were measured (Ehrt 2003, Strasburger 1991). A first series of measurements was done with unfiltered stimuli (Fig. 1, left). In the second part of the study the Landolt-target and flanks were individually digitally bandpass filtered (mid frequency 0,6 cycles per Landolt to 10 cpl, Fig. 1 mid and right). Contrast thresholds for the discrimination of the orientation of the C were determined.

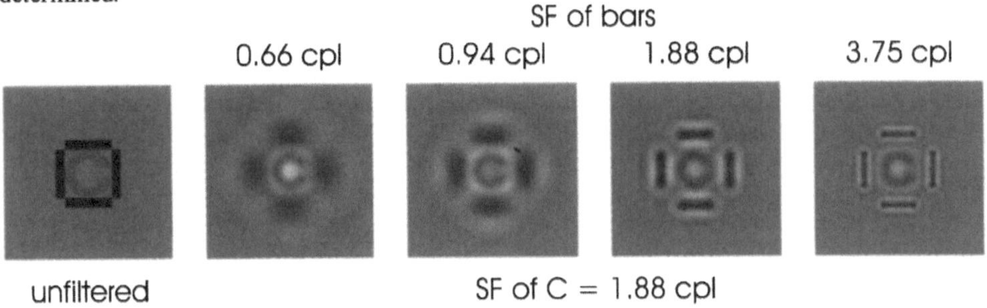

Figure 1. Sample stimuli of unfiltered Landolt - C flanked by abutting bars and bandpass filtered Landolt - C flanked by more distant (2 gap) bars filtered with different centre frequencies.

1.2 *Subjects*

Five normal subjects and five amblyopes (2 strabismic, 2 anisometropes, 1 mixed; VA 0.2 - 0.8 with single optotypes) participate in the study.

2 RESULTS

2.1 *Detection versus discrimination*

Detection thresholds for unfiltered stimuli did not change more than 30% when bars were brought in. Detection data are presented as dashed lines in Figure 2 a-c). Discrimination thresholds (continuous line) were 50% higher for unflanked Landolt - Cs (right end of lines). When bars were brought in (moving left in Figures 2 a-c) discrimination thresholds id show different results depending on the stimulus size: for large Landolt - C (1.0°) they increased parallel to detection thresholds. For medium and small stimuli discrimination was more affected than detection and thresholds rose much higher.

These data are summarized in Figure 2 d). The ratio of discrimination threshold to detection threshold is plotted over flank separation. It rises when flanks approach the C in the case of small stimuli and does not change significantly for large stimuli.

In amblyopic eyes the size of the Landolt - C and the flanks was scaled to their single optotype visual acuity by reducing the viewing distance to the monitor. Although the stimulus size was much larger for amblyopic eyes they did show a rise of the discrimination / detection ratio, i.e. flanks affect discrimination more than detection (Fig. 3).

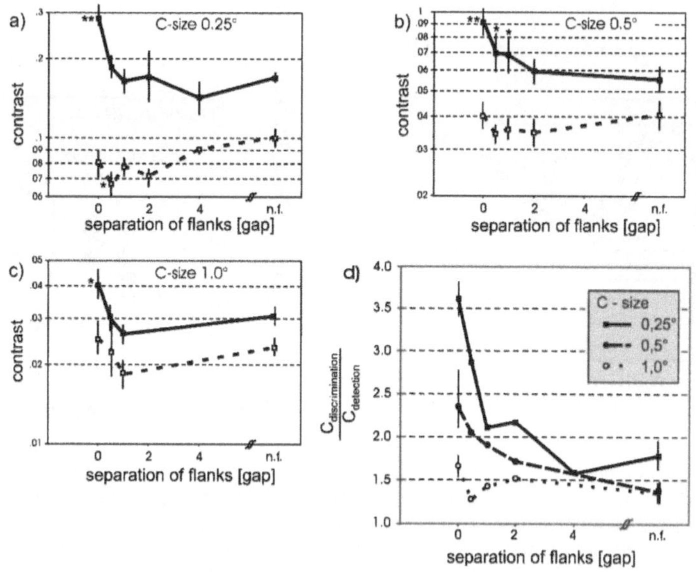

Figure 2. Detection and discrimination thresholds are plotted as dashed and solid lines over flank separation for three different stimulus sizes (a-c). Data represent the mean of 5 normal subjects, the vertical lines represent the 68% confidence intervals. In (d) the data are summarized and the ratio of discrimination threshold and detection threshold plotted over flank separation (n.f.: no flanks).

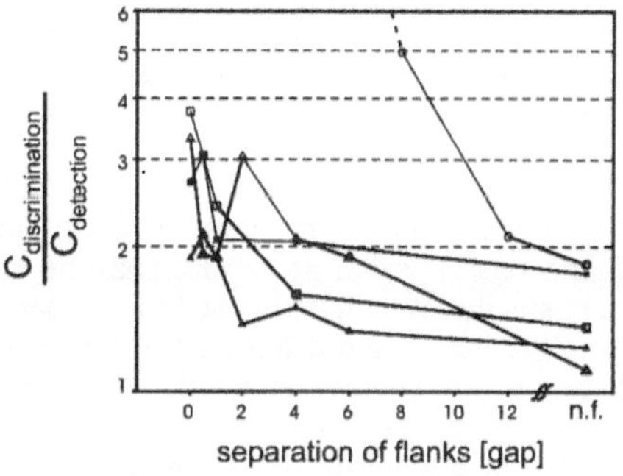

Figure 3. The ratio of discrimination and detection threshold is plotted over flank separation for 5 individual amblyopic subjects. The stimulus size was scaled to the single Landolt - C VA of the amblyopic eye.

2.2 *Spatial frequencies*

Landolt - Cs of three different spatial frequency filters (0.94, 1.88 and 3.75 cpl) were combined with flanks that were filtered from 0.6 to 10 cpl. The tuning curves for normal subjects is shown in Figure 4 a) for the medium spatial frequency. From this graph the spatial frequency for peak interaction is determined and entered in a plot that displays changes in peak frequencies of the flanks with respect to changes in the spatial frequency of the Landolt - C (Fig. 4 b).

The dashed line represents unity, i.e. the interaction is maximal when spatial frequency of bars and the Landolt - C coincide. This is to be expected in the case of contrast masking.

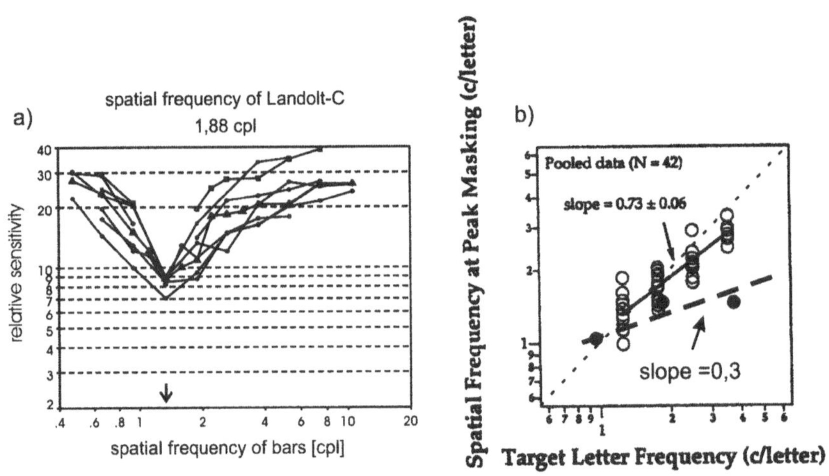

Figure 4. a) Tuning curves of all normal subjects. The SF of the Landolt - C was held constant and the relative sensitivity (1 / contrast threshold) was plotted for different filter frequencies of the bars. In b) the bar frequencies at peak interaction (arrow in a) show a rather flat correlation with the spatial frequency of the Landolt - C. Data of this study (slope 0.3) are presented together with a plot from Chung (2001).

3 CONCLUSIONS

Low level contrast masking was defined by the effect flanks have on the detection of the central Landolt - C. Contour interaction was defined by the effect flanks have on the discrimination of the Landolt - C orientation.

For large stimuli both contrast thresholds change in parallel. Thus contrast masking determines the amount of "contour interaction". This result is in agreement with findings by Levi et al. (2002) who used large stimuli only and concluded that "foveal contour interaction is simple contrast masking".

With smaller stimuli and in amblyopia however discrimination thresholds are affected much more than detection. Under these circumstances masking alone can not account for the contour interaction. Higher level mechanisms of visual processing may be involved. Again this result agrees with other studies where smaller stimuli were used to compare masking and contour interaction and significant differences were found (Chung 2001, Palomares (1999), Parkes 2001).

The tuning curves too do show that contour interaction is unlike masking. The maximal masking effect would be expected when the spatial frequencies of target and mask are equal. This was not the case for contour interaction in this study and similar in Chung's experiment with crowding letters (Chung 2001).

Two clinical applications may arise from these results: Limiting the SF-contents to medium frequencies may help to design vision chart that show strong contour interaction and hence crowding. This may be helpful for amblyopia screening and follow-up on treatment. The inverse approach may help to improve reading text e.g. for patients with central scotomas as they suffer from crowding as well. An image processing algorithm that reduces the medium spatial frequencies (notch-filter) that are most relevant for contour interaction may facilitate reading for these patients.

4 REFERENCES

Bouma, H. 1970. Interaction effects in parafoveal letter recognition. *Nature* 226: 177-178.

Chung, S.T.L., Levi, D.M. & Legge, G.E. 2001. Spatial-frequency and contrast properties of crowding. *Vision Res.* 41: 1833-1850.

Ehrt, O., Hess, R.F., Williams, C.B. & Sher, K. 2003. Foveal contrast thresholds exhibit spatial frequency- and polarity-specific contour interactions. *J Opt Soc Am A.* 20: 11-17.

Flom, M.C., Weymouth, F.W. & Kahneman, D. 1963. Visual resolution and contour interaction. *J Opt Soc Am.* 53: 1026-1032.

Hess, R.F., Dakin, S.C. & Kapoor, N. 2000. The foveal 'crowding' effect: physics or physiology? *Vision Res.* 40: 365-370.

Leat, S.J., Li, W. & Epp, K. 1999. Crowding in central and eccentric vision: the effects of contour interaction and attention. *Invest Ophthalmol Vis Sci.* 40: 504-512.

Levi, D.M., Klein, S.A. & Hariharan, S. 2002. Suppressive and facilitatory spatial interactions in foveal vision: Foveal crowding is simple contrast masking . *J Vision.* 2: 140-166.

Palomares, M., LaPutt, M. C. & Pelli, D.G. 1999. Crowding is unlike masking. Invest Ophthalmol Vis Sci 40 (Suppl 4): 351

Parkes, L., Lund, J., Angelucci, A., Solomon, J.A. & Morgan, M. 2001. Compulsory averaging of crowded orientation signals in human vision. *Nat Neurosci.* 4: 739-744.

Strasburger, H., Harvey, L.O., Rentschler, I. 1991. Contrast thresholds for identification of numeric characters in direct and eccentric view. *Percept Psychophys.* 49: 495-508.

Toet, A. & Levi, D.M. 1992. The two-dimensional shape of spatial interaction zones in the parafovea. *Vision Res.* 32: 1349-1357.

Transactions 28th Meeting European Strabismological Association, de Faber (ed.)

Rapid monocular adaptation of saccade amplitude in constant strabismus

H.J. Griffiths, D. Buckley & J.P. Whittle
Academic Unit of Ophthalmology and Orthoptics, University of Sheffield, Sheffield, UK

ABSTRACT: This study investigated fast disconjugate adaptations in subjects with bifoveal BSV and subjects with long-standing, small angled strabismus who clinically demonstrated no BSV (normal or abnormal). Eye movements were recorded using an infrared technique. An electronic feedback system, in which the calibrated eye movement position signal could be scaled by a factor (the feedback gain) to move the target visible to one eye during binocular viewing, was used to induce saccade disconjugacy. In all BSV subjects and three of six subjects with constant strabismus, saccadic adaptation occurred rapidly such that under conditions of visual feedback saccades became increasingly disconjugate. These disconjugacies persisted when normal viewing conditions were restored. The presence of an adaptive mechanism to adjust the binocular co-ordination of saccades, in the presence of constant strabismus with suppression and no clinically demonstrable BSV, has been demonstrated.

KEYWORDS: Saccades, Strabismus, Disconjugate adaptation

1 INTRODUCTION

Horizontal saccades are naturally disconjugate, with abducting saccades being faster and slightly larger than adducting saccades (Kapoula et al. 1987, Collewijn et al. 1988, de Faber et al. 1994). This gives rise to relative divergence of the eyes. In normal binocular single vision (BSV) this is small where typically, for horizontal saccades of <20° from the primary position, the two eyes differ by <0.5° (Collewijn et al. 1988). Binocular vision requires images to fall on the foveae of each eye and therefore precise control over ocular alignment is essential. To maintain control, saccades are under an adaptive control system to compensate for short or long term changes to the visual system. Adaptive control monitors performance and adjusts parameters to improve accuracy and behaviour where required. As saccades are ballistic in nature, on-going feedback is not possible, therefore saccade adaptation is achieved by a learning process.

Studies of symmetric saccadic adaptive control in subjects with normal BSV have been carried out experimentally by techniques such as intra-saccadic step (Deubel et al. 1986) and electronic feedback systems (Albano & King 1989).

Saccades may also adapt disconjugately, such that saccades become unequal in the two eyes. Lemij & Collewijn (1991) investigated the time course of disconjugate saccade adaptation in normal subjects using short-term wear of anisometropic spectacles. These spectacle lenses resulted in visual images that were differently sized for the two eyes. Disconjugate saccades occurred with anisometropias ranging from 2D to 8D, with the adaptations almost complete within one hour. More recent studies (Kapoula et al. 1995, Van der Steen & Bruno 1995) show that, under similar conditions where the image to one eye is magnified, disconjugacy occurs within a period of a few minutes and that it persists under monocular viewing. This indicates the presence of a fast learning mechanism.

As disconjugate adaptation sub-serves binocular vision, Kapoula et al. (1996) questioned whether foveal fusion is a prerequisite to achieve disconjugate adaptations. They studied three microstrabismic subjects who viewed a random dot pattern, which was 10% larger in one eye. Within 40 seconds, horizontal saccades became larger in the eye viewing the larger stimulus by 4 to 10%. The induced disconjugacy persisted under monocular viewing. This demonstrates that foveal fusion is not required for this mechanism and peripheral fusion is sufficient to drive adaptive changes.

Bucci et al. (1997) examined the degree of binocular vision necessary to stimulate disconjugate adaptation. They studied two subjects with small esotropia and peripheral fusion, two with intermediate esotropia, ARC and anomalous BSV and four subjects with large esotropia and no demonstrable binocular vision. The conclusions were that subjects with peripheral binocular vision, and those with anomalous BSV, were able to demonstrate disconjugate changes of the binocular coordination of their saccades appropriate for the induced disparity. However, subjects without binocular vision made disconjugate changes to the amplitude of saccades, but these were not in the direction appropriate for the induced disparity. This indicates that binocular vision (normal or anomalous) is required to simulate the appropriate mechanism of saccade adaptation.

In the experiment outlined above all subjects without potential BSV had their angle of deviation corrected, or partially corrected, with base out prisms, ranging from 2 to 22Δ, placed over the deviating eye. The reason stated for this was to render disparities similar in all subjects. This may have led to the anomalous responses found in the larger angled strabismus with no demonstrable binocular vision, as points stimulated in each eye were significantly altered to those normally stimulated without correction of the deviation. It may be that with their 'normal' ocular alignment, the disparity would have been detected and hence an appropriate disconjugate adaptation of saccades could be triggered.

This study therefore investigates disconjugate saccade adaptation in normal BSV and in strabismus with no demonstrable binocular vision without correction of the angle of strabismus. The method used to induce retinal disparity of targets was an electronic feedback system.

2 METHOD

Fourteen adult subjects participated in this experiment, eight with normal bifoveal BSV (mean age 29.3 years ±9.6) and six with manifest strabismus (mean age 34.0 years ±15.7). The group with normal BSV were all right eye dominant and had corrected visual acuity of at least 6/6 Sn and no ocular motility defects. The subjects with strabismus all had constant suppression and no clinically demonstrable BSV, their details are summarised in Table 1.

Table 1. Characteristics of subjects with strabismus and no BSV.

Subject	Age	VA (log MAR)		Cover Test	PCT	Onset	Surgery
	(years)	RE	LE			(years)	(age and type of strabismus)
1	42	-0.1	0.0	LXT	12Δ	2.0	Age 4 ET & Age 4 XT
2	19	-0.1	0.6	LXT	8Δ	1.5	Age 4 ET
3	23	0.0	-0.1	RET	8Δ	1.0	None
4	21	-0.1	0.0	LXT	18Δ	1.5	Age 4 ET
5	59	-0.1	0.2	LET	2Δ	<0.5	Age 53 XT
6	40	0.4	-0.1	RET	18Δ	<0.5	Age 2 ET & Age 34 XT

The subjects were seated comfortably 114cm from a flat back projection screen. The subject's head was stabilised using a chin and cheek rest, ensuring close fitting of cheek rests against the cheek bones and instructing the subject to remain firmly in position.

Two modified Kodak carousel slide projectors projected identical sized targets. The targets consisted of a cross, subtending 2° of luminance 18cd/m^2. These were projected so that they overlaid each other to appear as a single target and they could be moved by mirror galvanometers. Four liquid crystal polymer (LCP) shutters, one positioned in front of each projector lens and one in front of each eye and all operating at 80Hz, were set such that one target was visible to each eye. A blurred random dot stationary background of luminance 4 cd/m^2 was back projected by a third projector, and was constantly visible to both eyes.

Horizontal eye movements were recorded using a Skalar IRIS 6500 infrared limbal tracker. The calibrated eye movement position signal could be scaled by a factor (the feedback gain) and used to move one of the targets. Feedback gain, calculated by dividing target velocity by eye velocity, could be instantaneously adjusted between -1 and +1 in 0.05 steps. Zero feedback gain represented normal viewing conditions. When the feedback gain was >0 the target moved in the same direction as the eye; at +1 the target moved at the same speed as the eye. If feedback gain was <0, the target moved in the opposite direction to the eye (not used in this experiment). Feedback could be applied to one of the targets, visible to one eye only, to induce saccade disconjugacy.

Each eye movement recording session consisted of three phases: the pre-adaptation phase (60 trials); the adaptation phase (210 trials) and the post adaptation phase (60 trials). Each phase was run in series directly after each other with no break. The pre- and post-adaptation phases were the same and consisted of a single target step of 5° from the central fixation point and back. The adaptation phase consisted of two different conditions; +0.1 feedback gain applied to the target visible to one eye, and a control condition in which there was no feedback applied. The same gaze direction and eccentricity was maintained for all trials in the session to facilitate fast adaptation.

The eight subjects with normal BSV attended two sessions: one session where the feedback condition was performed and another for the control condition. All subjects were right eye dominant, four had feedback applied to the dominant eye and four had feedback applied to the non-dominant eye. The six subjects with constant strabismus attended three sessions; feedback to the fixing eye, feedback to the strabismic eye and the control condition. The order of testing these conditions was randomised.

Subjects were instructed to look at the centre of the target cross and move their eyes to follow it at all times as quickly and accurately as possible. They were told not to move their eyes until they actually saw the target appear in the eccentric position. They were also asked to try to keep the target single and clear. The subject was informed of the gaze direction prior to commencing the experiment. Each experimental session lasted approximately 30 minutes. Calibration of eye movements was performed prior to each phase.

The two identical overlapping targets appeared in the centre of the screen and, after a randomised time delay (500 to 1500ms), jumped 5° to the right or left of centre. Following a randomised period (500 to 1500ms) the targets would both return to the centre. In the feedback condition adaptation phase, both targets would jump from the centre to 5° eccentricity, when the eye with feedback moved to fixate the target, the dissociated target visible to that eye moved in the direction of the eye movement by a feedback gain of +0.1, producing retinal disparity. This therefore created a stimulus to induce disconjugate saccade adaptation.

The pre- and post-adaptation phases were performed with monocular fixation by closing the LCP shutter in front of the non-preferred eye. The adaptation phase was performed with LCP shutters to both eyes open.

3 RESULTS

The mean gain of saccades in each eye was calculated. The gain of the eye without feedback was subtracted from the eye with feedback to determine the saccade gain disconjugacy in the pre- and post-adaptation phases. Saccade gain disconjugacy in the pre-adaptation phases was subtracted from the post-adaptation saccade gain disconjugacy to give the magnitude of the adaptation effect. When no feedback was applied during the adaptation phase, there was no significant change in disconjugacy of saccades between the pre- and post-adaptation phases in any of the subjects (t-test $p>0.05$). The feedback, applied during the adaptation phase, induced appropriate saccade disconjugacy in all eight subjects with normal BSV. The results for all BSV subjects were pooled and the mean and range of results are shown in Figure 1. In the strabismic group examination of individual subject data reveals variable results as also shown in Figure 1. Five of the six subjects demonstrated adaptive changes to saccade disconjugacy following the adaptation phase when feedback was applied to a target visible to one eye. Three subjects (1, 2 and 3) showed increased disconjugacy appropriate in direction for the stimulus and two subjects

(4 and 5) demonstrated disconjugacy in an inappropriate direction. One subject (6) showed no change in saccade disconjugacy following the adaptation phase.

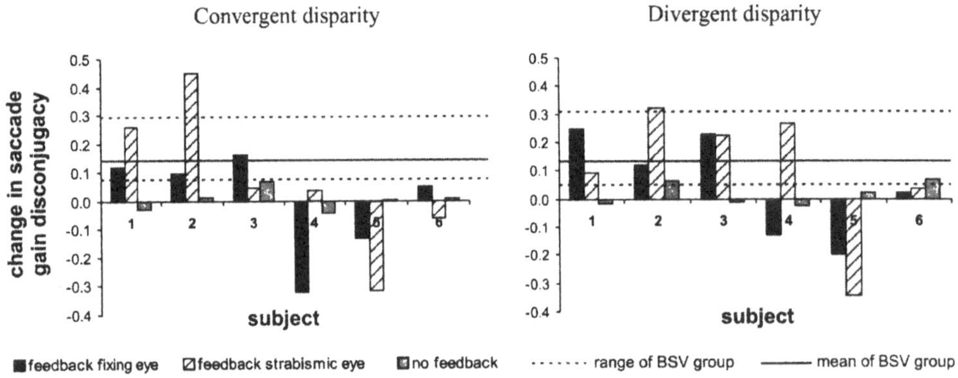

Figure 1. Change in saccade gain disconjugacy in the post-adaptation phase compared to the pre-adaptation phase. Results of individual strabismic subjects are plotted. The mean change in disconjugacy for the BSV subjects is represented by the solid black line.

4 DISCUSSION

The electronic feedback system applied to a target visible to one eye produced rapid disconjugate saccade adaptation in eight subjects with normal bifoveal BSV. The aim of this study was to determine whether subjects with manifest strabismus and no demonstrable BSV, normal or anomalous, could produce disconjugate saccades under such test conditions. The results demonstrated that three of the six strabismic subjects studied were able to produce appropriate disconjugate adaptations despite no clinically detectable binocular co-operation. The three subjects who adapted in the appropriate direction had small angled deviations (8Δ esotropia, 8Δ exotropia and 12Δ exotropia). These could therefore be considered likely candidates for development of abnormal retinal correspondence and anomalous binocular vision. Extreme care was taken clinically to investigate the subjects with detailed questioning for binocular tests requiring subjective responses and a complete investigation, with a full range of tests employed. Bucci et al. (1997) have demonstrated disconjugate adaptations in intermediate strabismus with abnormal binocular vision. They describe such adaptations in two subjects with 18 and 21Δ esotropia who had positive responses for Bagolini striated glasses, failed to demonstrate stereoacuity in free space (TNO and Titmus test) but demonstrated a stereoacuity of 3600 seconds of arc on the synoptophore.

The level of VA in the strabismic eye did not appear to prevent adaptation, as the target was clearly visible to the strabismic eye in all subjects. Subject 2 adapted in the appropriate direction (although by a larger amount than the normal BSV group) despite having the lowest VA of the group (0.6 logMAR). The age of onset of strabismus appeared to have been a significant factor as subject 5, who demonstrated constant anomalous adaptation responses, and subject 6, who had no response, had onset of strabismus before six months of age.

The maximum angle of deviation in which an appropriate adaptation response was found was 12Δ (one subject with esotropia of 12Δ and one subject with exotropia of 12Δ). The two subjects with strabismus measuring 18Δ had no response at all and a variable response. This finding is compatible with the results of Bucci et al. (1997) who failed to find normal saccadic adaptation in four subjects with no demonstrable BSV and esotropia of between 14 and 30Δ. The differences between the present study and Bucci et al. (1997) were the method of inducing disconjugacy and the subjects reported by Bucci et al. (1997) were corrected with prisms either fully or partially, to present the disparities close to the fovea of the deviating eye. The subjects reported in this current study did not have the strabismus corrected to determine how they would respond when in their 'normal' sensory state. It was shown that the two subjects with angles of deviation >12Δ did not demonstrate normal saccade adaptation with their 'normal' strabismic angle.

The mechanism for the resulting difference in primary saccade amplitude in each eye in BSV would appear to be due to re-scaling of the pulse step signal based on the post-saccadic disparity, with the primary aim of maintaining BSV. A mechanism in the strabismic subjects who adapted normally or abnormally is less clear.

In the absence of fusion there could be a purpose in ensuring that the retinal image stimulating the deviating eye is maintained in a reasonably constant position. This might be to ensure that it remains within the suppression area and to avoid diplopia. If no adaptation, or inappropriate adaptation, occurred then the location of the image in the deviating eye would no longer stimulate retina equal to the angle of deviation possibly causing symptoms. The pathway to drive such a response is also unclear. It is possible that, despite a lack of cortical perception of suppressed images, information from the strabismic eye sub-cortically leads to adaptation of saccades to avoid diplopia.

This present study found anomalous disconjugacy in two subjects with small angled strabismus. Bucci et al. (1997) found anomalous disconjugacy only in subjects with large angle strabismus and no fusion. They proposed that this might be driven by monocular visual inputs occurring to improve fixation of each eye and not to reduce binocular disparity. They suggest that the movements of the two eyes are controlled independently, so-called utrocular vision (or vision with each eye separately), as described by Schor (1991). This is a primitive form of binocular vision found in vertebrates with complete decussation of the visual pathways. Bucci et al. (1997) suggested that this form of independent eye control could allow avoidance of diplopia, but not establishment of a true binocular linkage.

5 CONCLUSION

Using LCP shutters for dissociation and an electronic feedback system to induce disparity, five out of six subjects with no clinically demonstrable BSV responded to stimuli within the suppression area by changing the amplitude of saccades in one eye. Three of these subjects demonstrated rapid disconjugate adaptation of saccades in an appropriate direction for the induced disparity and two subjects demonstrated adaptations in an inappropriate direction. This suggests that in constant strabismus with no clinical evidence of binocular co-operation, the eyes may have rudimentary linkage allowing gross co-ordination. A mechanism and purpose for such results has been discussed.

REFERENCES

Albano, J.E, King, W.M. 1989. Rapid adaptation of saccadic amplitude in humans and monkeys. Investigative Ophthalmology and Visual Science, 30: 1883-1893.

Bucci, M.P, Kapoula, Z, Eggert, T, Garraud L. 1997. Deficiency of adaptive control of the binocular coordination of saccades in strabismus. Vision Research, 37:2767-2777.

Collewijn, H., Erkelens, C.J., Steinman, R.M. 1988. Binocular co-ordination of human horizontal saccadic eye movements. Journal of Physiology (London) 404:157-182.

de Faber, J.T.H.N., van Rijn, L.J., Collewijn, H. 1994. Dynamics of saccades in strabismus and amblyopia.; In H. Kauffmann (ed.) Transactions of the 21st European Strabismological Association: 303-308.

Deubel, H, Wolf, W, Hauske, G. 1986. Adaptive gain control of saccadic eye movements. Human Neurobiology, 5:245-253.

Kapoula, Z, Hain, T.C, Zee, D.S, Robinson, D.A. 1987. Adaptive changes in post-saccadic drift induced by patching one eye. Vision Research, 27:1299-1307.

Kapoula, Z, Eggert, T, Bucci, M.P. 1995. Immediate saccade amplitude disconjugacy induced by unequal images. Vision Research, 35: 3505-3518.

Kapoula, Z., Bucci, M.P., Eggert, T., Zamfirescu, F. 1996. Fast disconjugate adaptations of saccades in microstrabismic subjects. Vision Research 36:103-108.

Lemij, H.G, Collewijn, H. 1991. Short-term nonconjugate adaptation of human saccades to anisometropic spectacles. Vision Research, 31: 1955-1966.

Schor, C.M. 1991. Binocular sensory disorders. In D. Regan (ed) Vision and visual dysfunction: vol. 9: Binocular vision. London. Macmillon Press. pp179-223.

van der Steen, J, Bruno, P. 1995. Unequal amplitude saccades produced by aniseikonic patterns: effects of viewing distance. Vision Research, 35: 3459-3473.

Transactions 28th Meeting European Strabismological Association, de Faber (ed.)
© 2004 European Strabismological Association, ISBN 90 265 1965 6

Synkinesis of vergence and accommodation in accommodative esotropia

M. Dostálek
Department of Ophthalmology (Ortoptic Section), City Hospital, Litomyšl, Czech Republic

ABSTRACT: The study deales with some properties of the dynamics of vergence and accommodation during the first second after step change of the fixation target's distance. We analyze two phenomena: saccadic contributions to vergence reactions and undulation of accommodation plots. The typology of reactions to the approaching of the fixation target in both refractive, and non-refractive accommodative ET were nearly similar to comparable reactions in the controls. ET was related to the significant reduction of purely vergent reactions to the removal of the fixation target. In patients with higher values of non-refractive component (esodeviation higher at near than at distance fixation) of accommodative esotropia, the higher values of refractive power instability (undulation of accommodation plots) were documented.

KEYWORDS: accommodative esotropia, saccadic contribution, accommodation instability.

1 INTRODUCTION

The static properties of horizontal eye vergent position and accommodation of squint patients were studied extensively. The measurements of AC/A ratio at clinical praxis is used nearly routinely. Little is known about early dynamic properties of the synkinesis. The objective of our pilot study was to describe the dynamics of duction and accommodation during the first second after step change of the fixation target's distance to the subject. Three signals are present if the synkinesis is stimulated from the real visual space: disparity, blur and proximity cues (Ciuffreda & Kenyon 1983). Our experiments manipulated some of these.

2 METHODOLOGY AND SUBJECTS

As a stimulus we used step change at the midline distance of the fixation target. The first type of stimulus, marked D→P, was the approximation of the target (Fig. 1). The second was a vice versa type of stimulus, marked P→D, involving the removal of the target.

The stimulus executed by our experiemental device was the step shift of the mother's face caught on live video between two monitors. Both monitors were placed at the midline of the experiemental subject. Both monitors were of identical angular subtense and approximately idential luminance (Fig. 1). For detailed information, please refer to our second transact (Dostalek, M., Dusek, J.: E.M.A.N. (Eye Movement and Accommodation Analyzer) device for vergence accommodation synkinesis recording and analysis).

All subjects were measured with the best correction to the distance. Measurements of the dominant eye were performed for both types of stimulation on the monocular (non-dominant eye occluded) and binocular conditions of viewing.

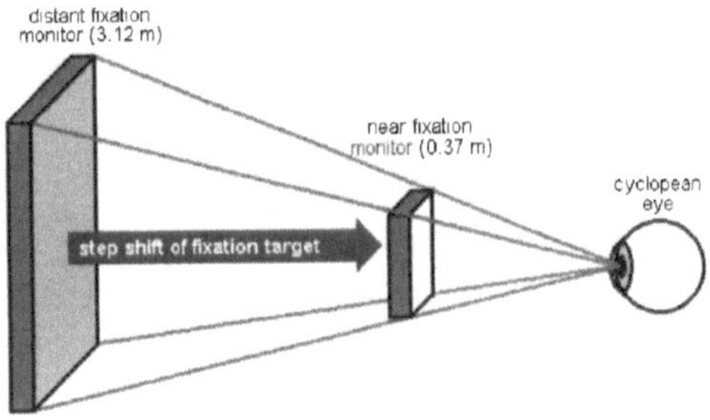

Figure 1. Stimulus D→P, step approximation of the target. Spatial properties of stimulating (fixating) video-circuit monitors

For quantitative analysis of the instability of the achieved degree of refractive power during accommodation reactions, we created a quantitative parameter describing the degree of undulation. Parameter U is defined as an average decay of refractive power between two consecutive measurements. The record of accommodation reaction is before the selection (Fig. 2) and averaging of the value of decays filtered from artificial oscillations. Increases between two measurements were nullified for parameter U's calculation. Calculation is performed from the start of accommodation to the end of the record.

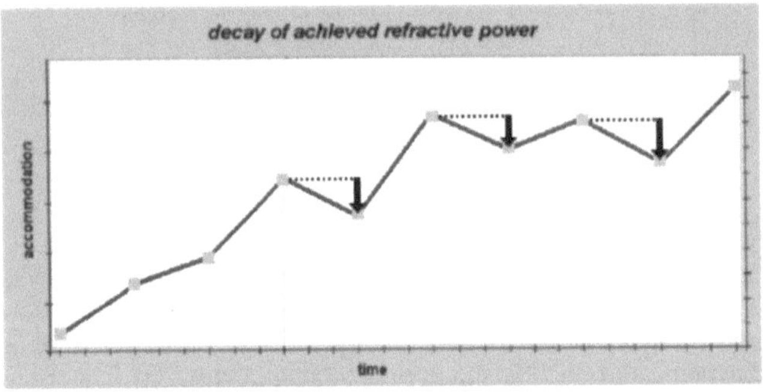

Figure 2. Schema of first step at calculation of parameter U: selection of particular decays between two consecutive measurements (black arrows indicate the particular decays between some couples of measurement)

For our clinical study, we have constituted a control group of fifteen ophthalmologically healthy children (mean age 7.25 years) and two experimental groups. The group of refractive accommodative esotropes consisted of thirty subjects (mean age 9.50 years) with esodeviation completely or nearly compensated (residual esodeviation <10 Δ) by hyperopic spectacle correction (>3.0 D). The group of non-refractive accommodative esotropes consisted of seventeen patients (mean age 8.50 years) wearing bifocal spectacle lenses because of their greater esodeviation at near than at distance fixation („sgital incommitance" > 15 Δ).

3 RESULTS

The main descriptions of both accommodation and duction reaction dynamics (mean latencies, accommodation speeds, saccadic and vergence speeds, time constants, etc.) of all the groups reached values comparable to previously published data. Besides this expected result we have documented two remarkable phenomena: saccadic contributions to vergence reactions and undulation of accommodation plots.

We have differenciated two types of saccadic contributions. The first type (Fig. 3a) is interposed to the course of vergent movement. The start of duction reaction has a dynamics of vergence. Saccadic fragment contributes incompletely to the whole movement reaction. The second type of saccadic contribution (Fig. 3b) represents complete movement which foveates new target positions in the dominant eye (Kenyon 1980). The ineffective initial saccadic movement of the non-dominant eye is consequently corrected by vergent movement.

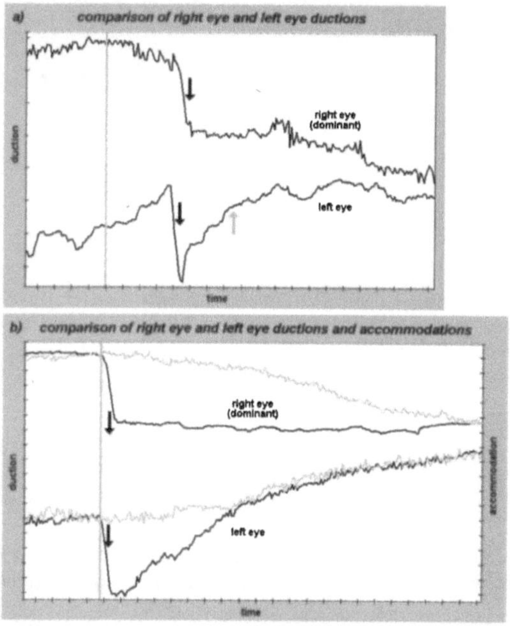

Figure 3. Types of saccadic contributions to vergent reactions: a) type I., b) type II. (parallel arrows = saccade, inverted arrows = vergence)

The diagrams in Figure 4 illustrate the frequency of purely vergent reactions (black parts of the columns) and the distribution of saccadic contribution of both types (white and grey parts of the columns) of the control and experimental groups during monocular and binocular conditions.

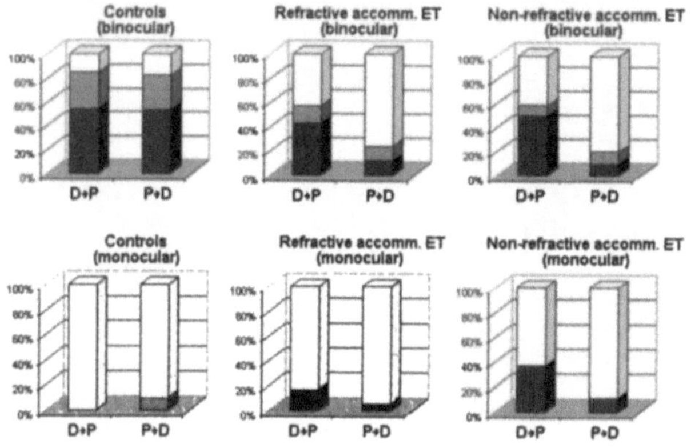

Figure 4. Typology of duction reacions (black = pure vergent reaction, grey = type I. saccadic contribution, white = type II. saccadic contribution, D→P = stimulation by fixation target aproximation, P→D = stimulation by fixation target removal)

The following graphs illustrate the second described phenomena: the undulation of accommodation plots. Figure 6a documents the instablility of the achieved degree of refractive power during refixation of the approximated target position in the patient with non-refractive accommodative esotropia. The similar undulation of the accommodation records was documented even in patients without non-refractive components of esotropia (Fig. 6b).

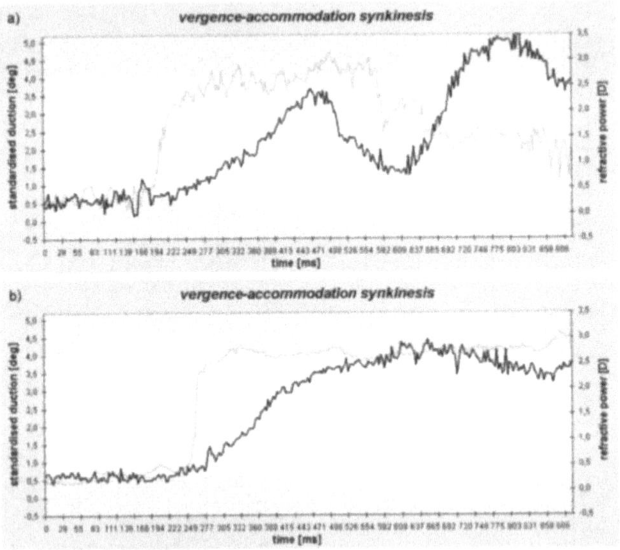

Figure 6. Undulation of accomodation: a) in patients with non-refractive accommodative esotropia (stimulation D→P), b) in patients with refractive accommodative esotropia (stimulation D→P) (black plot = accommodation, grey plot = duction)

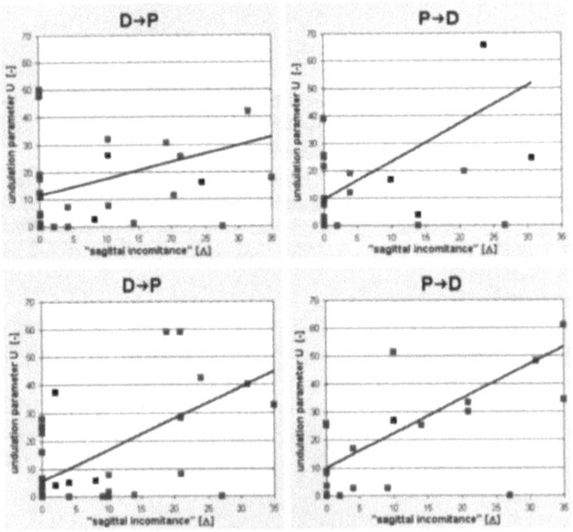

Figure 7. Trend to higher value of undulation parameter in patients with higher difference of esodeviation at distance and near (i.e. „ sagittal incommitance"): diagrams above: monocular conditions (non-dominant eye occluded) of viewing, diagrams below: binocular conditions of viewing. (Patients from refractive and non-refractive groups are pooled on the charts, D→P = approaching of the fixation target, P→D = removement of the fixation target)

The data documents the trend to higher values of undulation parameters in patients with highter difference of near and distance esodeviation. Figure 7 shows the pooled values of patients from the refractive and non-refractive accommodative esotropia groups.

4 DISCUSSION

Saccadic contributions to duction reactions was seen previously by Kenyon, Ciuffreda & Stark (1980, 1981). Our set of data describes differences of saccadic contributions typology between controls and both esotropia groups. The duction reaction on monocular conditions have nearly always saccadic initial dynamics as expected (Fig. 4, lower charts). The remarkable fraction of reactions with saccadic fragments in normal subjects on binocular conditions (Fig. 4, upper left chart) was unexpected. We ascribe this to our experimental conditions with reduced proximity cues. The typology of reactions to the approaching of the fixation target (stimulation D→P) in both esotropia groups (Fig. 4, upper central and right charts, left columns) were nearly similar to comparable reactions in the controls. The influence of strabismus could be seen only at the significant reduction of purely vergent reactions of esotropes to the removal of the fixation target (stimulation P→D) (Fig. 4, upper central and right charts, right columns) Our hypothesis for further research is that the defective disparity sense of esotropes fails in substitution of more profound proximity cues reduction in the second type of stimulation.u

The study of the second phenomena, undulation accommodation plots, documented significant differences between non-refractive accommodative esotropes and the rest of our subjects. In patients with higher values of non-refractive components of accommodative esotropia, the higher values of accommodation reaction instability were present. This trends were not remarkably influenced by manipulation with disparity information by the means of occlusion, but the trends were rather more evident in the binocular conditions. The direction of stimulation did not change the trend significantly. The type of stimulation, i.e. step approaching (stimulation D→P) or removal (stimulation P→D), had no remarkable influence to the slopes of regression lines. Because of the fact that the undulation was present in children with monofocal correction (subjects from refractive accommodative esotropia group), this phenomena could not be ascribed to the adaptation to bifocals. Probably, the ineffective decay of refraction was the result of the incapability of the step component of the step-pulse neural controller of accommodation. We hypothesize the slow intergrator (Judge 1996) could be the compromised controlling segment. Analogical fluctuations of accommodation at steady-state phase of reaction to step change at the distance of the fixation target were described at accommodative disfacility associated with intermittent exotropia (Stark 1984).

REFERENCES

Ophthalmol Vis Sci 19(1): 60-74.

Kenyon, R.V., Ciuffreda, K.J. & Stark, L. 1981. Dynmic vergence eye movements in strabismus and amblyopia: assymetric vergence. *Br J Ophthalmol* 65(3): 167-176.

Stark, L., Ciuffreda, K.J., Grisham, J.D., Kenyon, R.V., Liu, J. & Polse, K. 1984. Accommodative disfacility presenting as intermittent exotropia. *Ophthal* Ciuffreda, K.J. & Kenyon, R.V. 1983. Accommodative vergence and accommodation in normals,
amblyopes, and strabismics. In C.M. Schor & K.J. Ciuffreda (eds.), *Vergence Eye Movements: Basic and Clinical Aspects:* 101-173, Boston: Butterworths.

Judge, S.J. 1996. How is binocularity maintained during convergence and divergence. *Eye* 10: 172-176.

Kenyon, R.V., Ciuffreda, K.J. & Stark, L. 1980. Dynamic vergence eye movements in strabismus and amblyopia: symmetric vergence. *Invest Physiol Opt* 4(3): 233-244.

Transactions 28th Meeting European Strabismological Association, de Faber (ed.)
© 2004 European Strabismological Association, ISBN 90 265 1965 6

Isometric force development of single horizontal eye muscles in esotropia and exotropia

C. Schiavi (1), R. Bolzani (2), G. Lennerstrand (3), S. Tian (3), M.G. Benassi (2), N. Longo (4) & E.C. Campos (1)
Department of Ophthalmology, University of Bologna, Bologna, Italy (1)
Department of Psychology, University of Bologna, Bologna, Italy (2)
Department of Ophthalmology, Karolinska Institutet, Stockholm, Sweden (3)
Department of Anesthesiology, University of Bologna, Bologna, Italy (4)

ABSTRACT: A comparison was done between force development in the medial and lateral rectus muscles during saccadic movements in 8 adult patients, 2 with esotropia and 6 with exotropia who underwent surgery under topical anesthesia. Five medial rectus muscles and 8 lateral rectus muscles were studied. Isometric muscle tension was recorded with a strain gauge system from the detached muscle. Patients made saccadic eye movements with the non recorded eye. In the tension signals produced by saccades, peak tension (Fp) and steady tension (Fs) were measured. The values of Fp and Fs at different amplitudes of the saccadic eye movements were compared in the lateral and the medial rectus muscles of patients with esotropia and exotropia. There were no consistent statistical differences between values of Fp and Fs obtained in the two strabismus conditions. The force development was the same in both horizontal eye muscles of patients with esotropia and exotropia.

KEYWORDS: Isometric muscle tension, horizontal eye muscles, esotropia, exotropia

INTRODUCTION

Measurements of isometric force development in eye muscles are of value in studies of strabismus of different types and can also supply data for planning surgery. Studies on extraocular muscle forces have been performed mainly with non-invasive techniques. Tension measurements with suction-contact lenses-strain gauge systems, have shown that the characteristics of saccadic velocity and force development in congenital and acquired superior oblique palsy are different and measurements of isometric force development is helpful in differentiating the subtypes of superior oblique paralysis (1). For patients with exotropia, the measurements of the horizontal movements have shown imbalances of isometric force production and saccadic velocity with different patterns in patients with intermittent exotropia and constant exotropia (2). Increased muscle tension was found in severe and longstanding dysthyroid ophthalmopathy but not in the early disease (3,4). Measurements of actively developed horizontal muscle forces in normals by means of non-invasive length-tension forceps have shown that the active force developed at extreme gaze is greater for the medial rectus than for the lateral rectus (5). In the present study, we have compared tension values measured intraoperatively at the tendon from horizontal muscles during saccadic movements in patients with esotropia and exotropia.

MATERIAL AND METHODS

Eight patients were examined during surgery under topical anesthesia. Of them, 2 had non-alternating comitant esotropia and 6 non-alternating comitant exotropia. Patient's age ranged from 20 to 48 years. Refractive errors of the fixating eyes did not exceed +/- 1 dioptre and did not cause obstacle to fixation during the task. The angle of deviation ranged from +25 to +30 prism dioptres (PD) in esotropia patients and from –20 to –45 PD in exotropia patients. Ocular motility examination revealed slight medial rectus overaction in the deviated eye in esotropia patients and slight lateral rectus overaction in the deviated eye in exotropia patients. A total of 13 horizontal rectus muscles, 5 medial and 8 lateral, were studied. None of the muscles examined had been operated before. Isometric muscle tension was recorded with a strain gauge system. The eye was anesthetized with Oxibuprocaine 0.2% supplemented with Lidocaine 4% when needed. A 5-0 silk suture was applied to the tendon of the detached muscle and tied around the strain gauge probe. An initial tension of 10g was applied with the muscle relaxed. The fixation targets were small red light-emitting diodes (LEDs) which were positioned on the ceiling 180 cm in front of the patient's head. Patients made saccadic eye movements with the non-recorded eye, either by fixating LEDs in the centre and at 10, 20, and 30 degrees horizontally to each side (step movements), or by fixating LEDs in a sequence from 30 degrees in the off-direction of the muscle to 30 degrees in the on-direction (continuous movements). Tension data sampling and data analyses were carried out by a special program (3). In the tension signals produced by saccades from the centre, peak tension (Fp) and steady-state tension (Fs) were measured. Diagrams of eye position against tension were calculated for Fp and Fs values, from the tension signals during a sequence of saccades from off- to on- direction. To analyse the pulse characteristics, the time constant value was evaluated by fitting the recorded data with an exponential decay curve. Statistical analysis was done with multivariate ANOVA.

RESULTS

The values of Fp and Fs at different amplitudes of the saccadic eye movements were compared in the lateral and medial rectus muscles of patients with esotropia and exotropia. There were no consistent statistical differences between values of Fp and Fs obtained in the two strabismic conditions either in the continuous movements (fig.1, 2, 3, and 4) or in the step movements (fig. 5, 6, 7, and 8). The time constant of pulse decay obtained for the medial rectus resulted shorter than that of the lateral rectus, i.e., a faster tension decay was seen in the medial rectus. Graphs of tension versus eye position show a typical hysteresis loop, during continuous saccades. To analyse this curve, the area enclosed in the loop was evaluated. The medial rectus seemed to have a larger hysteresis area than the lateral rectus, both for Fp and Fs values (fig. 1, 2, 3, and 4).

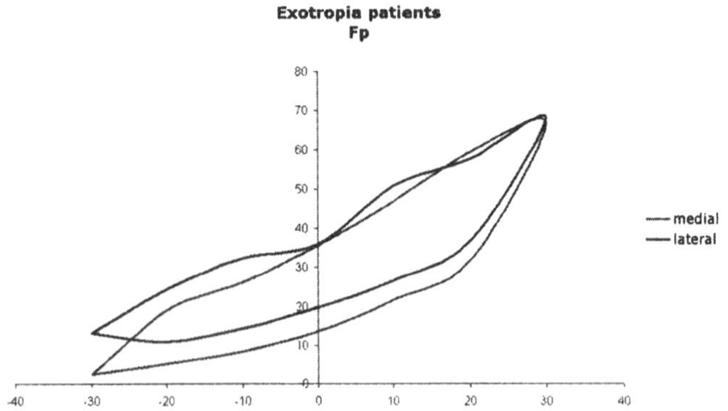

Fig.1: Fp values from recordings of continuous saccades in exotropia patients.

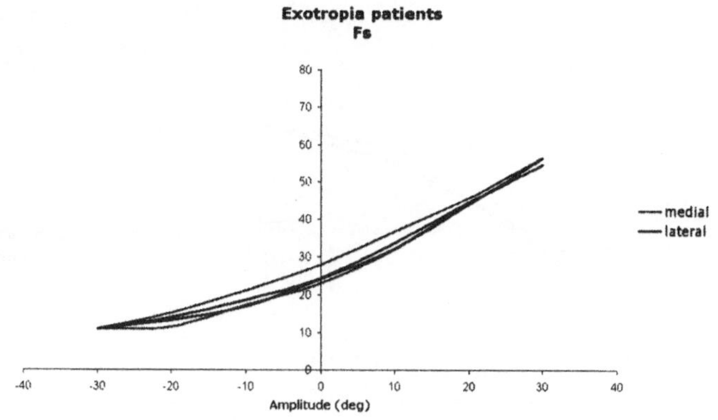

Fig. 2: Fs values from recordings of continuous saccades in exotropia patients.

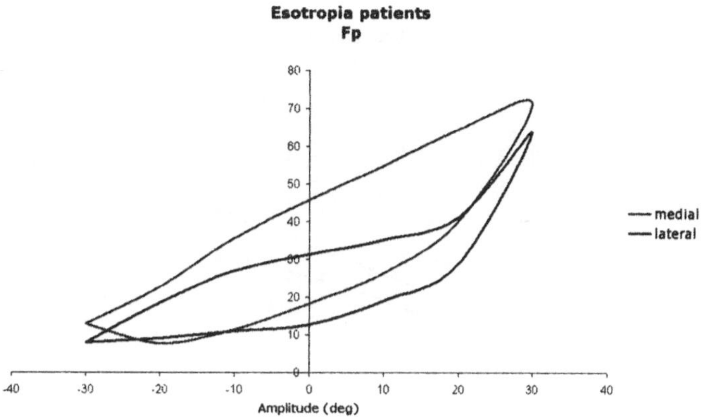

Fig. 3: Fp values from recordings of continuous saccades in esotropia patients.

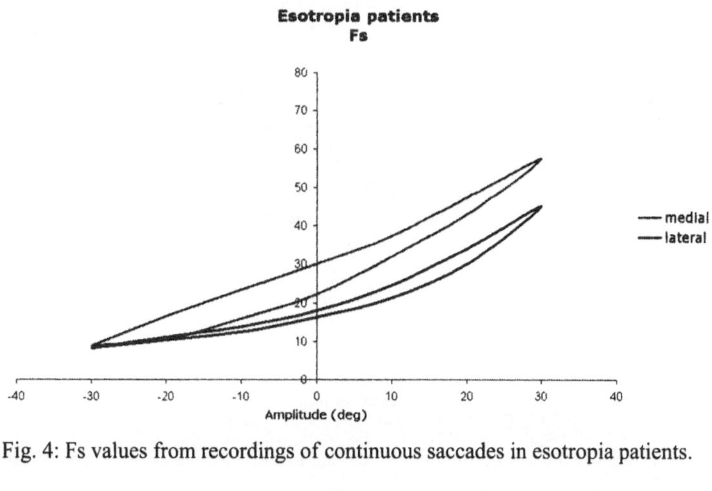

Fig. 4: Fs values from recordings of continuous saccades in esotropia patients.

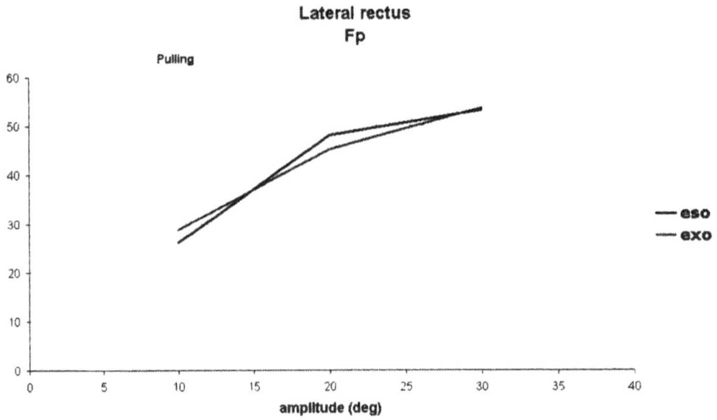

Fig. 5: Fp values from the lateral rectus muscle during step-wise saccades.

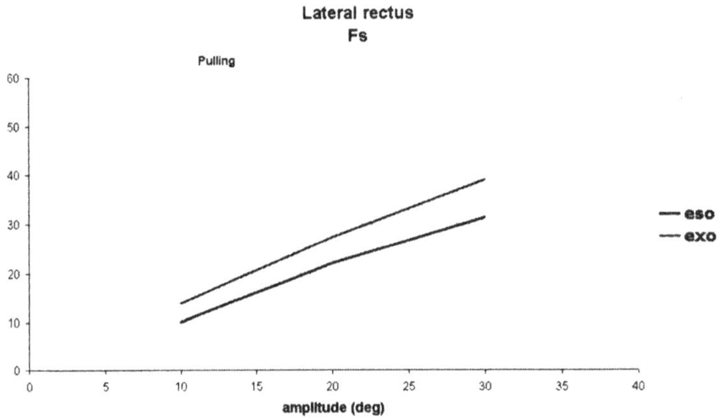

Fig. 6: Fs values from the lateral rectus muscle during step-wise saccades.

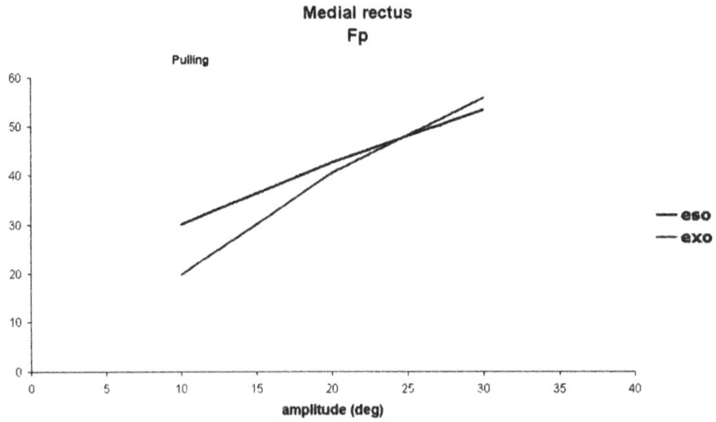

Fig. 7: Fp values from the medial rectus muscle during step-wise movements.

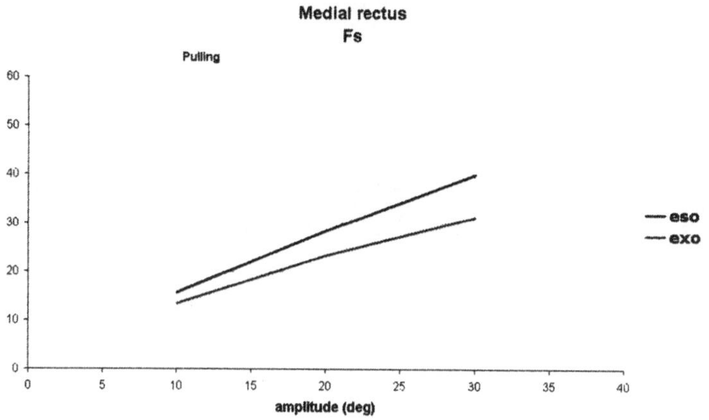

Fig. 8: Fs values from the medial rectus muscle during step-wise movements.

CONCLUSIONS

Measurements of the horizontal movements with non-invasive techniques have shown that isometric force in abduction is higher in patients with constant exotropia than in normals, while isometric force in adduction is higher in intermittent exotropia patients than in normals and constant exotropia patients (2). In the present study, intraoperative tension measurements during saccadic eye movements showed that the force development was the same in both horizontal eye muscles of patients with non-alternating esotropia and non-alternating exotropia. In exotropia patients, no differences were seen between the medial and the lateral rectus muscles. In esotropia patients, the medial rectus seemed stronger than the lateral rectus, but more data are needed to confirm that.

REFERENCES

1. Tian, S. Lennerstrand, G. 1994. Vertical saccadic velocity and force development in superior oblique palsy. *Vision Res.* 34:1785-1798.
2. Lennerstrand, G. Tian, S. 1995. Force development and velocity of saccadic eye movements in exotropia. *Neuro-ophthalmology*, 15:1-16.
3. Simonsz, H.J. Kommerell, G. 1989. Increased muscle tension and reduced elasticity of affected muscles in recent-onset Graves' disease caused primarily by active muscle contraction. *Doc. Ophthalmol.* 72:215-224.
4. Tian, S. Lennerstrand, G. 1995. Force development and saccadic velocity in dysthyroid ophthalmopathy. In: *Transactions of the 7th Orthoptic Congress*, Kyoto, pp. 129-133.
5. Collins, C.C. Carlson, M.R. Scott, AB. Jampolsky, A. 1981. Extraocular muscle forces in normal human subjects. *Invest. Ophthalmol. Vis. Sci.*, 20:652-664.

Transactions 28th Meeting European Strabismological Association, de Faber (ed.)
© 2004 European Strabismological Association, ISBN 90 265 1965 6

Introduction of the 2003 ESA Lecturer Professor Gunnar Lennerstrand

Emilio C. Campos, MD
Professor and Chief of Ophthalmology, University of Bologna, Bologna, Italy

The ESA lecture was established in 1993, after prolonged discussions on whether it should bear the name of a distinguished strabismologist. In order not to hurt the feelings of any Country, I suggested the present definition. The first ESA Lecturer was Professor Joseph Lang from Zuerich, who gave his lecture in 1995 during our Cambridge Congress. I am extremely honoured of having been one of the lecturers myself. I am grateful to the ESA Council for having been requested to introduce to you today the 2003 ESA Lecturer, Gunnar Lennerstrand. This is a great privilege and pleasure for me.

The interest in strabismology has been growing in Europe over the years. Yet, approaches and new insight have been limited to clinical aspects. Gunnar Lennerstrand has had a special role in our small family of Euroepan Strabismologists. He deserves our gratitude for having been instrumental in filling the gap between basic scientists interested in vision and ocular motility and clinicians. This was accomplished because of his unusual cultural background.

Gunnar was born in Stockholm some years ago and started to travel quite early, following as an adjunct his father in London, were they both earned a fellowship at the Lister Institute. After having received both his M.D. and Ph.D at the Karolinska Institute he started his career in ophthalmology first at Karolinska and then in Linkoping. This brought him to become Professor and Chief in Umea for one year (you should realize that this fostered his capability as cross-country ski expert). Then back to the Alma Mater, where he eventually became professor and Chief, first of the Department of Ophthalmology at Huddinge Hospital and then of the Department of Clinical Sciences of the Karolinska Institute.

Gunnar Lennerstrand started his career as a scientist with mentors as Professors Granit and von Euler. He then pursued his studies on muscle functions at the McGill University of Montreal and the Smith Kettlewell Institute of San Francisco, collaborating with the world experts of the time in muscle physiology, personalities of the calibre of Paul Bach-y-Rita, Carter Collins, Arthur Jampolsky and Alan Scott.

In Gunnar's bibliography it is possible to find basic contributions: you will be surprised to know that his first papers are in Italian! He then turned his attention to his life-time interest in the sensitive innervation of extra-ocular muscles first of animals and then of humans. An area of great importance has been the study of contractile properties of the muscles and eventually of their forces. He has also been interested in amblyopia and analysis of binocular interaction with visual evoked potentials. Gunnar's bibliography is extremely rich and accounts around 180 publications and editing of books. All this brought him to become a world expert in muscle function with the insight of a clinician. As a consequence he has acquired a great reputation in Scandinavia from where he attracts patients for consultations.

One of the big achievements of Gunnar Lennerstrand's is the organization of several memorable symposia on ocular motility and amblyopia at the Wenner Gren Center in Stockholm. Speakers of these events have been the world leading experts of the field. For this reason, the Proceedings of these meetings are still a land-mark in the literature. I am sure, however, that although recognition is given to Gunnar for these symposia, nothing could have been achieved without the invaluable help and organizational capabilities of Gun, his lovely wife who, in her quite and modest way, has always stayed on his side: we have not to forget that the organization of the first of these symposia created the opportunity for Gun and Gunnar to meet!

I have started to be closer to Gunnar in the mid eighties, when Gunnar, Gunter von Noorden and I decided to organize together a symposium in Stockholm on Ocular Motility and Strabismus. This was a real memorable event, which took place in June 1987. We met numerous times for the preparation of the meeting (at that time the electronic mail system was not yet effective). I vividly remember an afternoon in Brussels of November 1986. The three of us got together to work on the symposium in the hall of the hotel of one us. Before starting the meeting, Gunnar asked for the key of the room and reappeared shortly thereafter. At the end of the meeting, it turned out that he put in the refrigerator a bottle of Aquavit, of which we got rid in a very short time, feeling relived and in excellent mood. Our collaboration (not just in drinking!) has continued and is still very active. At the present time we are involved in the recording of muscle forces in patients and this brings to the pleasure of periodical meetings in Stockholm and Bologna, which have created strong ties also between our collaborators and our Institutions, with a definite increase in business for the Aquavit dealers, at least from my side.

Gunnar has the merit of having fostered along the years younger scientists from all over the world (many of his post-docs came from Europe, China and Japan) and was instrumental in establishing the Sigvar & Marianne Bernadotte Research Foundation for Children's Eyecare.

Our ESA Lecturer has devoted also a lot of energies not only in glass collection – of which he is a real expert, who goes so far as to blow the glass by himself! – and in taking care of his beautiful summer house in Oland, but in serving in numerous scientific Organizations, among which ESA (of which he has been Council member and Vice-President) and ISA (of which he was Editor and Vice-President).

Gunnar is an easy-going and friendly person and I have never found one single colleague who has shown bad feelings in his direction. This is a further quality in his favour and shows the joy of all his friends for today's recognition. Ladies and Gentlemen, let me introduce to you the 2003 ESA Lecturer, Professor Gunnar Lennerstrand.

Transactions 28th Meeting European Strabismological Association, de Faber (ed.)

What can eye muscle studies tell us about strabismus?

Gunnar Lennerstrand,
Department of Ophthalmology, Karolinska Institutet
S:t Erik's Eye Hospital and Huddinge University Hospital,
S-141 86 STOCKHOLM, Sweden

INTRODUCTION

I feel very honored to be invited to present the 6th ESA lecture, joining such prominent strabismus researchers and ESA-lecturers as Joseph Lang, Peter Fells, Gunter von Noorden, Emilio Campos and Guntram Kommerell. I have chosen to speak about eye muscle studies and how they relate to strabismus. In the incomitant strabismus, i.e. the paralytic and mechanic types, eye muscle function is clearly affected. However, in the common types of concomitant strabismus any changes in eye muscle structure and function are less obvious. I will review my own and others research on eye muscles over a couple of decades up to the present time, to see if the results can shed some light on issues concerning particularly the concomitant strabismus.
The human extra ocular muscles (EOM) show morphological and functional properties that are different in many aspects from ordinary skeletal, striated muscles in the human body. The traditional fiber type classification cannot be applied to the EOM, and the assumptions concerning their structure and function can only partly be based on data from other skeletal muscles. These differences are probably of importance in explaining why the eye muscles are involved in some diseases where other skeletal muscle is spared, and vice versa, but this is outside the topic of this presentation.
The eye muscles participate in motor acts that are not only among the fastest in the body, the saccadic eye movements, but also among the most sustained of all motor activity, in gaze fixation and in vergence eye movements. It is not yet quite clear how these actions are connected with different EOM fiber populations, how the labor of eye movements are divided between different muscle fiber and motor unit types, and how this may be related to strabismus.
The maturation process of contractile structures and properties of EOM in animals has been found to be closely related in time to the development of monocular and binocular visual function, and can be modified to some extent in defects of these functions. Visual demands can also modify eye muscle function in some strabismus conditions as shown for the adult human ocular motor system.
The eye muscles contain muscle receptors that are structurally similar to those in skeletal muscle, but their function in the motor control seems to be quite different. Most of the previous research had been done in animals, but lately also studies on sensory functions of human EOM have been presented, suggesting that the proprioception participates in space localization and that the functions may differ in normal and strabismic subjects.

MOTOR FUNCTION OF EYE MUSCLES

Gross anatomy

The improvements of imaging techniques have allowed more detailed studies of eye muscles and other tissues in the orbit. The size of the different eye muscles has been calculated from MRI measurements and the volume of normal adult muscle is about 500 mm3 for all the rectus muscles, but only about 270 mm3 for the superior oblique and about 170 mm3 for the inferior oblique muscle.
EOM in paralytic strabismus may be atrophic (Demer et al. 1994, Sato M et al. 1997), but there are no indications that muscle volume is different from normal values in concomitant strabismus. Analysis of EOM function can be done by measuring the muscle width with MRI in different directions of gaze, since gaze activation of the muscle will increase the cross sectional diameter of the muscle belly in a normal muscle, but not in a paretic muscle (Demer et al. 1994).

In Thyroid Associated Ophthalmopathy (TAO) the muscle volume is increased in all eye muscles except possibly the inferior oblique (Nishida et al. 2001), and the volume change is the first sign of the TAO, before the disease is clinically obvious (Lennerstrand et al. 2002).

Muscle layers and pulleys

The EOMs are divided into an inner, global layer that runs from the origin to the tendon, and an outer, orbital layer that extends over a restricted part and inserts on the so called pulley of the rectus muscles (see below). In the human EOM, the mean number of fibers in the global layer is 10 000– 13 000 in all rectus muscles from childhood to adult age. In the orbital layer the number is higher in the medial rectus (about 11 000), than in the other rectus muscles (7 000 – 9 000) (Oh et al 2001 a).

As revealed by detailed MRI observations, the rectus eye muscles are surrounded by distinct fibroelastic pulleys that maintain EOM position relative to the orbit (Demer 2000, Demer 2002). The pulleys contain collagen, elastin and smooth muscle. In the smooth muscle there is evidence of noradrenergic and cholinergic innervation, as well as for nitric oxide as a neurotransmitter. This will allow tension on the pulleys to be varied in a slow fashion and such tonic effects of eye muscle function may be important in some types of strabismus, particularly in phorias. It has been suggested that the orbital layer inserts on the pulleys and not directly on the globe like the global fibers (Demer 2002). The orbital layer is more vascularized than the global, which also correlates with greater metabolic activity (Oh et al 2001 b). The proposition has been made that the orbital layer would be mainly responsible for positioning the globe, and that in looking for muscle mechanisms behind strabismus, attention should be focused on structure and function of the orbital layer fibers and the balance between orbital layers of the individual muscles in a muscle pair.

No pulley abnormalities seem to occur in the common forms of strabismus. On the other hand, surgical treatment of strabismus may affect the pulley actions, by altering the relationship between EOM insertions and pulleys, and the action of the orbital layer on their pulleys (Demer 2000). Further, primary abnormal pulley location could lead to abnormal muscle actions and subsequently to strabismus. This has been demonstrated in some cases of A- and V-patterns that did not respond to oblique muscle surgery. It has also been shown that the structural abnormalities and displacements of the pulleys occurring in Marfan´s syndrome, can lead to strabismus (Demer 2002).

Muscle fibers and motor units

The important functional characteristics of muscle fibers are contraction speed and fatigue resistance, and they have correlates in muscle fiber structure. The present understanding of the different eye muscle fiber types, their morphological characteristics, innervation, histochemistry and distribution within the eye muscle, have recently been described (Porter et al. 1995). In a large variety of animal species including man, the orbital layer would consist of singly innervated fibers (SIF) making up about 80% of the fiber population, and multiply innervated fibers (MIF) in 20%. The global layer SIFs are of three types: Red SIF in 33%, Intermediate SIF in 25% and White SIF in 32%, and one type of MIF in 10%.

The speed of contraction of the fibers is indicated by the type of myosine heavy chain isoforms (MHCI) they contain. The distribution of MHCI types in EOM fibers are outlined in Table 2. The orbital fibers, both SIF and MIF, show a distribution of MHCI with the fast type IIA in the innervational zone. However, outside the innervational zone the MHCI is of a slower type, only seen in embryonic/neonatal muscle, and not in other adult mammalian muscle. The global SIF types contain MHCI of fast type IIB, found also in skeletal muscle , but the MIF fiber contain a slow type of MHCI seen in heart muscle. There is no counterpart to this fiber type in any other human skeletal muscle.

The fiber content of mitochondria (MI) is an indicator of the fatigue resistance (FR). The types of MHCI and the MI content in the different types of EOM fibers are shown schematically in Table 1.

The speed of contraction and the fatigue properties of EOM are reflected in the properties of the smallest functional units of the muscle, the motor unit, consisting of the motoneuron in the brain stem and the muscle fibers it innervates in the muscle itself. All fibers in an EOM motor unit are most likely of the same type. Studies of EOM motor units have been performed mainly in the cat, and to a smaller extent in the squirrel monkey, by recording the mechanical and electrical responses in the muscle to stimulation of single motoneurons or their axons (Lennerstrand 1975, Goldberg, Lennerstrand & Hull 1975, Goldberg & Shall 1999). In Table 2 the functional characteristics of the different types of EOM fibers are outlined, measured as speed of contraction (speed) and fatigue resistance (FR).

Table 1. Structural and functional characteristics of EOM fibers.

	Orbital layer		Global layer			
Fiber type	SIF	MIF	Red SIF	Intermed SIF	White SIF	MIF
MHCI	2A + Embr	1 + Embr	2A	2B	2B	Alpha-Cardiac
Mito	many	intermed	many	intermed	few	intermed
Contraction						
Speed	fast	slow (twitch)	fast	fast	fast	slow (non-twitch)
FR	high	high	high	intermed	low	high

For abbreviations see the text.

The orbital SIF are considered the major contributors to sustained EOM force in fixation in primary or deviated positions. It is also the fiber type that is most affected by denervation, be it by damage to the motor nerve or to the end plate function by Botulinum toxin (Spencer & Mc Neer 1988).

The MIFs are not seen in the accessory extraocular muscles such as the levator palpebrae and the retractor bulbi, indicating that the MIFs are involved in the finer control of fixation, and in the smooth and finely graded eye movements particularly in vergence control.

In the early studies of single motor units in the cat EOM it was possible to identify only 2 or 3 types of motor units, i.e. twitch units and multiply innervated twitch and slow units (Lennerstrand 1975, Goldberg, Lennerstrand & Hull 1976). The fibers of these units were processed with electron microscopy and identified as singly and multiply innervated fibers, respectively (Lennerstrand 1975). Later, Goldberg and his group have studied tetanic tension and fatigue properties of the motor units with a more elaborate technique, and have been able to differentiate 5 types of motor units (Goldberg & Shall 1999).

Studies of single motor units in human EOM can be conducted with EMG, but no serious attempts have been made to differentiate EOM fiber types by this method. For example, the amplitude of the EMG action potentials would be lower in the smaller than in the larger fibers, and the speed of propagation of the action potential would be slower in the multiply innervated and smaller muscle fibers than in the singly innervated and larger fibers. No studies of these types have been performed in concomitant strabismus.

Recruitment of motor units

EOM are employed in different types of eye movements: vestibulo-ocular, optokinetic, pursuit, saccadic and vergence movements. In addition the EOM are active in steady fixation.

It is generally held that all types of motor units are participating in all types of eye movements (Robinson 1978). However, a grading with respect to motor units and fiber properties has been suggested (Goldberg & Shall 1999). When the eye is in the primary position a majority of the fatigue-resistant units of the orbital and global layers are recruited for the fine and sustained gradation of force needed for fixation and binocular vision. The increasingly faster, but fatiguing fibers are recruited when the eye moves into the direction of gaze with maximal contraction of the muscle.

Recordings of EMG with multiple electrodes in human EOM have supported the view that EOM units can be separately recruited in slow and fast eye movements (Scott & Collins, 1975). EMG from the orbital layer did not show any marked pulse in the firing rate of the units, indicating that these fibers are not responsible for the force needed to accelerate the globe in a saccadic movement. This activity would instead be derived from the global layer fibers, which is in support of the active pulley hypothesis, predicting that motor neurons preferentially innervating fibers in the orbital layer should exhibit step but no pulse change in activity during saccades (Demer 2002). Many motor neurons firing tonically with no initial pulse have been found in the abducens and oculomotor nuclei, in addition to phasically discharging units. EMG from single fibers in human EOM could be very useful in elucidating the recruitment pattern of different types of motor units, but the technique has been used to a very limited extent.

EOM fibers in strabismic animals and humans

The structural composition of eye muscles in animals with innate strabismus have been studied in the Siamese cat (Lennerstrand 1979). The distribution of fiber types, determined histochemically, were not affected, but most fibers were smaller in size in the Siamese cat than in cats with normal eye position. Further the capillary network was reduced in the Siamese cat eye muscles, particularly in the orbital layer. Studies of EOM motor units have not been performed in strabismic animals and we do not know if the distribution of motor unit types may vary depending on the type of strabismus etc.

Previous studies of histopathology of human strabismic extraocular muscle have revealed a constellation of structural abnormalities, most of which are rather non-specific (Spencer & McNeer 1988). The examination of human extraocular muscle is usually done in muscle samples obtained in resection procedures, which limits the sampling to the distal portion of the muscle. It does not include an entire cross-sectional profile of the muscle, particularly not the orbital layer and the region on motor innervation. The orbital layer fibers, inserting on the muscle pulleys, are very difficult to reach in surgery. As noted previously, it is believed that fibers in the orbital layer are involved in the parts of ocular motility that include slow and tonic components and therefore are most likely involved in strabismus.

Postnatal development of eye muscle

The postnatal development of the cat inferior oblique muscle has been studied with physiological and histochemical techniques (Lennerstrand 1982). Fatigue resistance of the muscle reached adult levels at about 6 weeks of age, while speed of contraction continued to increase into adulthood. In other skeletal muscle the speed of contraction reached adult levels at about 10 weeks of age in the cat. With histochemical methods five EOM muscle fiber types could be identified. All fiber types were recognized already in newborn kittens and no age related changes were observed in their relative proportions. Variations with age in muscle contractile properties and in fiber size indicate that the slow fiber systems of eye muscle matured earlier than fast fiber systems. This might be related to the need for slow eye motor activity in the development of binocular visual functions and visual resolution. There was also a considerable increase in mitochondrial content. Thus there existed a strong correlation between the structural basis for fatigue resistance in the eye muscles and the increasing reliance upon fixational and vergence eye movements in the visual development.

There are no data in children to relate the findings in speed of contraction of EOM to the development of saccadic velocity. However, in humans the need for vergence control in binocular vision and sustained EOM activity would seem to emerge gradually from age 4 –6 months (Hainline & Riddell 1996).

In the EOM nearly all known striated muscle myosin heavy chain isoforms are found. Studies of rat EOM have shown that some fiber types continue to express embryonic and neonatal isoforms (Brueckner, Itkis & Porter 1996). Human EOM has also very complex patterns of myosin heavy chain isoforms, both in the prenatal stage (Pedrosa-Dommelöf et al. 2000) and in the adult muscle (Kjellgren et al. 2003). The retention of embryonic myosin observed in the orbital singly innervated fibers, but not in its close counterpart in the global layer (the global red singly innervated fibers), is probably related to differing muscle force dynamics for the two layers. The maintenance of sustained extraocular muscle force levels at a minimum of 10 g, even in extreme off-direction gaze positions, is most likely due to the continuous activity of singly innervated orbital fibers. Other factors to influence the fiber phenotype could be the existence of multiple innervation of some fiber types and motoneuron discharge rates that are an order of magnitude higher than those seen for other skeletal muscle.

The altered visual processing in monocular deprivation would be expected to change the firing patterns of oculomotor motoneurons for the slow and sustained types of eye movements, and this would effect EOM fiber development. Cats with defects of binocular vision, due to surgically induced strabismus and monocular occlusion with lid suture from age 2 – 3 weeks in domestic cats, or to a genetic defect in Siamese (albino) cats, showed slower contractions and lower fatigue resistance of their eye muscles than normal domestic cats (Lennerstrand 1982). No variations in fiber types or in the relative proportions between types were observed. However, fibers of all types were smaller and the capillary density per fibers was lower in cats with binocular defects than in normal cats. The developmental visual insult of monocular deprivation has been shown to interfere with EOM maturation sufficiently to change expression of the typical myosin heavy chain isoforms of the singly innervated orbital fibers (Brueckner & Porter 1998).

In guinea pig with poor binocularity also in the normal animals due to the lateral position of the eyes, no difference in contractile properties were recorded between normally pigmented and albino animals (Lennerstrand 1985). This finding lends support to the idea that variations in functional properties between normal cats and lid sutured or Siamese cats depended on the state of binocular vision, and might represent adaptations to the reduced demands for fusional movements in cats with binocular deficiencies.

Thus, there may be a critical period during development when alterations in visual activity have significant consequences for the eye muscle phenotype. Studies of myosin heavy chain isoforms of EOM fibers in the human have begun and should be continued. It might be possible that the maturational state of the EOM must be considered in the design of therapies for congenital ocular motility disorders.

Effects of denervation and Botulinum toxin

Denervation of EOM via nerve transsection and subsequent reinnervation produced less atrophy than would be expected in a skeletal muscle. Denervation also reduced the amount of mitochondria in the orbital singly innervated fiber. In reinnervation the postparetic fiber type grouping that typifies reinnervated skeletal muscle was not seen in EOM (Spencer et al. 1992).

In typical skeletal muscle injection of botulinum toxin results in denervation atrophy of all muscle fiber types. When injected into extraocular muscle of monkey, botulinum toxin does not produce the generalized atrophy but instead causes specific effects of reduced cross-sectional area and mitochondrial content in the orbital singly innervated fibers (Spencer & McNeer 1988). The reduction in the functional capacity of the orbital singly innervated fiber, acting on the muscle pulley system, would produce the static position change in strabismus seen as a long term effect of Botulinum treatment. The consequences of toxin are more severe when used in infant and juvenile monkeys, indicating an influence on the postnatal development of the EOM fibers as discussed above.

Clinical studies on the effects of small doses of botulinum toxin have shown that eye alignment can be changed, probabaly due to denervation of orbital singly innervated fibers, but that there was no change in saccadic velocity and movement range, since these functions are subserved by other muscle fiber types, unaffected by the low dosis (Stahl et al. 1998). In larger doses of botulinum toxin dysfunction of all muscle fiber types is seen.

Contractile properties of normal and strabismic human EOM

Force measurements from horizontal eye muscles during normal eye movements have been performed in humans undergoing surgery for concomitant strabismus under topical anesthesia (Collins, O'Meara & Scott 1975, Lennerstrand et al. 2003). Extraocular muscles show a significant degree of activity even when the eye is directed well into the off-direction of muscle activity (Scott & Collins 1975). This would eliminate any slack in the muscle and permit it to operate within the linear region of muscle length-tension curves at all times. Recently it has been shown that force development in saccadic movements can be evaluated adequately with the muscles still attached to the globe (Lennerstrand et al 2003). This will allow extensive studies of contractile properties in different eye muscles during ophthalmic surgery under topical anethesia.

In a clinical setting force measurements can also be performed using a probe with strain gauges applied to a suction contact lens. The isometric force development in one eye is recorded, while the other eye is performing saccadic movements to fixation targets in different locations. With this method, various studies have been done in normal subjects during horizontal eye movements and vertical eye movements (Lennerstrand, Tian & Zhao 1993, Tian & Lennerstrand 1993). For the vertical components, measurements were performed in 20 degrees of abduction, in order to study force production in the vertical rectus muscles with reduced

interference from the oblique muscles. With the eye in 20 degrees of adduction, the activity of both oblique and rectus muscles were recorded. Tension reductions in the oblique muscles can be evaluated by this method, as shown in a study of force development in patients with superior oblique palsy of the congenital and the acquired types (Tian & Lennerstrand 1994). Force measurements have also been useful in evaluating muscle function in Thyroid Associated Ophthalmopathy (TAO), where the EOMs are significantly enlarged and restrictions of eye movements are noted, in combination with misalignment of the eyes and diplopia. The tension development in TAO was higher than normal in nearly all movement directions. This would indicate that there is no paresis of EOM, but rather a compensatory increase of muscle tension to overcome the restrictions of eye movements induced by the myopathy, in an attempt to normalize the saccadic movements in amplitude and velocity (Lennerstrand et al. 1995). When the myopathy was treated with steroids and retrobulbar irradiation, the eye motility improved and the tension development was normalized.
As mentioned before, studies on eye muscle function in animals indicate that the properties of eye muscle are changed after disruption of binocular vision by strabismus induced at an early age. This was thought to be due to lower neural demands for fusional vergence movements. It is not known if adaptations of eye muscle function and changes of contractile properties can be found also in human eye muscle as a result of binocular deficiences. Force production was compared in orthophoric subjects with full vision and stereoacuity, in adult patients with intermittent exotropia (IXT), and in adult patients with constant exotropia (CXT) (Lennerstrand & Tian 1995). Patients with IXT showed normal binocular functions when fixating at near. They were constantly exercising motor fusion for near in order to overcome the exodeviation, which would lead to an increase in medial rectus contractile force in relation to the lateral rectus, and an increase in adduction force also during versional movements. In patients with CXT, the eyes were always misaligned and little or no motor fusional activity was at hand. Force developed in adduction was found to be higher in IXT patients than in normal subjects and CXT patients. Saccadic velocity, however, did not show a significant difference between groups. Thus, the force developed by the medial and the lateral rectus muscles are balanced differently in patients with intermittent exotropia, in comparison with normal subjects and patients with constant exotropia.

Summary of motor function and concomitant strabismus

It is not generally believed that concomitant strabismus is due to a primary abnormality of the eye muscles or the ocular motor system. The gross anatomy of EOM including the shape and position of the eye muscle pulleys was not changed in strabismus. The histology of the EOM fibers was also basically the same, but changes have been observed in the cellular and biochemical machinery of the fibers, most notably in the singly innervated orbital fibers. Functionally this was seen as slower contractions and reduced fatigue resistance of EOM in animals with strabismus and defects of binocular vision. Most likely the changes represented an adaptation to modified visual demands on the ocular motor control, due to the defects of binocular vision in strabismus from an early age. Adaptation of EOM function to visual demands could be seen also in the adult human ocular motor system, but here the effects can be reversed with treatment in some conditions. However, it is not known if the developmental modifications of EOM function seen in animals are reversible or represent an insurmountable obstacle to treatment of strabismus.

SENSORY FUNCTION OF EYE MUSCLES

Structure and functional properties of muscle receptors

Sensory information from EOM derive from muscle spindles with an intricate machinery of sensory endings and specialized motor control, and from tendon organs, so called palisade endings, with a simpler structure and response pattern (Ruskel 1999, Donaldson 2000). Functionally, tendon organs react to muscle tension changes, since they are coupled in series with the muscle fibers, while the spindles react to changes in muscle length, due to their position in parallel with the ordinary muscle fibers. However, there are no data on the physiological properties of the palisade endings, and they seem to be missing in human infant

EOM (Bruenech & Ruskell 2000). The functional characteristics of muscle spindles would seem to be the same as in other skeletal muscle (Lennerstrand & Bach-y-Rita 1974). Vibration of the muscle tendon is an effective way of activating the muscle spindle afferents. The primary endings of the human muscle spindle will respond with one or more pulses per vibration cycle in the frequency region of 10-120 Hz (Roll & Vedel 1982). The signals are interpreted centrally as a continuous stretching of the muscle either passively or as a result of contraction in an opposing muscle.

Afferent pathways and central connections
The afferent signals from EOM muscle receptors travel to the brain stem through the trigeminal complex (Ruskell 1999, Donaldson 2000). The cell bodies of the first order neurons are in the semilunar ganglion and the second order neuron somas in the descending part of the spinal trigeminal nucleus. Further projections have been found to many different parts of the CNS: superior colliculus, vestibular nuclei, pontine nuclei, central gray matter dorsal to the third nerve nucleus, cerebellum, and even to the frontal cortex and the visual cortex. In many of these sites, the EOM proprioceptive input has been shown to interact with visual as well as vestibular inputs. However, there are very few reports on any direct connections between muscle receptor afferents and EOM motoneurons, and the existence of an EOM stretch reflex is strongly questioned (Donaldson 2000).

Proprioception and the visual system
Recent studies have demonstrated that eye and neck muscle proprioception plays an important role in the development of monocular and binocular vision (Buisseret 1995). In order for normal orientational sensitivity to develop in the visual cortex, the visual signals must associated with proper eye movement signals mediated through EOM receptors. The extraretinal proprioceptive signals coupled to gaze movements would act as a gating factor for a response to a visual stimulus. Further it has been shown in animal experiments that surgical immobilization of one eye, proprioceptive EOM deafferentation or destruction of proprioceptive afferents from the neck, resulted in marked reduction in the number of binocular cells in specific regions of the visual cortex and in impaired binocular visuo-motor behaviour. Possibly suppression of EOM proprioceptive signals could impair neural processing of binocular disparity, the basis of depth perception. Unbalanced inflow of proprioceptive information due to unilateral lesions are the most deleterious in this respect (Buisseret 1995).

Proprioception and space localization
Experiments in humans using vibration of muscles have shown that there is an influence from proprioceptors in the postural, neck and eye muscles on the perception of target localization in space (Roll, Vedel & Roll 1989, Weir 2000). Illusions of target movement could be induced by vibration of eye muscles and neck muscles with head and body fixed. Thus, there is a change in egocentric localisation when proprioception is activated. Under conditions of subdued ambient illumination and no visual references except a faint visual orientation target, the apparent displacement of the target is referred to as a visual illusory movement. The direction of the perceived movement is related to the EOM or neck muscle group vibrated. Under conditions of normal visual stimulation these EOM proprioceptive effects are more or less ignored.
The illusory movements induced by eye muscle vibration have been quantified and the interaction between retinal and extraretinal signals have been analyzed (Velay et al. 1994, Han & Lennerstrand 1999). The direction of the illusory movements was determined by the vibrated eye muscle. For example, the effect of inferior rectus vibration is perceived as an upward movement of the target, as if the inferior rectus muscle had been stretched during elevation of the eye. For lateral rectus vibration the direction of the illusory movement was to the side opposite to the vibrated muscle.

Proprioceptive reflexes in strabismus
The accuracy of egocentric localization in strabismus patients was measured by pointing to a covered target. No change was seen unless the muscles in charge had been reoperated. No change was noticed in testing with the non-operated eye (Campos et al. 1989, Steinbach 1987).

This suggests a central integration of afferent messages from both eyes in an egocentric map of motor programs used for pointing tasks.
Stretch induced activity in EOM of humans with strabismus has been reported (Mitsui & Tamura 1986). Small adductive forces applied to the dominant eye in patients with manifest exotropia, and abductive forces applied to the lateral rectus in esotropia, were observed to cause a corrective movement of the other eye, which eventually reached an orthophoric position (but never went beyond that point). It was suggested that abnormal proprioceptive impulses, originating from the dominant eye were the basis for the exodeviation of the non-dominant eye. It should be noted, however, that these ideas are not widely accepted, since in these experiments the motor reaction could have been elicited by a shift of the retinal image rather than by proprioceptive input.

Effects of vibration of EOM on eye position and pointing
The spindle function in strabismus was studied by means of eye muscle vibration, measuring pointing behavior and eye position in subjects with normal vision, and in patients with exotropia. The strabismus was either of the intermittent type with normal binocular vision for near, or of the constant exotropia type, with normal monocular but disrupted binocular vision both for near and distance. The methods have been described by Lennerstrand, Tian & Han (1997) and Han & Lennerstrand (1999).
In vibration of the inferior rectus muscles, the direction of eye movements and past pointing was mainly upwards in both normal and exotropic subjects. During lateral rectus vibration in normal subjects and in patients with intermittent exotropia the covered, non-dominant eye deviated in the temporal, abducting direction. However, in the patients with basic exotropia the covered, strabismic eye deviated in the nasal, adducting direction. The directions of the eye deviations, summarized in Table 2, were the same as the pointing directions during eye muscle vibration. The results indicate that proprioceptive information plays a part in the gaze directing mechanisms, but that the information is used differently for horizontal gaze in normal and strabismic subjects, and probably related to the state of binocular vision.

Table 2. Effects of eye muscle vibration on eye position

Vibration of one eye	Effects on the other eye Normals	Exotropia
Inferior rectus	Elevation	Elevation
Lateral rectus	Abduction	Adduction

This type of sensory adaptation occurs most likely at a central (cortical) level. In subjects with normal binocular vision, proprioceptive input from the eye muscles has access to the mechanisms that are used in the calculation of the direction of gaze. As a result the motor output of the gaze system is modified in such a way that the eye position is shifted. This re-direction of gaze is dependent on which muscles are activated, and in the direction to stretch the particular muscle whose proprioception was activated. This is also the direction of the illusory movement that is perceived and the direction of past-pointing, as an effects of the vibration.
In the exotropic patients, with disrupted binocular vision, the direction of eye movements and past-pointing were the same as in normal subjects for muscles that move the eye vertically. However, when muscles that move the eye to the side were activated, the eye movement and illusory movements were in the opposite direction to that seen in normal subjects. The reactions to eye muscle vibration would imply that the coupling between the proprioceptive input from the lateral rectus muscle and the visual gaze functions is different in exotropic and normal subjects, probably depending on the condition of the binocular functions.

Summary of sensory function and concomitant strabismus
It is not known how EOM proprioception is used more specifically in ocular motor control, but a clear influence on space localization and eye position can be demonstrated with vibratory stimulation of the eye muscles, presumably activating muscle spindles. Results of inferior rectus

activation were the same in normal subjects and in adult patients with strabismus but the effects of lateral rectus activation were not. This could be interpreted as if the sensory input from EOM in patients with concomitant strabismus and poor binocularity was handled differently, in much the same fashion as the visual input, i.e. binocular connections are disrupted by suppression from the non-dominant eye. Such an interaction would most likely occur in the visual cortex, and not in the ocular motor system. Further studies of proprioceptive mechanisms, during the postnatal developmental stage and in adult comitant strabismus may shed light on the mechanisms of childhood strabismus and may in this respect be a more fruitful avenue for further research than eye motor studies.

ACKNOWLEDGEMENTS

The research reported from the authors′ laboratory has been supported by grants from the Swedish Medical Research Council (No. 4751), the Funds of Karolinska Institutet, and the Sigvard & Marianne Benadotte Research Foundation

REFERENCES

Brueckner JF & Porter JD (1998) Visual system maldevelopment disrupts extraocular muscle-specific myosin expression. J Appl Physiol, 85: 584 – 592.

Brueckner JK, Itkis O & Porter JD (1996) Spatial and temporal patterns of myosin heavy chain expression in developing rat extraocular muscle. J Muscle Res Cell Biol. 17: 297 – 312.

Bruenech R & Ruskell GL (2000) Myotendenous nerve endings in human infant and adult extraocular muscles. Anatomical Record 260:132 - 140.

Buisseret P (1995) Influence of extraocular muscle proprioception on vision. Physiol Rev 75: 323 – 338.

Campos EC, Bolzani R, Schiavi C, Fanti MR & Cavallini GM (1989) Further evidence for the role of proprioception in space perception. Doc Ophthalmol 72: 155 – 160.

Collins, C.C., O′Meara, D. and Scott, A.B. (1975) Muscle tension during unrestrained human eye movements. J. Physiol. (Lond) 245, 351-369.

Demer JL (2000) Orbital connective tissue in binocular alignment and strabismus. In Lennerstrand G & Ygge J (eds) Advances in Strabismus Research: Basic and Clinical Aspects. Portland Press.

Demer JL (2002) The orbital pulley system: A revolution in concepts of orbital anatomy. Ann. N.Y.Acad.Sci 956: 17 – 32.

Demer JL, Miller JM Koo EY & Rosenbaum AL (1994) Quantitative magnetic resonance morphometry of extraocular muscles: a new diagnostic tool in paralytic strabismus. J Pediatr Opthalmol Strabismus 31: 177 – 188.

Donaldson IML (200) The functions of the proprioceptors of the eye muscles. Phil Trans R Soc Lond B 355:1685 – 1754.

Goldberg SJ & Shall MS (1999) "Motor units of extraocular muscle:recent findings. In: MD Bender (ed) "Progress in Brain Research, Vol 123, pp 221 – 232, Elsevier Science BV

Hainline L & Riddell PM (1996) Eye alignment and convergence in young infants. In :Infant Vision, Eds. Vital-Durand F, Atkinson J & Braddick OJ, EBBS Publications Series – 2, Oxford University Press, pp 221 – 247.

Han,Y. and Lennerstrand, G. (1999) Changes of visual localization induced by eye and neck muscle vibration in normal and strabismic subjects. Graefe′s Arch. Clin. Exp. Ophthalmol. 237, 21-28.

Lennerstrand G & Tian S (1995). Force development and velocity of saccadic eye movements in exotropia. Neuro-ophthalmology, 15: 1 - 16.

Lennerstrand G, Schiavi C, Bolzani R, Tian S, Benassi M, Longo N and Campos C (2003) Isometric force development in human horizontal muscle, attached to or detached from the globe. IOVS, Abstracts ARVO 2003 (in Press).

Lennerstrand, G. (1975) Motor units in eye muscles. In "Basic mechanisms of ocular motility and their clinical implications". (Lennerstrand, G. and Bach-y-Rita, P., eds.), pp 119-143, Pergamon Press, Oxford

Lennerstrand, G. (1982) Postnatal development of eye muscle function. An experimental study in cats with normal and impaired binocular vision. In "Functional Basis of Ocular Motility Disorders". (Lennerstrand, G., Zee, D. and Keller, E., eds.), pp 39-47, Pergamon Press, Oxford & New York

Lennerstrand, G. (1988) Motor and sensory functions of normal and strabismic extraocular muscle. In "Strabismus and Amblyopia". (Lennerstrand, G., von Noorden, G.K. and Campos, E.C., eds.), pp 47-63, Macmillan Press, Great Britain
Lennerstrand, G. and Bach-y-Rita, P. (1974) Spindle responses in pig eye muscles. Acta Physiol. Scand. 90, 795-797
Lennerstrand, G., Tian, S. and Han, Y. (1997) Effects of eye muscle proprioceptive activation on eye position in normal and exotropic subjects. Graefe´s Arch. Clin. Exp. Ophthalmol. 235, 63-69
Lennerstrand, G., Tian, S. and Zhao, T.X. (1993) Force development and velocity of humans saccadic eye movements. I. Abduction and adduction. Clin. Vision. Sci. 8, 295- 305.
Lennerstrand,G (2000) Functional properties of eye muscles: motor and sensory adaptation in strabismus. In: Advances in Strabismus Research: Basic and Clinical Aspects, Eds G Lennerstrand & J Ygge, Portland Press, London.
Mitsui, Y. and Tamura, O. (1986) Strabismus and the sensorimotor reflex. Clinical practice Series no 30, Excerpta Medica, Amsterdam
Oh SY, Poukens V & Demer JL (2001) Quantitative analysis of rectus extraocular muscle layers in monkey and humans. Invest Ophthalmol & Visual Science, 42:10 – 15
Oh SY, Poukens V, Cohen MS & Demer JL (2001) Structure-Function Correlations of laminar vascularity in human rectus extraocular muscles. Invest Ophthalmol & Vis Sci, 42: 17 – 22.
Pedrosa-Dommelöf F, Holmgren Y, Luca CA, Hoh JFY and Thornell L-E (2002) Human extraocular muscles: unique pattern of myosin heavy chain expression during myotube formation. Invest Ophthalmol Vic Sci, 41:1608- 1616.
Porter, J.D., Baker, R.S., Ragusa, R.J. and Brueckner, J.K. (1995) Extraocular muscles: Basic and clinical aspects of structure and function. Surv. Ophthalmol. 39, 451-484
Robinson DA (1978) The functional behavior of the peripheral ocular motor apparatus: a review. In “Disorders of Ocular Motility”, (Kommerell G ,ed.), pp 43 – 61, Bergmann, Munich..
Roll, J-P. and Vedel, J-P. (1982) Kinesthetic role of muscle afferents in man, studied by tendon vibration and microneurography. Exp. Brain. Res. 47, 177-190
Roll, J-P., Vedel, J-P. and Roll, R. (1989) Eye, head and skeletal muscle spindle feedback in the elaboration of body reference. In "Afferent control of posture and locomotion", (Allum, J.H.J. and Hulliger, M., eds.), Progr. Brain Res. 80, 113-123
Ruskell GL (1999) Extraocular muscle proprioceptors and proprioception. Progress in Retinal and Eye Research, 18:269 – 291.
Sato M, Yagasaki T, Kora T & Awaya S (1997) Comparison of muscle volume between congenital and acquired superior oblique palsies by magnetic resonance imaging, Jpn J Ophthalmol, 42: 466 - 470.
Scott, A.B. and Collins, C.C. (1973) Division of labor in human extraocular muscle. Arch. Ophthalmol. 90, 319-322
Spencer RF, Tucker MG, McNeer KW & Porter JD (1992) Experimental studies of pharmacological and surgical denervation of extraocular muscles in adult and infantile monkeys. In: The Mechanics of Strabismus: A Symposium on Oculomotor Engineering. Ed. A B Scott. San Francisco, CA: Smith-Kettlewell Eye Research Institute, pp 207 – 227.
Spencer, R.F. and McNeer, K.W. (1988) Morphology of the extraocular muscle in relation to the clinical manifestation of strabismus. In "Strabismus and Amblyopia". (Lennerstrand, G., von Noorden, G.K. and Campos, E.C., eds.), Macmillan Press, Great Britain
Spencer, R.F. and Porter, J.D. (1988) Structural organization of the extraocular muscles. In "Reviews in Oculomotor Research, Vol 2, Neuroanatomy of the Oculomotor System, (Buttner-Ennever, J.A., ed.), pp 33-79. Elsevier, New York
Stahl JS, Averbuch-Heller L, Remler BF & Leigh RJ (1998) Clinical evidence of extraocular fiber-type specificity of botulinum toxin. Neurology, 51: 1093 – 1099.
Steinbach MJ (1987) Proprioceptive knowledge of eye position. Vision Res 27: 1737 – 1744.
Steinbach, M.J. (1987) Proprioceptive knowledge of eye position. Vision Res. 27: 1737- 1744
Suna T, Nishida Y, Isberg B & Lennerstrand G (2000) MRI measurements of normal extraocular muscles and other orbital structures. Graefe´s Arch Clin Exp Ophthalmol. 23:393– 404
Tian S & Lennerstrand G (1994) Vertical saccadic velocity and force development in superior oblique palsy. Vision Res. 34: 1785-1798.
Tian S, Lennerstrand G, Nishida Y & Tallstedt L (2003) Eye muscle force development and saccadic velocity in thyroid associated ophthalmopathy. Graefe´s Arch Clin Exp Ophthalmol. (In Press).
Tian, S. and Lennerstrand, G. (1993) Force development and velocity of human saccadic eye movements. II. Elevation and depression. Clin. Vision. Sci. 34, 305-317

Weir CR (2000) Spatial localisation: does extraocular muscle proprioception play a role? Greafe's Arch Clin Exp Ophthalmol 238: 868 – 873.
Velay. J-L., Roll, R., Lennerstrand, G. and Roll, J-P. (1994) Eye proprioception and visual localization in humans: influence of ocular dominance and visual context. Vision Res. 34, 2169 -2176.

Session 3
Vision/Refraction/Nystagmus/Stereopsis

Transactions 28th Meeting European Strabismological Association, de Faber (ed.)
© 2004 European Strabismological Association, ISBN 90 265 1965 6

Effect of off-axis retinoscopy on objective refractive measurement

E.A. Paysse M.D., D.W. Jackson M.D., K.R. Wilhelmus M.D., M.A.W. Hussein M.D., G. Rosby C.O., D.K. Coats M.D.
Cullen Eye Institute, Baylor College of Medicine, Departments of Ophthalmology and Pediatrics, Texas Children's Hospital, Houston, Texas, United States

Purpose: On-axis retinoscopy is believed to be necessary for accurate determination of refractive error. The purpose of this study was to determine the effect of off-axis retinoscopy on objective refractive measurement. Methods: Eight volunteers underwent cycloplegic retinoscopy of their right eye on-axis, and at 5, 10, 15, and 20 degrees off-axis in adduction. A masked examiner performed all retinoscopy with randomization of the patient and axis refracted. Results: The average spherical retinoscopic value at 0, 5,10,15, and 20 degrees of off-axis alignment was –0.4, -0.9, -1, -1.38, and –1.8 diopters, respectively. The average sphero-equivalent retinoscopic value for each axis position was –0.02, -0.59, -0.45, -0.64, and –0.98 diopters, respectively. Cylinder power increased by an average of 3% for each degree of off-axis retinoscopy. Conclusion: Objective refractive measurement by retinoscopy is significantly altered by off-axis retinoscopy. KEYWORDS: retinoscopy, axis, refraction

1. INTRODUCTION

Retinoscopy often provides the only assessment of refractive error in pediatric patients and is frequently a key determinant in therapeutic decisions. While frequently stated in optics textbooks that on-axis retinoscopy is necessary for an accurate determination of a subject's refractive error, there is little published information regarding the actual effect that off-axis retinoscopy has on the determination of refractive error in a clinical setting.[1-4] In addition, most studies began the measurement of peripheral refraction at 20 degrees of eccentricity along the horizontal meridian, a situation not likely to be encountered clinically.[5,6,7] The purpose of this study was to determine the effect of off-the-visual-axis retinoscopy on objective refractive measurement using standard clinical techniques in a simulated clinical scenario.

2. METHODS

Eight cooperative adult subjects with a refractive error of +/- 2.50 diopters underwent cycloplegic retinoscopic evaluation of their right eye on-the-visual-axis, and at 5, 10, 15, and 20 degrees off-the-visual-axis in adduction. Adult subjects were used to assure steady fixation during retinoscopy. Each subject had a normal ophthalmologic examination except for the presence of a refractive error.

The patients were placed in a plus cylinder phoropter that had been modified for the study. A barrier at the nose separated the right and left eyes. A second barrier with fixation lights at zero, 5, 10, 15, and 20 degrees to the left of fixation was placed 40 cm in front of the patient's left eye. The study subjects were asked to direct the gaze of their left eye toward the illuminated fixation light and maintain fixation on the light until retinoscopy was complete. Cycloplegic refraction was performed by a single masked examiner at a constant working distance of 66 cm. Retinoscopy at all 5 gaze positions was completed within 1 hour on each subject. Patient order and eccentric gaze position tested were randomized.

3. RESULTS

Each patient's cycloplegic refraction correlated well with his or her manifest refraction when aligned on-the-visual-axis. The spherical equivalent also showed an increasing myopic shift with increasing eccentricity of gaze. (Figure 1) The average spherical equivalent measured on-the-visual-axis and at each position of off-axis alignment is shown in Figure 2. The mean spherical equivalent retinoscopic value measured for 0, 5, 10, 15, and 20 degrees was –0.02, -0.59, -0.45, -0.64, -0.98 diopters, respectively.

Off-axis retinoscopy also resulted in an induced cylindrical error that increased by an average of 3% for every degree of eccentricity (p=0.009). Figure 3 shows the linear regression plot, with 95% prediction band. The actual cylindrical values obtained are displayed in the Table.

Table: Retinoscopic plus cylinder obtained on-axis and 5, 10, 15, and 20 degrees off-ais in adduction

Patient #	On-Axis	5^0	10^0	15^0	20°
1	0.50 X 089	Sphere	Sphere	0.50 X 180	1.25 X 167
2	0.75 X 025	Sphere	1.00 X 178	0.25 X 175	2.25 X 019
3	1.00 X 003	1.00 X 003	1.75 X 005	1.75 X169	2.75 X 003
4	2.25 X157	2.25 X 155	3.50 X 160	3.75 X 159	2.25 X 155
5	1.00 X 095	1.00 X 126	Sphere	0.50 X 155	0.50 X 118
6	0.25 X 010	0.25 X 012	1.25 X 010	2.25 X 020	2.25 X 002
7	Sphere	0.75 X 005	1.00 X 178	1.75 X 180	1.50 X 175
8	1.00 X 077	0.25 X 089	0.25 X 175	1.00 X 085	0.50 X 004

4. DISCUSSION

Accurate retinoscopy is a key component of pediatric ophthalmologic examination. Optics text-books have repeatedly stated that the accuracy of retinoscopy is improved when performed on-the-visual-axis.[1-3,10] Uncooperative children, unsteady fixation, and problems with eye position during examination under anesthesia can make it difficult, if not impossible, to refract on-the-visual-axis.[4] The true impact of eccentric retinoscopy in clinical situations has received little attention.

In the few in-vivo studies that demonstrate the effect of refracting the peripheral retina, the purpose was mainly to determine the state of the peripheral vision.[7,8,9] Situations not likely to be encountered in a clinical situation were studied, and cycloplegia was not used.

Our results confirm that accuracy of the retinoscopic measurement is reduced during off-axis retinoscopy. The induced errors are potentially clinically significant, even with small degrees of eccentricity likely to be encountered in clinical practice, but are higher with increasingly eccentric gaze. An average myopic shift of 5% for each degree off axis was noted in the spherical equivalent, while "induced" cylinder power increased by an average of 3% for every degree of eccentricity.

The refractive power of the eye is essentially related to three variables: corneal curvature, axial length, and power of the crystalline lens. Corneal curvature flattens from apex to limbus and becomes less spherical.[11-13] Likewise, the axial length of the normal eye is longest on the visual axis. Both of these factors should induce a hyperopic error.[14] On the other hand, when light rays strike the crystalline lens obliquely, a myopic and oblique astigmatic error is induced, a finding very similar to our off-axis retinoscopy results.[12,15-16] It has been demonstrated that tilting an intraocular lens en vitro 7, 11, or 15 degrees using a Gullstrand model eye induced a –0.30, -0.77, and -1.47 diopter myopic refractive error, respectively.[12] The human crystalline lens is likely to behave in a similar fashion.

Our findings concur with others that the accuracy of retinoscopy decreases proportionally with the degree of eccentricity of the incident light beam from the visual axis. Even small degrees of eccentricity can result in significant errors in refractive error determination.

5. REFERENCES:

Safir A. Refraction and clinical optics. Harper & Row, Publishers Inc, Hagerstown, Va. 1980;174.
Abrams D. Duke-Elder's practice of refraction tenth edition. Churchill Livingstone, New York, NY, 1993; 164.
Michaels DD. Visual optics and refraction a clinical approach, third edition. The C.V. Mosby Company, St. Louis, Mo, 1985; 305.
Saunders RA, Andrews CJ. Refractive Changes in Children under general anesthesia. J Pediatric Ophth Strabismus. 1981;18:38-41.
Lotmar W, Lotmar T. Peripheral astigmatism in the human eye: Experimental data and theoretical model predictions. J Opt Soc Am. 1974;64 (4):510-513.
Millodot M, Lamont A. Refraction of the periphery of the eye. J Opt Soc Am. 1974;64(1):110-111.
Rempt F, Hoogerheide J, Hoogenboom WPH. Peripheral Retinoscopy and the Skiagram. Ophthalmologica. 1971;162:1-10.
Ferree CE, Rand G, Hardy C. Refraction for the peripheral field of vision. Arch Ophthalmol.1931:5717-731.
Ferree CE, Rand G. Interpretation of refractive conditions in the peripheral field of vision. Amer J Ophthal. 1932;15:513-522.
Benjamin W. Borish's Clinical Refraction. Philadelphia, Saunders W.B.; 1988:582.
Holladay JT, Waring GO. Optics and topography of radial keratotomy. Edited by G.O. Waring in Refractive Keratotomy for myopia and astigmatism. Mosby Year Book, 1992;47-51.
Erickson P. Effects of intraocular lens position errors on postoperative refractive error. J Cataract Refract Surg 1990:16;305-311.
Bogan SJ, Waring GO, Ibrahim O. classification of normal corneal topography based on computer-assisted videokeratography. Arch Ophthalmol, 1990; 108:945-949.
Berges O, Puech M, Assouline M, Letenneur L, Gastellu-Etchegorry M. B-mode-guided vector-A-mode versus A-mode biometry to determine axial length and intraocular lens power. J Cataract Refract Surg.1998:24;529-535.
Korynta J, Bok J, Cendelin J, Michalova K. Computer modeling of visual impairment caused by intraocular lens misalignment. J Cataract Refract Surg 25:100-105;1999.
Lakshminarayanan V, Enoch JM, Raasch T, Crawford B, Nygaard RW. Refractive changes induced by intraocular lens tilt and longitudinal displacement. Arch Ophthalmol, 1986:104;90-92.

Transactions 28th Meeting European Strabismological Association, de Faber (ed.)
© 2004 European Strabismological Association, ISBN 90 265 1965 6

Interrelation of optokinetic nystagmus response and recognation visual acuity.

Sibel Oto MD,Altu_Çetinkaya MD,Ahmet Akman MD,Yonca Akova MD
Baskent University School of Medicine,Ankara,Turkey

Objective:Optokinetic nystagmus (OKN)response is a useful method for objective assess-ment of visual acuity in the preverbal infants.The aim of this study was to investigate thecorrelation between recognition visual acuity and OKN response elicited by different bar si-zes with varying contrast.

Methods:Two groups were studied .The first group consisted of 44 eyes of 22 normal chil-dren (age:4-10)with binocular recognition visual acuities 0,1 logMAR unit and better.The se-cond group consisted of 30 children with uncorrected refractive errors with recognition visualacuity between 0.2 to 1 logMAR unit.Recognition visual acuity was evaluated using Snellenletters or numbers and Lea Hyvarinen charts.Optokinetic nystagmus (OKN)was elicited withstandardized OKN stimulator program of computerized Ophthimus device.Consecutive blackand white stripes moving at 7 pre-determined bar size and rate levels (480-60 pixel/sec),in30 different contrast units were shown to the children sitting 60 cm to a 27,5 x 20,5 cm scre-en.First,the narrowest stripes eliciting the OKN response was assessed then at this bar sizethe minimum contrast level was established starting from 30 units (dark bar =1 cd/m2,whitebar=80 cd/m2)by a reduction of 5 units until OKN response was undetectable.

Results:In 40 of 42 eyes of the first group OKN response was detected as 60 pixel/sec (mi-nimum bar size)and in 2 eyes as120 pixel/sec and the contrast levels were 5 unit and betterin 6-10 years old group and 15-30 units in three children aged 4-5 years.None of these eyesrevealed any nystagmus asymmetry.In the second group the minimum OKN response was 120 pixel/sec with 1-15 unit contrastlevel and no correlation was found between the level of visual acuity and the threshold ofspatial frequency.However the contrast level varied with the child 's age and attention.

Conclusions:The spatial frequency threshold quantitatively detected by OKN program ofOphthimus device was not found as correlated with recognition visual acuity.

Transactions 28th Meeting European Strabismological Association, de Faber (ed.)

Observational analysis of nystagmic oscillations by two-dimensional video-oculography

R.Frosini,L.Frosini,P.Linari,S.Frosini,S.Brogelli and G.Alfieri
Department of Oto-Neuro-Ophtalmological Surgical SciencesUniversity of Florence,Italy

Objective:To study nystagmic oscillations of ophthalmological interest by means of 2DVOG TM(two-dimensional video-oculography),a recently introduced technology which has shown to be useful in monitoring patients affected by oto-vestibular illnesses.

Design : Prospective observational non-masked clinical study
Method : Preliminary validation phase of the study is ongoing through acquisition and processation of clinical data obtained and recorded by means of a commercial 2DVOG system. Protocol of examination is currently under development.

Results : The first series of 10 observed clinical cases will be discussed.

References:
1.Frosini R,Boschi MC,Grasso Canizzo P:Studio bidimensionale della cinetica oculare insoggetti normali ed in alcuni quadri patologici.Atti della Fondazione Giorgio Ronchi1983;38:304-318.
2.Frosini R,Campa L:Analisi dei movimenti oculari mediante digitalizzazione di immagini televisive.Audiovisivo n.150.Centro Didattico Televisivo dell'Università di Firenze.1987.
3.Wassill KH,Kaufmann H:Binokulare dreidimensionale Videookulographie.Ophthalmologe2000;97:629-632.

Transactions 28th Meeting European Strabismological Association, de Faber (ed.)
© 2004 European Strabismological Association, ISBN 90 265 1965 6

Stereoacuity norms for the Frisby Davis Distance stereotest at different distances

H. Davis, J. P. Frisby, J. Hoole & L. Baker
University of Sheffield United Kingdom

J. Hoole

Leeds Teaching Hospitals United Kingdom

L.Baker

Manchester Royal Eye Hospital United Kingdom

Stereoacuity is routinely measured for the detection of abnormality. It is important that we establish normative data. This study was a repeated measure design in which data from normal subjects for the Frisby Davis Distance (FD2) stereotest for 6metres and 3metres were compared to results of the Frisby near stereotest (FNS). Mean FD2 stereoacuities were similar to those of previous studies. There were significant correlations between all test distances. The difference between 6metres and near was statistically significant. However this difference was only 6" of arc and may not be clinically important.

Stereoacuity, FD2, distance stereopsis, Frisby stereotest

1. INTRODUCTION

There has been conflicting evidence as to whether stereoacuity changes from near to distance. We report a study using tests of real objects. Two previous studies have used alignment of real objects at different distances. Lit & Flynn (1976) had two subjects and used distances of 0.2 to 1.5metres. The results were similar but the range of distances was small. Kaye et al (1999) had 63 normal subjects and tested at 6metres, 3metres and 1metre for which the mean stereoacuities were 9", 14" and 32" of arc respectively.

2. METHODS

The FD2 was used at 6metres and 3metres. It is a test of real depth, it cannot be learned and at 6metres has a range of 50" to 5" of arc. The 6metres norm for young adults is approximately 10" of arc (Frisby & Davis 2003). The FNS was used for near. It is also a test of real depth and cannot be learned. In this study the smallest disparity tested was 5" of arc to achieve comparability with the FD2. Frisby & Davis (2003) found the FNS mean for normal young adults was approx 30" of arc when testing to a limit of 20" of arc (as per instructions). This limit was achieved for the FD2 at 3metres by using additional more closely spaced markings on the rods.

All subjects had a distance and near visual acuity of 6/9 or better and no deviation or a well controlled heterophoria. There were 71 subjects with an age range of 6-62yrs and a mean of 34yrs. There were 29 males and 42 females.

The FD2 was tested in a counter-balanced order at 6 or 3metres. Near stereoacuity was tested using FNS in between the FD2 presentations. In all cases 2 out of 3 correct responses were required for a positive response.

For the FD2 the largest disparity was presented first, i.e. 50" at 6metres, which translates to 200" at 3metres. The disparities were then halved, e.g. 50" to 25" etc, until an incorrect response was produced. The disparity was then increased, e.g. 10" to 15" etc, until threshold or the limit of 5" of arc was reached.

For the FNS the 3 plates were tested at 40cms, then the distance of the thinnest plate was increased to produce disparities of 20", 15", 10" and 5" of arc (80, 95, 115 and 165cms distances)

3. RESULTS

Three subjects were excluded as outliers because their FNS result was more than 9 s.d. from the mean. The group means of the remaing subjects (N=68) were very similar with only 6" of arc being the maximum difference.

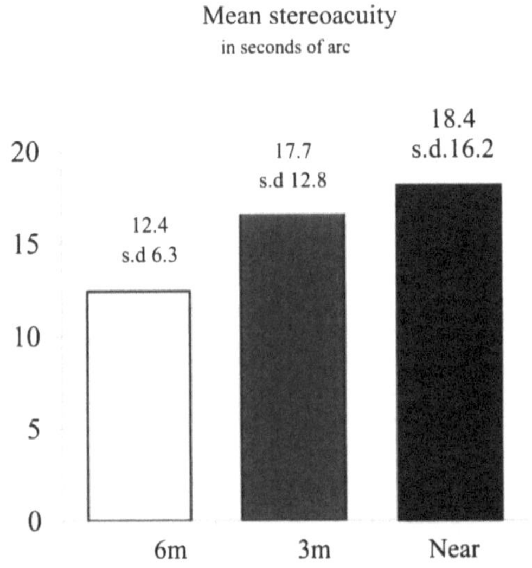

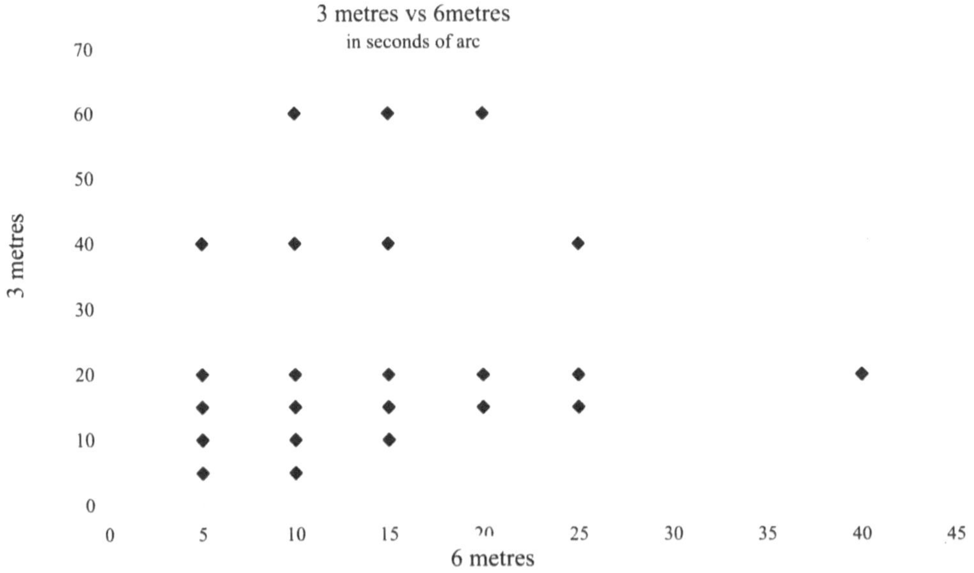

Spearman Rank Correlation p<.01 rho=.453

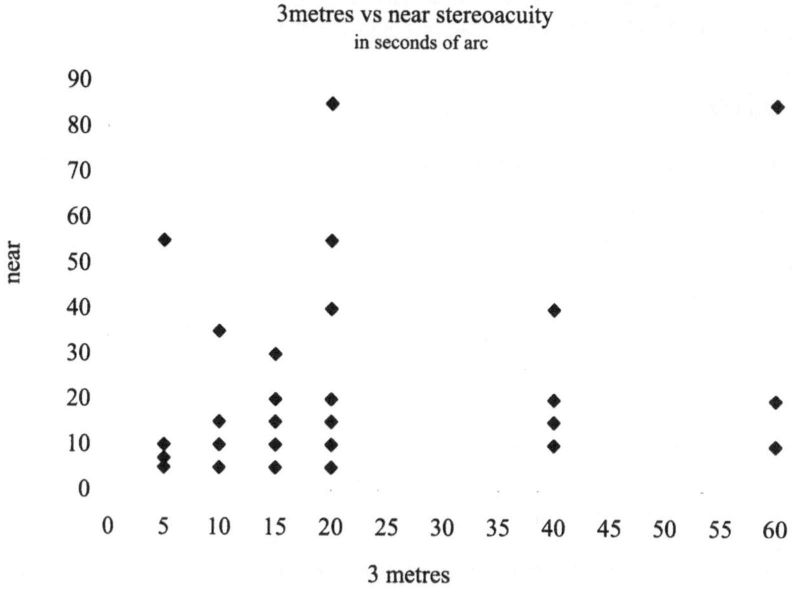

Spearman Rank Correlation p=.01 rho=.436

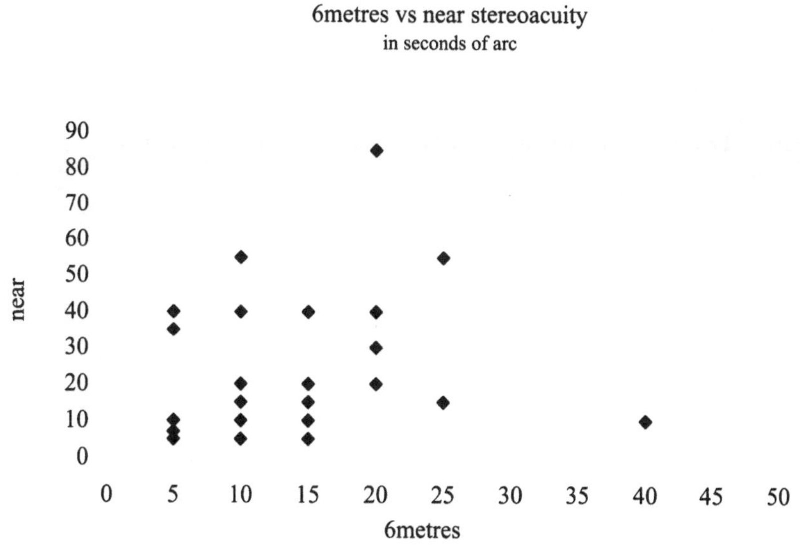

Spearman Rank Correlation <.01 rho .489

Although the group means were very similar the difference was significant (Friedman test $p<0.01$).

Multiple comparisons between group means showed a significant difference ($p<.01$) between 6metres and near. The 6metres vs 3metres difference was not significant but it was only just above the $p<.05$ limit. The 3metres vs near was not significant.

4. DISCUSSION

In agreement with Kaye et al this study demonstrated better stereoacuity at 6metres were compared to near. In order that the FNS could be tested to a limit of 5" of arc the thinnest plate was moved back to 165cms. This increase in test distance may have affected the results. Ideally a reduction in plate thickness would have been more appropriate but this was not technically feasible.

Whilst there was a statistically significant difference between 6metres and near, the difference between the means was 6" of arc and the clinical relevance of this small difference has yet to be established.

5. CONCLUSIONS

The mean stereoacuity of the FD2 at 6metres was 12" of arc, which is close to Frisby & Davis's (2003) previously published test norm of approximately 10" of arc. The mean FD2 at 3metres was 18" of arc.

When testing to a 5" limit the mean near stereoacuity using the FNS was 18" of arc, but this entailed using the FNS at up to 165cms.

There were significant correlations between all test distances. Whilst there was a significant difference between 6metres and near this was only of the order of 6" of arc and may not be clinically important.

REFERENCES

Frisby JP, Davis H 2003 2003 Clinical Tests of distance stereopsis:state of the art Transactions of the 9th International Strabismological Association Sydney 187-90

Lit A, Finn JP 1976 Variability of depth-discrimination thresholds as a function of observation distance. J Opt Soc Am 6;66:740-2

Kaye SB, Siddiqui A, Ward A, Noonan C Fisher AC, Green JR, Brown MC, Wareing PA, Watt P 1999 Monocular and binocular depth discrimination thresholds. Optom Vis Sci 76:770-82

Transactions 28th Meeting European Strabismological Association, de Faber (ed.)
© 2004 European Strabismological Association, ISBN 90 265 1965 6

Stereoacuity is not always the best measure of control.

J.E.S.White
Sussex Eye Hospital, Brighton, UK.

ABSTRACT: The aim of this study was to assess how accurate stereoacuity is as a measure of control. A retrospective review was carried out of 50 patients with either an intermittent heterotropia, symptom producing heterophoria or convergence insufficiency. In the Orthoptic reports particular note was taken of the Prism Fusion Range, Binocular Visual Acuity, Stereoacuity and Prism Cover Test. The Prism Fusion Range and Binocular Visual Acuity showed reductions which mirrored the deterioration of control of a deviation and they were also a better indicator of the outcome of treatment. Stereoacuity was not shown to reduce with decreasing control of a deviation nor to improve with treatment. Stereoacuity though shown, in previous studies to be linked to the size of a deviation does not show improvement when the angle of deviation is reduced or when a heterophoria is no longer symptom producing.

KEYWORDS: Stereopsis, Prism Fusion Range

1 INTRODUCTION

Stereopsis is appreciated due to the disparity of similar objects. Stereoacuity is a measure of the disparity discriminated to appreciate stereopsis. It has been shown that stereoacuity is affected by visual acuity, anisometropia and the presence of a manifest deviation (Brown 2001). Age has also been shown to affect levels of stereoacuity. Parks (1969) found that the average stereoacuity was 24" of arc in adult patients with normal BSV and for young children no better than 60" of arc .There is discussion in the literature as to whether stereoacuity is affected by heterophoria (Harwerth 1995 & Saladin 1995). If stereoacuity is not affected by size of the vergence disparity it could be argued that it is therefore not the best measure of control in patients with intermittent heterotropia or heterophoria. The aim of this study was therefore to assess whether stereoacuity is an accurate measure of control of a deviation.

2 METHOD

A retrospective study was carried out looking at the case notes of patients attending the authors clinic. The inclusion criteria were that the patient had an intermittent heterotropia, a decompensating heterophoria or a convergence insufficiency, and had had either conservative or surgical treatment. The Orthoptic reports pre- and post-treatment were reviewed and particular note was taken of the Prism Fusion range, Binocular Visual Acuity (BVA), Stereoacuity and the Prism Cover Test measurements.

3 RESULTS

66 case notes were reviewed and a total of 50 included in the study. There were 27 female and 23 male with a mean age of 6 years (range 2-39 years) at first attendance. The differential diagnoses can be seen in Table 1, the majority of cases having Distance Exotropia or Convergence Insufficiency.

Diagnosis	Number of Cases
Near Exophoria	6
Distance Exophoria	7
NonSpecific Exophoria	8
Distance Exotropia	11
NonSpecific Exotropia	5
Convergence Insufficiency	13

Table 1: Differential Diagnoses of cases reviewed. (n=50)

All patients had undergone treatment. The main treatment option, as can be seen in Table 2, was Orthoptic exercises closely followed by surgery.

Treatment	Number of Cases
Orthoptic Exercises	25
Prisms	1
Surgery	21
Glasses	2
Occlusion	1

Table 2: Treatment of cases reviewed. (n=50)

All patients had corrected visual acuity of 6/9 Snellens or better, their level of stereoacuity could therefore not be significantly influenced by their visual acuity. All patients had symptoms or parents had concerns about their child's eyes prior to commencing treatment. Post treatment 44 patients (88%) were asymptomatic.

It can be seen in Table 3 that in all diagnostic categories there is an improvement post-treatment in the mean positive fusion vergence both at 1/3m and 6m.

Diagnosis	Pre-Treatment 1/3m PBO	Post-Treatment 1/3m PBO	Pre-Treatment 6m PBO	Post-Treatment 6m PBO
Near Exophoria	10	17	6	10
Distance Exophoria	13.5	19	1	4.5
NonSpecific Exophoria	21	22	7	11
Distance Exotropia	14	29	10	13
NonSpecific Exotropia	14	23	3	19
Convergence Insufficiency	21	28	9	15

Table 3: Mean Positive Fusion Vergence (Base Out Fusion Range) Pre- and Post-Treatment. (n=50)

The deviation also shows a reduction post-treatment as is seen in Table 4.

Diagnosis	Pre-Treatment PCT 1/3m	Post-Treatment PCT 1/3m	Pre-Treatment PCT 6m	Post-Treatment PCT 6m
Near Exophoria	17	11	6	5
Distance Exophoria	11	7	28	12.5
NonSpecific Exophoria	24	12	22	14
Distance Exotropia	18	8	26	9
NonSpecific Exotropia	38	8	34	4
Convergence Insufficiency	6	5.5	2	1

Table 4: Deviation measured by Prism Cover Test Pre- and Post-Treatment. (n=50)

The data for the Binocular Visual Acuity was not sufficient to analyse for each diagnostic category, mainly due to the age of the patient and their being to young to read. The data which was obtained did however mirror the improvements seen on positive fusion vergence.

When looking at stereoacuity for each diagnostic category it can be seen, on Table 5, that there is a wide variation of values. The variation pre-treatment could be attributed to age, as Distance Exotropia with the worst mean stereoacuity pre-treatment had a mean age of first attendance of 4 years where as NonSpecific Exotropia with the best mean stereoacuity pre-treatment had a mean age of 11 years. The mean measurements post-treatment were erratic, two groups showed an improvement, two groups were unchanged and two groups showed a reduction in stereoacuity. There was no correlation between stereoacuity and the size of the deviation either pre- or post-Treatment.

Diagnosis	Pre-Treatment	Post-Treatment
	Near Stereoacuity	Near Stereoacuity
Near Exophoria	121"	110"
Distance Exophoria	205"	350"
NonSpecific Exophoria	93"	427"
Distance Exotropia	400"	340"
NonSpecific Exotropia	90"	90"
Convergence Insufficiency	106"	106"

Table 5: Mean Near Stereoacuity, measured in seconds of arc, Pre- and Post-Treatment. (n=50)
4

5 CONCLUSIONS

The results show that Positive Fusion Vergence measurements and the BVA mirrors a decrease in the deviation and the patients symptoms. Stereopsis did not demonstrate any correlation with the size of deviation or symptoms, nor did show the improvement seen in the Positive fusion Vergence and BVA. It is therefore concluded that in patients with an intermittent heterotropia, a symptom producing heterophoria or convergence insufficiency that Fusion Vergence is a better indicator of binocular control than Stereoacuity.

There were inherent problems with the study design as it was a retrospective study. Firstly there was a lack of complete data in some of the case notes, this could in many cases be attributed to the age of the patients reviewed. The results could also be argued to be affected by the fact that there were a variety of stereotests employed, the majority of patients were tested using the Frisby stereotest but Titmus, TNO and Lang stereotests were also used. A correlation between the control at distance and stereoacuity could not be carried out as stereoacuity had not been measured at distance, as a free space distance stereotest has not been readily available in the UK until recently. To address some of these issues it would be interesting to carry out a prospective study.

REFERENCES

Brown,S.et al. 2001. Assessment of adult stereopsis using the Lang 1 Stereotest: a pilot study. *Binocul.Vis.Strabismus.* Summer; 16(2):91-8

Harwerth,R.S. et al. 1995. Behavioural studies of local stereopsis and disparity vergence in monkeys. *Vision Res.* Jun;35(12):1755-70

Parks,M. 1969. Monofixation syndrome. *Trans. Am. Ophthalmol.* 67;584-587

Saladin,J.J. 1995. Effects of heterophoria on stereopsis. *Optom.Vis.Sci.*Jul;72(7):487-92

Session 4
Exotropia/Eye movements

Transactions 28th Meeting European Strabismological Association, de Faber (ed.)
 ISBN 90 265 1965 6

Latent Nystagmus: Is the Eye an Accessory Vestibule?

M.C. Brodsky
University of Arkansas for Medical Sciences, Little Rock, Arkansas, USA

R.J. Tusa
Emory University, Atlanta, Georgia, USA

ABSTRACT:

Introduction: Latent nystagmus is a binocular horizontal ocular oscillation that is evoked by unequal visual input to the two eyes.

Methods: Examination of subcortical neuroanatomical pathways producing latent nystagmus and nasotemporal asymmetry of optokinetic nystagmus during monocular viewing.

Results: In lateral-eyed animals, each eye has a nasalward bias for visual detection of optic flow. This monocular nasotemporal asymmetry promotes binocular stabilization of the frontal visual world during forward navigation and monocular stabilization of the lateral visual world during horizontal body rotation, allowing the animal to frontalize, inspect, and ingest nutrients. In humans with congenital strabismus or early monocular visual loss, this primitive monocular nasalward bias modulates horizontal muscle tonus to produce the slow phase of latent nystagmus.

Conclusions: Latent nystagmus is a visuo-vestibular tonus imbalance that is driven by unbalanced input from the two eyes to the vestibular system. Latent nystagmus is the ocular counterpart of peripheral horizontal vestibular nystagmus. Its emergence in humans with congenital strabismus attests to the primitive role of the eye as an accessory vestibule.

Transactions 28th Meeting European Strabismological Association, de Faber (ed.)
© 2004 European Strabismological Association, ISBN 90 265 1965 6

Saccadic eye movements in thyroid associated ophthalmopathy

Hermann Dieter Schworm[1,2], Jan Ygge[1], Roberto Bolzani[1,3], Suna Tian[1], Leif Tallstedt[1], Agneta Rydberg[1], Gunnar Lennerstrand[1]
[1]*Dept. of Ophthalmology, Karolinska Institutet, Stockholm, Sweden,*
[2]*Eye Hospital of the City of Dessau, Germany,*
[3]*University Eye Hospital Bologna, Italy*

ABSTRACT
The aim of the present study was to find out whether saccadic eye movements of patients with different stages of thyroid associated ophthalmopathy (TAO) differ from those of healthy individuals. Horizontal and vertical saccades with an amplitude of 10°, 20°, 30° and 40° of 4 groups of 36 patients with different stages of TAO and 10 control subjects were recorded using the induction scleral search coil technique. Two constants of the main sequence (V_0 and α) were calculated for each eye. Statistic analysis of the two constants revealed changes of saccadic properties in all stages of TAO. The changes were more pronounced in patients with severe acute and longstanding restrictive disease; they were less pronounced in those with early mild disease. To our surprise, however, patients without TAO but proven auto-immune thyroiditis revealed the most characteristic changes. Our results suggest that recordings of rapid eye movements and main sequence analysis of saccades could well contribute to the clinical assessment of TAO, especially when in doubt about existing TAO in thyroiditis.

Key words: thyroid associated ophthalmopathy – disease stages – saccades – induction scleral search coil – main sequence constants

1. INTRODUCTION

A number of studies has been published during the past decades reporting on saccade dynamics in patients with thyroid associated ophthalmopathy (TAO). However, the results compared to normal individuals were contradictory. While some authors detected decreased saccade velocity [1,2], others observed an increase of saccade velocity [3] or an absence of significant changes [4]. To further analyze the underlying causes for the differing results and to establish whether or not different stages of TAO lead to different changes of saccade dynamics, we designed a prospective clinical study on patients with well defined different stages of TAO. If significant changes in patients were to be detected, we aimed to find out whether analysis of rapid eye movements could serve as an additional diagnostic tool for early detection of inflammatory activity in TAO.

2. METHODS

Thirty-six patients with TAO and 10 age- and sex-matched control subjects were investigated. According to the stage of the disease, the patients were divided into 4 groups: 1. early mild disease (n=10), 2. early severe disease (n=10), 3. longstanding restrictive disease (n=10), and 4. proven auto-immune thyroid disease without any signs of TAO (n=6). Horizontal and vertical saccades with an amplitude of 10°, 20°, 30° and 40° were recorded binocularly using the induction scleral search coil technique. Two constants of the main sequence were calculated for each eye according to the formula as described by Bahill et al. [5]: V_0, describing the asymptotic maximum velocity, and α, characterizing the steepness of the amplitude dependent change of velocity. The two parameters V_0 and α served as dependend variables in a repeated measures analysis of variance (General Linear Model, GLM) to test for differences between different gaze directions, eyes and groups. As between group factor the five groups of subjects were used and as within subjects factors we used up- and downgaze, abductional and adductional movement direction. Applying V_0 and α to the main sequence formula, the average main sequence curves of the different groups were reconstructed. The SPSS statistical package version 10 was applied for statistical evaluation. GLM procedure was used to perform the analysis of variance for repeated measures.

3. RESULTS

The statistical analysis of the differences between groups and directions is shown in Table 1. In horizontal saccades, significant differences were found only between groups (P=0.05). There were no significant differences between ab- and ad-ductional saccades. No significant interaction was found between groups and ab- and adduction. In vertical saccades, the differences between groups and the interaction between groups and up- and down-gaze saccades were statistically significant (P=0.036).

Significances	**Test**	**Horizontal**	**Vertical**
Multiv Test, Group	Wilk's Lambda	0.05	0.04
Multiv Test, Direct*Group	Wilk's Lambda	ns	0.003
Univ Test, Direct*Group	F-Test	V0: ns α: ns	V0: 0.002 α: ns
Contrast Level 2 vs prev.	F-Test	V0: ns α: ns	V0: ns α: ns
Contrast Level 3 vs prev.	F-Test	V0: ns α: ns	V0: ns α: ns
Contrast Level 4 vs prev.	F-Test	V0: ns α: ns	V0: ns α: ns
Contrast Level 5 vs prev.	F-Test	V0: 0.008 α: ns	V0: 0.005 α: ns

Table 1

Constant	**Group**	**Mean**	**Mean**	**Mean**
		Horizontal	Upgaze	Downg.
V0	Volunteers	438,1	377,3	468,4
	No sign (4)	500,9	499,4	413,8
	Mild (1)	455,6	451,6	446,2
	Severe (2)	417,5	437,6	372,8
	Longstanding (3)	376,6	372,4	321,7
α	Volunteers	8,09	8,78	11,1
	No sign (4)	8,81	10,2	9,47
	Mild (1)	9,03	10,5	8,65
	Severe (2)	8,68	12,3	9,34
	Longstanding (3)	8,98	11,0	8,34

Table 2

The data of the calculated mean values of V_0 and α are listed in Table 2. Because of the absence of statistical significance of the differences, horizontal gaze directions were not differentiated. The reconstructed main sequence curves obtained by drawing the main sequence function using the mean values of V_0 and α compared to the volunteers showed reduced velocity of the patients with severe and longstanding disease and increased velocity of the patients with mild and no eye disease. The difference was more pronounced in the longstanding group and in the no eye disease group, respectively.

Due to the differences concerning gaze directions, the vertical saccades were divided into up- and downgaze movements. The reconstructed main sequence curves are illustrated in Fig. 1. Whereas the volunteers showed higher velocity on downgaze saccades than on upgaze saccades (Fig. 1a), the opposite behaviour was found in the patients with severe (group 2, Fig. 1c) and longstanding disease (group 3, Fig. 1d) as well as in the patients with no apparent orbitopathy (group 4, Fig. 1e). The patients with mild disease (group 1, Fig. 1b) showed almost no difference between up- and downgaze saccades. To our surprise, the difference compared to the gaze dependent velocity pattern was most pronounced in the patients of group 4 (no clinically visible TAO).

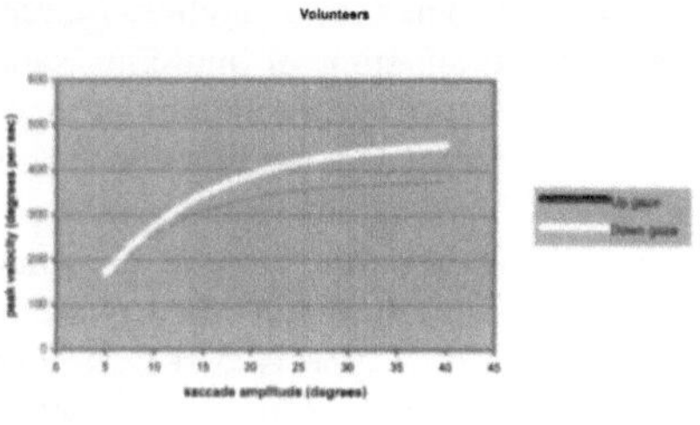

Fig. 1a: Volunteers

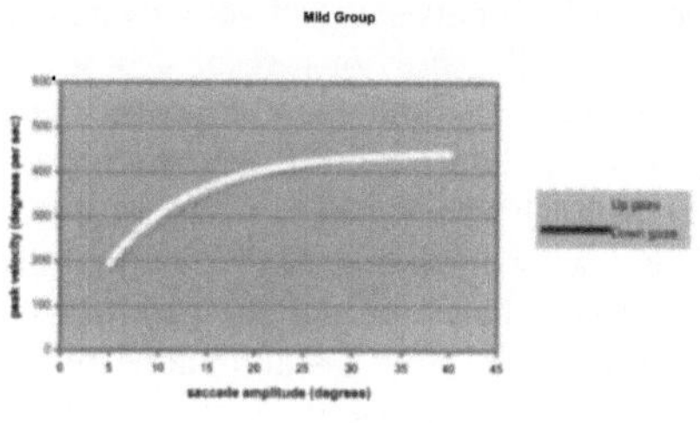

Fig. 1b: Group 1

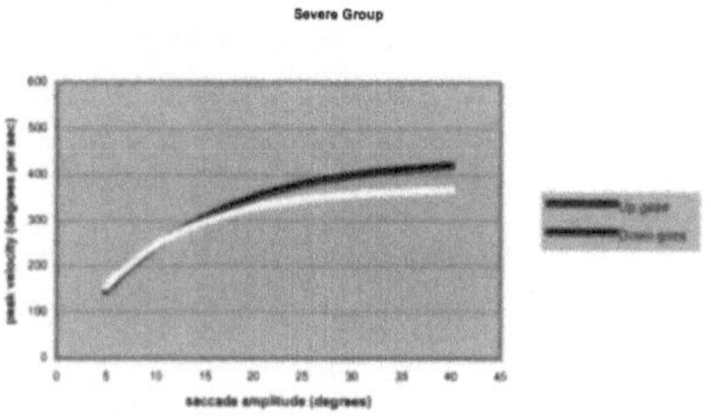

Fig. 1c: Group 2

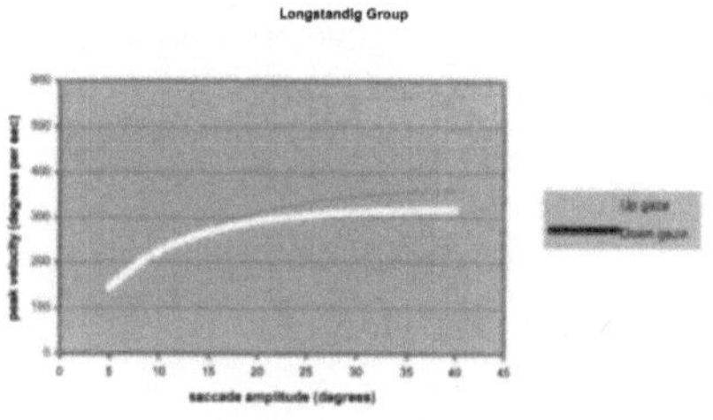

Fig. 1d: Group 3

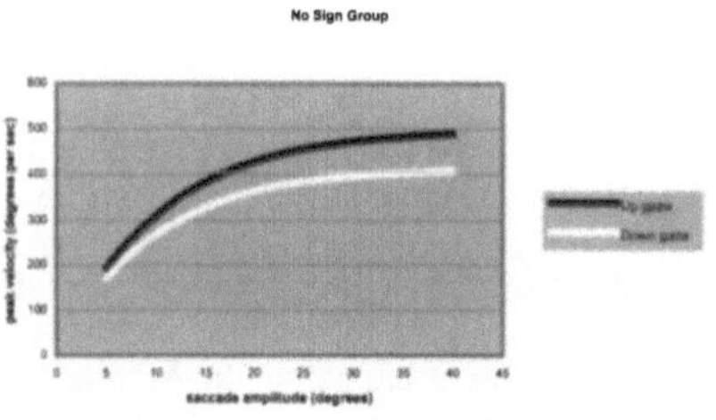

Fig. 1e: Group 4

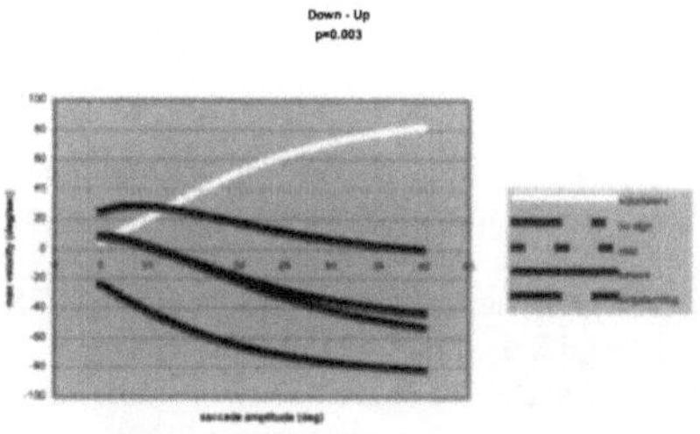

Fig. 2: Downgaze minus Upgaze

To further elaborate the differences between up- and downgaze saccades, upgaze velocity was subtracted of downgaze velocity and a graph was constructed based on the subtraction values (Fig. 2). Looking at the characteristics at high amplitude saccades, this figure impressively illustrates the clear difference between the healthy individuals and the patients who all showed the opposite behaviour. While the value of the volunteers increased with increasing amplitude, it decreased among all groups of patients, again most pronounced among those of group 4.

4. CONCLUSIONS

In addition to our preliminary results [6], the final results of our prospective study clearly differentiating between different stages of TAO demonstrated that analysis of the two main sequence constants V_0 and α and subsequent mathematical reconstruction of the amplitude/velocity curves sensitively reveal changes of saccade dynamics that otherwise remain undetected. Unlike previous results based on the mere evaluation of multiple saccade parameters [4], analysis of the main sequence curve enabled us to detect alterations of saccadic properties in all patients with TAO. An unexpected and most fascinating finding was that even those patients who clinically had no signs of orbitopathy showed marked changes of saccadic velocity characteristics, pointing to the fact that the extraocular muscles were already affected by the disease. These findings may add further information to the question whether a patient with laboratory test proven autoimmune thyroiditis of the Basedow type is at risk to develop TAO. Apparently, compared to clinical investigation, saccade analysis is a more sensitive parameter in early detection of TAO than traditional clinical investigation methods. However, since induction scleral search coil recordings and main sequence analysis are complex and time consuming techniques, it can not yet be recommended for routine screening investigation. Our ongoing studies are designed to search for easier but as well accurate recording techniques suitable for application on a larger study population. We further aim to find out whether saccade analysis can help to identify patients with autoimmune thyroid disease who are at risk to develop TAO.

5. ACKNOWLEDGEMENTS

This study was supported by a scholarship from the International Research Foundation for Children's Eyecare, Inc., New York, and by the Karolinska Insitutet Foundation.

REFERENCES

Feldon SE, Levin L, Liu SK. Graves' ophthalmopathy. Correlation of saccadic eye movements with age, presence of optic neuropathy, and extraocular muscle volume. Arch Ophthalmol. 1990; 108:1568-1571.

Wouters RJ, van den Bosch WA, Lemij HG. Saccadic eye movements in Graves' disease. Invest Ophthalmol Vis Sci. 1998; 39: 1544-1550.

Kirsch A, Rüssmann W, Konen W. Vertikale Sakkaden bei endokriner Orbitopathie. In: Mühlendyck H, Rüssmann W, eds. Augenbewegung und visuelle Wahrnehmung. Stuttgart: Enke; 1990:147-150.

Schworm HD, Heufelder AE, Kunze A, Welge E, Boergen K-P. Clinical significance of saccade analysis in early active Graves' ophthalmopathy. Invest Ophthalmol Vis Sci. 2000; 41:1710-1718.

Bahill AT, Clark MR, Stark L. The main sequence, a tool for studying human eye movements. Math Biosciences. 1975; 24:191-204.

Schworm HD, Ygge J, Rydberg A, Tian S, Bolzani R, Lennerstrand G. Extraocular muscle changes in Graves' ophthalmopathy – Saccadic eye movements. *Invest Ophthalmol Vis Sci* 2000; 41: S416.

Author's address

Prof. Dr. H.D. Schworm
Department of Ophthalmology
City Hospital Dessau
Auenweg 38
D-06847 Dessau

Email: schworm@uke.uni-hamburg.de

Transactions 28th Meeting European Strabismological Association, de Faber (ed.)

Classification of Control in Intermittent Exotropia

B.G. Mohney & J.M. Holmes
Mayo Clinic, Rochester, Minnesota, USA

ABSTRACT: INTRODUCTION: There is no widely accepted method for quantifying control in intermittent exotropia. METHODS: Twenty-nine intermittent exotropic patients less than 11 years of age were prospectively evaluated with a new scale to measure level of control for both the distance and near angle of deviation. Twenty (69%) were re-evaluated 2 to 12 months later using the same scale. RESULTS: In all but one of the 29 patients, the level of control at distance fixation was worse than or the same as the level of control at near. Among the 20 patients who had 2 or more exams, 7 demonstrated a worsening of control, 7 improved, and 6 showed no change. CONCLUSIONS: Our control scale for intermittent exotropia is useful in categorizing level and longitudinal changes of control. Our data suggest that approximately one-third of children with intermittent exotropia will demonstrate an improvement in control within the first year of follow-up.

KEYWORDS: Intermittent exotropia, natural history, control of deviation

Intermittent exotropia is the most common form of childhood exotropia[1] and may be more prevalent than esotropia in some populations.[2] Although common, the natural history of intermittent exotropia has not been rigorously studied. Jampolsky has stated that, with rare exceptions, exodeviations begin as an exophoria that may deteriorate into intermittent and constant exotropia as suppression develops.[3] However, there are no longitudinal prospective studies and only a few retrospective studies of untreated intermittent exotropia.[4-6]

One of the primary challenges in studying the natural history of intermittent exotropia is in quantifying the level of control of the deviation. Currently, there is no widely accepted method for assessing control in intermittent exotropia. The primary objective of this study was to prospectively test the feasibility of a new scale of control in children with intermittent exotropia.

1. METHODS

We prospectively identified all patients with intermittent exotropia less than 11 years of age presenting to Mayo Clinic from January 1, 2002, through February 28, 2003. Each child underwent a comprehensive medical history and ocular examination. The occurrence of premature birth, family history of strabismus, and the age at onset were recorded on all patients. The ophthalmologic examination included visual acuity or fixation assessment, ocular deviation in prism diopters (PD), ocular rotations, sensory testing (whenever possible), cycloplegic refraction, and evaluation of the anterior and posterior segments.

Control of the intermittent exotropia was evaluated for each patient at both distance and near using the following scale:

5 = Constant exotropia
4 = Exotropia > 50% of the exam before dissociation
3 = Exotropia < 50% of the exam before dissociation
2 = Never exotropia unless dissociated, recovers in > 5 seconds
1 = Never exotropia unless dissociated, recovers in 1-5 seconds
0 = Never exotropia unless dissociated, recovers in < 1 second (phoria)

Fixation targets were standardized: a TV screen at 3 meters for distance and a Lang near viewing stick or similar accommodative target for near. Levels 5 to 3 could be assigned while observing the patient during the first several minutes of the history and examination before any dissociation. The cover uncover test was used to assign levels 2 to 0. For each examination, the worst level of control was recorded for both distance and near fixation.

Twenty (69%) of the 29 children had 1 or more follow-up exams 2 or more months after their enrollment into the study. The return examinations were identical to the initial evaluations except that a dilated fundus exam and cycloplegic refraction were not repeated.

2. RESULTS

A total of 29 patients with intermittent exotropia were prospectively enrolled during the study period. The median age of the patients at their initial examination was 54 months (range, 14 months to 10 years) and 17 (59%) were female. Four (13.8%) of the 29 patients were born before 37 weeks gestational age and a family history of strabismus was recorded as positive in 10 (34%) of the 29 study patients. One child had mild developmental delay, a second had cerebral palsy, and the remaining 27 children were developmentally normal. The median age at onset of the exodeviation, by parent history, was 24 months (range, 2 months to 8 years). Two of the 29 children had previously undergone bilateral lateral rectus recessions.

A history of amblyopia, defined as an intraocular difference of at least 2 logMAR lines, was present in 3 (10.3%) patients. However, none of the patients required treatment during the study period. Two of the 3 patients with amblyopia were felt to be due to anisometropia while the third was due to a nearly constant exodeviation. The median angle of deviation at the enrollment examination was 25 prism diopters (range, 12 PD to 40 PD) at distance. Stereoacuity at near was measured using the Titmus fly and circles or the Preschool Randot test in 19 patients, and was found to range from 40-3000 arc seconds with a median of 50 arc seconds. The anterior and posterior segments of all patients were entirely normal. The median cycloplegic refraction for the 29 patients was +1.00 spherical equivalent with a range from -.50 to +3.25.

The level of control could be classified using our 6-point scale at distance and near for all 29 patients. As expected in patients with intermittent exotropia, the level of control at distance fixation was worse than or the same as the level of control at near in all but one patient. The level of control for the distant deviation at the initial evaluation ranged from 1 to 5 with a median of 2. The level of control for the near deviation at the initial evaluation ranged from 0 to 4 with a median of 1. Combining the level of control at distance and near yields a minimum score of 0 (phoric distance and near) and a maximum of 10 (constantly tropic distance and near). In the 29 patients with intermittent exotropia in this study, the combined control score ranged from 1 to 8 with a median of 3.

Twenty (69%) of the 29 patients had 1 or more follow-up examinations at 2 or more months after their initial examination. The mean duration of follow-up was 6.5 months (range, 2 months to 12 months). A change in control over time was defined as an increase or decrease of 1 level or more in the 6-point scale from the first to the last exam. At distant fixation, 4 patients demonstrated an improvement in control over time, 3 patients a worsening of control, and the remaining 13 patients remained unchanged. At near, 4 patients demonstrated an improvement in control, 5 patients a worsening of control, and the remaining 11 patients remained unchanged. Because there were no systemic differences between the distance and near changes in control, the values at the 2 distances were combined. Using this overall control score (0-10) for our 20 patients who were examined on at least 2 occasions, we found an improvement in control in 7 patients, a worsening of control in 7 patients, and no change in the remaining 6 patients (Figure 1).

Figure 1:
Change of Control in 20 Patients with 2 or More Examinations

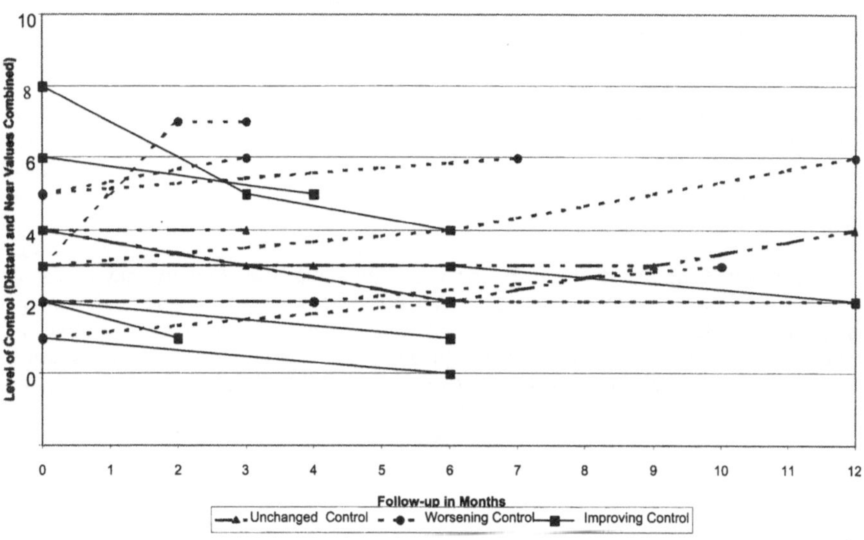

3. DISCUSSION

In this prospective study of intermittent exotropia in children, we found our new scale (0-5 at both distance and near) useful in quantifying control of the exodeviation. The values at distance and near can then be combined to create an overall control score ranging from 0-10. Using this system in longitudinal follow-up, we found that approximately one third of children with intermittent exotropia will demonstrate an improvement in control within the first year of follow-up.

It is commonly believed that a worsening of control in intermittent exotropia is an indication for surgical intervention and that, without intervention, there will be further deterioration with loss of fusion and stereopsis. Several methods for measuring control in intermittent exotropia have been advocated. Von Noorden describes a number of clinical features that indicate worsening of control in intermittent exotropia: 1) the development of a secondary convergence insufficiency, 2) an increase in size of the basic deviation, 3) development of suppression as evidenced by absence of diplopia during the manifest phase of the strabismus, or 4) a decrease in stereoacuity.[5] Wright argues that progression should be monitored by recording the size, frequency or duration of the tropia phase.[7] Nevertheless, precise quantitative criteria for "progression" have not been established.

Questioning the family regarding the control of the deviation and the occurrence of monocular eye closure in bright light have also been promoted as signs of progression. However, these historical clues are dependent upon the observation and memory of non-professional observers.

Stathacopoulos et al[8] have advocated the serial measurement of distance stereoacuity as a measure of control in X(T). Using the Mentor B-VAT II BVS to test distance stereoacuity, they reported significantly worse distance stereoacuity among 44 patients with X(T) compared with 50 normal subjects ($p < 0.001$). The authors compared the use of the B-VAT Monitor system with 3 other measurements: an office-based evaluation of control, a home-based report of control, and monocular eye closure in bright light.

Although Stathacopoulos[8] and co-investigators could not demonstrate a *statistical* correlation between distance stereoacuity by the B-VAT system and the 3 other subjective measures of control, they observed that office control tended to correspond with the objective findings of distance stereoacuity. Subsequent work has demonstrated that distance stereoacuity can improve in up to 75% of patients who undergo successful strabismus surgery.[9] Yildirim et al[10] demonstrated an improvement in distance stereoacuity in 15 (58%) of 26 consecutive patients who underwent surgical correction.

Walsh and coauthors[11] have suggested that poor distance stereoacuity in patients with intermittent exotropia is due to reduced binocular visual acuity, caused by increased accommodation. They advocated the measurement of distance binocular vision as a simple method of quantifying fusional control in patients with intermittent exotropia. To date, this method has not been widely used.

Although the evaluation of distance stereopsis and binocular visual acuity may be useful in assessing control in intermittent exotropia, the B-VAT system is not available to all clinicians who manage this disorder. We therefore believe that there is a need to establish a simple yet valid and reliable office-based classification system to quantitatively describe the level of control in intermittent exotropia. Hence, the development of our control scale for patients with intermittent exotropia which yields a score that ranges from 0 to 10.

4. CONCLUSION

Our control scale is useful in categorizing level of control in patients with intermittent exotropia and may become an important outcome measure for future clinical studies. Our prospective data suggest that approximately one third of children with intermittent exotropia will demonstrate an improvement in control within the first year of follow-up.

REFERENCES

Mohney BG, Huffaker RK. *Common forms of childhood exotropia.* Ophthalmology: In press.

Yu Cbo, Fan Dsp, Wong VWY, Wong CY, Lam DSC. *Changing patterns of strabismus: a decade of experience in Hong Kong.* Br J Ophthalmol 2002;86:854-856.

Jampolsky A. *Ocular deviations.* Int Ophthalmol Clin 1964;4:567

Hiles Da, Davies D, Costenbader F. *Long-term observations of unoperated intermittent exotropia.* Arch Ophthalmol 1968;80:436-442.

Von Noorden GK & Burian HM: *Exodeviations in Binocular Vision and Ocular Motility. Theory and Management of Strabismus*, pp356-376. CV Mosby, St Louis, 2002.

Kii T, Nakagawa T. *Natural history of intermittent exotropia – statistical study of preoperative strabismic angle in different age groups.* Nippon Ganka Gakkai Zasshi 1992;96:904-9.

Wright K. Exotropia. In: Wright KW, editor. *Pediatric ophthalmology and strabismus.* St Louis: Mosby;1995. P. 195-202.

Stathacopoulos RA, Rosenbaum AL, Zanoni D, Stager DR, McCall LC, Ziffer AJ, Everett M. *Distance stereoacuity. Assessing control in intermittent exotropia.* Ophthalmology 1993;100:495-500.

O'Neal TD, Rosenbaum AL, Stathacopoulos RA. *Distance stereoacuity improvement in intermittent exotropic patients following strabismus surgery.* J Pediatr Ophthalmol Strabismus. 1995;32:353-7.
Yildirim C, Mutlu FM, Chen Y, Altinsoy HI. *Assessment of central and peripheral fusion and near and distance stereoacuity in intermittent exotropic patients before and after strabismus surgery.* Am J Ophthalmol 1999;128:222-230.
Walsh LA, LaRoche GR, Tremblay F. The use of binocular visual acuity in the assessment of intermittent exotropia. J AAPOS 2000;4:154-7.

Transactions 28th Meeting European Strabismological Association, de Faber (ed.)
© 2004 European Strabismological Association, ISBN 90 265 1965 6

The Evaluation of Office Control in X(T): A Systematic Approach

Judy L. Petrunak, CO, COT, Rajesh C. Rao, M.D. & John D. Baker, M.D.
Children's Hospital of Michigan, Detroit, Michigan, United States of America

ABSTRACT: Background and Purpose: The clinical assessment of control in childhood intermittent exotropia is difficult to characterize and document. Yet, the quality of control often dictates when to proceed with treatment for X(T). Methods: A prospective method to evaluate and document control in children with X(T) is presented, utilizing the timeliness of the recovery of fusion after brief and prolonged binocular dissociation. Conclusion: This assessment provides a method to systematically observe, describe, and document the control of X(T) in an office setting.

KEYWORDS: Intermittent exotropia, control, assessing control, documenting control

X(T) is one of the most common forms of childhood strabismus. It has been classified by Duane, Burian, and Kushner. (von Noorden, 1985 & Kushner, 1988) There is wide opinion in the literature regarding the most appropriate age for optimal surgical outcome. (Abroms et al, 2001, Edelman et al, 1988, Richard et al, 1983, Pratt-Johnson et al, 1977) Recurrence of X(T) after surgery makes long-term success a challenging task for the treating physician, in part because cortical suppression of the deviated eye is a large obstacle to good fusional control. The characterization of this control is elusive, and in a direct sense, seemingly clinically immeasurable. Yet it is often the quality of control that dictates when to proceed with treatment.

Control in X(T) appears to be dependant on many known factors, including:

Range of viewing	Visual environment
Illumination	Binocular disruption
Fatigue	Visual alertness
Depth of suppression	Convergence amplitudes

The complex interdependency of these and other less-known factors precludes a thorough study and complete understanding of control in X(T).

Caregivers' observations of control may provide valuable longitudinal information that cannot be obtained from a single office visit by the examiner. Daily effects of fatigue and visual attention are important factors in appreciating control. However, sometimes parents' observations can be unreliable without any resemblance to the control observed in the office. We've all heard caregivers' responses such as, "I'm getting used to it," or "I really don't look for it," or "I never saw it in the first place, her grandma did."

The evaluation of X(T) control during an office examination tends to be highly subjective, difficult to characterize and document, and thus, may be variable between examiners.

In 1993, Stathacopoulos and colleagues, using the Mentor BVAT/Binocular Visual system, reported that patients with X(T) demonstrated significantly worse distance stereo acuity than a nonstrabismic group, suggesting that the measurement of distance stereo acuity is an objective assessment of control in X(T). (Stathacopoulos et al, 1993) Correlating observed office control to distance stereo acuity in their X(T) patients, using a three-point grading system for office control, they found that:

- Patients with "excellent" control, generally exophoric during examination, demonstrated good distance stereo acuity.
- Patients with "poor" control, spontaneously manifesting a tropia, demonstrated poor distance stereo acuity.
- Patients with control in between "excellent" and "poor" demonstrated a wide range of distance stereo acuity.

The investigators stated that this wide range of distance stereo acuity among patients with intermittent control may be an indication that their three-point scoring system for assessing observed office control is not adequately defined.

The evaluation and documentation of exo-deviation intermittence in the examination setting is a great challenge. In response, we have developed a methodical technique to evaluate and document intermittent control during the office exam by observing the time of "re-fusion" (the recovery of fusion), after dissociation.

1.1 *Materials and Methods*

Single Cover-Uncover Test (CT) Assessment

The evaluation begins with observing the effect of brief dissociation on the recovery of fusion. While fixing at 6-meters (distance), with visual attention controlled, a brief 1-2 second single Cover-Uncover Test is performed over the right eye (or the preferred eye, if known from previous exam).

Immediately after the cover is removed, the effect of dissociation is noted and reported as follows:

- Immediate re-fusion
- Without blink
- With blink
- Re-fusion in 1-5 seconds
- Without blink
- With blink
- Re-fusion in 6-15 seconds
- Without blink
- With blink
- No re-fusion within 15 seconds
- Re-fusion after near fixation
- No re-fusion after near fixation

A brief 1-2 second single CT is repeated, now over the left eye (or the non-preferred eye, if known from previous exam). Again, immediately after the cover is removed; the effect of dissociation on re-fusion is observed and recorded in the same fashion. The Single CT Assessment is repeated at 1/3-meter (near) range and similarly recorded.

1.2 *Prism Alternate Cover-test (PACT) Assessment*

The evaluation continues by observing the effect of prolonged dissociation on the recovery of fusion. While fixing at 6-meter range with visual attention controlled, the PACT is performed with the prism over the non-preferred eye, with a minimum of seven consecutive repetitions. The deviation is quantified. Immediately after the occluder is removed, the effect of dissociation on re-fusion is observed and recorded as previously described. The PACT Assessment is repeated at 1/3-meter range and similarly recorded.

1.3 *Fixation Preference*

In addition, fixation preference is graded by noting the time required to reestablish fixation of the preferred eye, after the preferred eye is occluded by the initial cover-test:

- Marked – fixation switched immediately (one second)
- Moderate – fixation switched within 5 seconds
- None/Mild – fixation not switched within 5 seconds

All data is recorded on a single form (See Figure 1.) which can be incorporated in the patient's record for that visit.

1.4 *Required Criteria*

Because the effects of dissociation by single CT and PACT are key to this assessment, patients must not receive any binocular dissociation by the examiner, such as monocular visual acuity or motility measurements, prior to the assessment of control. In addition, visual attention must be sustainable for a minimum of fifteen consecutive seconds with the aide of a visually appealing target such as a continuous-play cartoon/movie. Because the examiner is observing motor fusion movements after dissociation, the exo-deviation must be sizable enough to be visualized by the examiner, without confusion of tropic or phoric status. For this evaluation to be meaningful, a patient must be phoric at the onset of the assessment. An initial presentation of a constant tropia precludes any assessment of control, since control is not an analyzable factor when the deviation is constantly manifest.

1.5 *Discussion*

Over multiple visits, this systematic evaluation of X(T) may reveal a pattern of control that may be helpful in determining the timing of non-surgical or surgical treatment. In addition, it may prove beneficial in understanding aspects of X(T) presently not well understood, such as the natural course of untreated X(T), or the effect of occlusion therapy on X(T) control. Occlusion therapy as an anti-suppression treatment for X(T) has been reported in the literature. Some studies have demonstrated positive effects – specifically that patching can result in a decrease in the magnitude of the exo-deviation.(Berg et al, 1998, Freeman et al, 1989, Iacobucci et al, 1965, Spoor et al, 1979, Chutter, 1977) To our knowledge, effects of patching therapy specifically on fusional control in X(T) have not been reported, apart from general descriptions of control as simply phoric, intermittent, or constant.

By assigning a numeric grade to the various levels of control in this assessment, one can view trends of observed office control over time. The following five-point grading system assigns increasing numbers as the timeliness for re-fusion increases and observed control decreases:

Immediate re-fusion		Re-fusion in 6-15 seconds	
1	Without blink	3	Without blink
1.5	With blink	3.5	With blink
Re-fusion in 1-5 seconds		No re-fusion within 15 seconds	
2	Without blink	4	Re-fusion after near fixation
2.5	With blink	5	No re-fusion after near fixation

The following cases/graphs illustrate trends of observed office control using this evaluation and grading scale. They are not intended to draw conclusions about patching therapy, but rather show that in some patients, this systematic evaluation may be helpful in revealing patterns of control over time.

Intermittent control is a complex aspect of X(T) and the described assessment does not grasp its complexity. The office evaluation of control is highly limited by its environment, not accounting for the effects of outdoor illumination, varied visual environments, or fixation ranges greater than 6 meters.

Factors such as visual attention and fatigue are uncontrollable, yet can significantly influence office control in patients with X(T). The control of some patients may be sensitive to certain factors whereas other patients may be sensitive to other factors. Hence the relevance of the timeliness of re-fusion after dissociation may be variable from patient to patient, and the assigned levels of control in this assessment may be too broad, or not broad enough.

Furthermore, although we presently assess control in X(T) routinely by this method in children over 2-3 years of age, the testability of this assessment has not been formally evaluated on a large scale. We are committed to longer follow-up with a larger pool of patients to assist in validating the effectiveness of this prospective method. In addition, a proper analysis for reliability measures has not been carried out. Reliability testing in this assessment of X(T) control is particularly challenging because repeated dissociation often fatigues control in X(T), thereby altering it. Lastly, although presumptuously relevant in this assessment, the effects of a blink on the recovery of fusion after dissociation have not been fully explored and understood.

In summary, we present a systematic assessment of office control in X(T) based on the timeliness of re-fusion after brief and prolonged dissociation. This assessment provides a way to systematically observe, describe and document office control in X(T), and hence, allows for some common language and consistency between multiple examiners. It appears to be a practical assessment in the cooperative child when approached in a smooth and efficient manner.

Lastly, when repeated over multiple office visits, this assessment may reveal a pattern of control, which may in turn, be helpful in timing treatment for X(T).

References

Abroms AD, Mohney BG, Rush DP, Parks MM: Timely Surgery in Intermittent and Constant Exotropia for Superior Sensory Outcome. *Am J Ophthal* 2001; 131: 111-16.

Berg PH, Lozano MJ, Isenberg SJ: Long Term Results of Part-Time Occlusion of Intermittent Exotropia. *Am Orthopt J* 1998; 48: 85-89.

Chutter CP: Occlusion Tretment of Intermittent Divergent Strabismus. *Am Orthopt J* 1977; 27:80-84.

Edelman PM, Brown MH, Murphree AL, Wright KW. Consecutive Esodeviation...Then What? *Am Orthopt J* 1988; 38:111-116.

Freeman RS, Isenberg SJ: The Use of Part-Time Occlusion for Early Onset Unilateral Exotropia. *J Pediatr Ophthal Strab* 1989; 26:94-96.

Iacobucci I, Henderson JW: Occlusion in the Preoperative Treatment of Exo Deviations. *Am Orthopt J* 1965; 15: 42-47.

Kushner BJ: Exotropic Deviations: A Functional Classification and Approach to Treatment. *Am Orthopt J* 1988; 38: 81-93.

Pratt-Johnson JA, Barlow JM, Tillson G: Early Surgery in Intermittent Exotropia. *Am J Ophthal* 1977; 84: 689-694.

Richard JM, Parks MM: Intermittent Exotropia: Surgical Results in Different Age Groups. *Ophthalmol* 1983; 90: 1172-1177.

Spoor DK, Hiles DA: Occlusion Therapy for Exodeviations Occurring in Infants and Young Children. *Ophthalmol* 1979; 86: 2152-2157.

Stathacopoulos RA, Rosenbaum AL, Zanoni D, Stager DR: Distance Stereoacuity: Assessing Control in Intermittent Exotropia. *Ophthalmol* 1993; 100: 495-500.

von Noorden GK. *Burian and von Noorden's Binocular Vision and Ocular Motility.* St. Louis: CV Mosby Co.; 1985. p. 304-305.

Transactions 28th Meeting European Strabismological Association, de Faber (ed.)
© 2004 European Strabismological Association, ISBN 90 265 1965 6

Exotropia in infancy: Management experience at Manchester Royal Eye Hospital, UK.

Badia Fahad, Sus Biswas, Chris Lloyd
Manchester Royal Eye Hospital, UK

OBJECTIVE /INTRODUCTION: Exotropia in infancy is believed to be associated with increased prevalence of neurological, ocular, and craniofacial abnormalities;however, the prevalence of coexistingocular and systemic disease in these patients is unknown.1 A large-angle incomitant exotropia maybe the presenting feature of congenital third nerve palsy, which is a rare condition and is often associated with ptosis and amblyopia.2 We present our experience of managing infants presenting with exotropia looking at the underlying causes and their management.

METHOD: Retrospective case review of 69 patients for the period between 1991 and 2000.Ocular, orthoptic and systemic evaluation including neurological examination was carried out in all patients. Neuroimaging was undertaken when appropriate.

RESULTS :Patients 'age at first visit ranged from 18 days to 17 years and 4 months. The degree of exotropia varied in severity. Orthoptic evaluation in all patients showed constant exotropia. Progression and management of cases was reviewed and will be presented. Follow up ranged from2 months to 7 years and 4 months. Exotropia presenting in infancy was difficult to evaluate and an accurate diagnosis was often notpossible at the first visit. Progression often occurs and continuous follow up was required. We looked at the different presentations of exotropia in infancy including congenital exotropia, third nerve palsy, Duane 's retraction syndrome, associated craniofacial abnormalities and systemic diseases. Associated systemic abnormalities were present in 13 patients, and other ocular features present in13 patients. The different management techniques including botulinum toxin injection and surgery will be discussed in detail.

CONCLUSION: Children presenting to the Manchester Royal Eye Hospital with early onset exotropia were likely to have co-existing ocular and systemic disease.Therefore, ophthalmologists should consider these children at risk, and refer them to a specialist centre for further evaluation and treatment. The percentages measured in this population may not be applicable to other practices because of referral bias.

REFERENCES

Hunter DG, Ellis FJ. Prevalence of systemic and ocular disease in infantile exotropia:comparison with infantile esotropia.Ophtalmol 1999;106 (10):1951-6

Lee V, Bently CR, Lee JP.Strabismus surgery in congenital third nerve palsy. Strabismus 2001Jun;9 (2):91-9

Transactions 28th Meeting European Strabismological Association, de Faber (ed.)

The accommodative-convergence complex – A review

R.L. Brautaset
Unit of Optometry, Karolinska Institutet, Stockholm, Sweden

J.A.M. Jennings
Department of Optometry and Neuroscience, UMIST, Manchester, UK

ABSTRACT: This article reviews the accommodation and vergence systems and their interactions. Clinical methods for cross-link interaction measurements and adaptation measurements are described, and average results with these methods, as found in young (mean age 25 years) subjects with normal binocular vision presented. Based on data from subjects operated binocularly for infantile cataract the question of whether cross-link interaction and adaptation are prerequisites for the development of normal binocular vision is raised.

KEYWORDS: Accommodation, Vergence, Cross-link interaction, Adaptation

1 ACCOMMODATION AND VERGENCE

1.1 *Introduction*

When binocular fixation of an object is required at varying object distances, three distinct oculomotor activities occur which are intrinsically linked. If the object of interest moves closer to a subject, accommodation increases, the eyes converge (by equal amounts if the object is equidistant from both eyes) and the pupils constrict. If the object moves away, the opposite occurs.
The synkinesis of the three systems controlling accommodation, convergence or divergence and pupil size to produce a focused image of the object of interest on the fovea has been termed the "near triad" (Burian & von Noorden, 1974). The effect of pupil size in relation to accommodation and vergence is outside the scope of this review.

1.2 *Accommodation*

Accommodation is the adjustment of the power of the eye. The adjustment of the power is made so that objects of interest at any distance from the eye can be focused on the retina. Some authors have suggested that the mechanism, which responds to blurring of the retinal image cannot determine the direction of the accommodative effort (see for example Stark & Takahashi, 1965). However, more recent investigations have shown that lateral chromatic aberration of the eye provides a directional cue for accommodation (for review see Charman (2000)). Accommodation has been described, analogous to the components of vergence discussed below, as having the following features (Heath, 1956): (1) Reflex accommodation, the part of accommodation response, which occurs solely in response to changes in the vergence of incident light. (2) Tonic accommodation, the resting state of accommodation that is assumed when the eye has no stimulus, e.g. in complete darkness or in a uniformly bright field of view. This resting state is determined by the balance of sympathetic and parasympathetic innervations (Culhane & Gilmartin,

1999, Winn et al., 2002, Gilmartin et al., 2002). (3) Proximal accommodation, the accommodation response stimulated by the awareness of an object being near. (4) Convergence accommodation (CA), the accommodation response that occurs due to changes in convergence. If the eyes are stimulated to make a vergence eye movement while viewing a stimulus in which all visual stimuli for accommodation have been removed, the eyes will show a change in the level of accommodation. The visual stimuli for accommodation can be removed most easily by viewing the target through pinhole to ensure a large depth of field. Preventing in this way the change in accommodation affecting the clarity of the retinal image is referred to as "open-looping" the accommodative system.

A noteworthy feature of the accommodation system is the ability to adapt to changing conditions. Following prolonged accommodative effort, for example viewing a near target, the eyes return much more slowly than normally to their tonic position when the stimulus is removed (see for example Miles, 1985, Rosenfield & Gilmartin, 1989). This effect is known as accommodative adaptation.

1.3 *Vergence*

Vergence eye movements (the common term for either convergence or divergence) are prerequisites of normal binocular vision. Vergence movements minimize retinal disparity and place the two retinal images of a single object on corresponding retinal points. Analogous to accommodation, vergence movements have been identified as containing the following four features (Maddox, 1886): (1) Fusional vergence, the part of the vergence movement necessary to achieve sensory fusion and avoid diplopia and which occurs in response to retinal disparity. Retinal disparity provides information about both direction and magnitude for the fusional vergence movement needed. (2) Tonic vergence, a continuous effort of convergence, which maintains the eyes in their physiological position of rest. (3) Proximal vergence, the part of the vergence movement initiated by an awareness of a near object. (4) Accommodative vergence (AC), the part of the vergence reflex that occurs solely due to changes in accommodation. If one eye is occluded so that there is no stimulus for vergence movements, and the other eye is presented with an accommodative stimulus, then the occluded eye will make a vergence movement. The process of removing vergence stimuli is referred to as making the vergence system "open-loop".

In a similar manner to the accommodation system, the vergence system exhibits adaptation (Henson & North, 1980, Miles, 1985, Schor, 1986).

2 MODLLING ACCOMMODATION AND VERGENCE

Control system models have been used to aid the understanding and analysis of the human accommodation and vergence systems. The accommodation and vergence systems have been modelled as a dual interactive negative feedback model in which both accommodation and vergence are negative feedback systems (Fig. 1). The accommodation controller is triggered by blur and the level of accommodation altered in order to eliminate blur. The vergence system strives to eliminate disparity. In both systems, the forward controllers are leaky integrators. This means that the input and output will never be perfectly balanced and that a steady state error exists. Fixation disparity is the steady state error of the vergence system, whereas the lag/lead of accommodation is the steady state error of the accommodation system. Together, the steady state errors provide continuous stimulation to assist in maintaining a given accommodation and vergence level.

The controllers for both the accommodation and vergence loops have fast and slow components. The fast component reacts quickly but fatigues when having to maintain innervation. The output of the fast component is the input to the slow component. The slow system reacts more slowly but does not fatigue easily. The longer time constant (the time for the exponential response to reach 63% of its final output) of the decay of the slow component causes the slow component to continue its innervation even after the stimulus has been removed. This may be observed by noting the esophoric shift in the phoria after measuring vergence with base-out prisms (Saladin, 1986). The slow component is responsible for allowing the system to adjust to changes over time (i.e. adaptation).

The accommodative loop and the vergence loop interact with each other. The AC/A and CA/C ratios are the measures of the interaction of the accommodative loop with the vergence and of the vergence loop with accommodation, respectively. However, as soon as the innervation is taken over by the slow component (i.e. after adaptation has occurred while continuing to fixate the same object) no cross-link (AC and CA) innervation is provided. There is likely to be a complementary relationship between the AC/A and CA/C amplitudes and the adaptation of accommodation and vergence, respectively (Schor & Kotulak, 1986). Accommodation is likely to be more adaptable in subjects with low AC/A ratios. Vergence is likely to be more adaptable with low CA/C ratios. Moderate AC/A ratios are balanced by moderate CA/C ratios. Whenever one of these ratios is high there is likely to be an imbalance between accommodative and vergence adaptability.

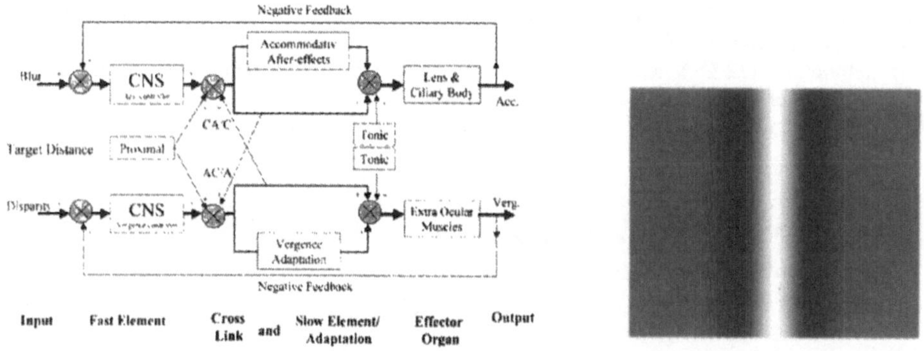

Figure 1. Descriptive model of the vergence and accommodation systems and their interaction (left) and an illustration of a DOG (Difference of Gaussian) target used to open-loop the accommodative system (right). Within the vergence and accommodation systems the fast element provides the immediate response to a change in disparity or blur. The slow element uses the output of the fast element to provide a slower adaptive adjustment of the level of accommodation and vergence. The fast elements also provide cross-link stimulation, whereas adaptation (i.e. the slow element) does not provide any cross-link stimulation since the cross-link interactions occur before the slow elements.

3 MEASUREMENTS OF THE AC/A AND CA/C RATIOS

3.1 *The AC/A ratio*

The synkinetic effect of accommodation and convergence can be readily measured using the AC/A and CA/C ratios. The accommodative convergence/accommodation (AC/A) ratio (Fry, 1939) measures the convergence produced per unit of accommodation (Δ/D). The two most common methods for measuring the AC/A ratio are the gradient and heterophoria methods. With the gradient method matched pairs of lenses of varying dioptric powers are placed in front of the eyes and the convergence produced is measured for each lens pair. The gradient of a graph of the convergence against the power of the lens yields the stimulus AC/A ratio. The heterophoria method is based on a comparison of the distance and near phoria, and the AC/A ratio determined using the formula:

$$AC/A = PD_{(cm)} + ((\text{near phoria} - \text{distance phoria})/D)$$

in which esophoria is positive and exophoria negative, the PD (pupillary distance) in centimetres (cm) and where D is the dioptric equivalent of the distance at which the near phoria was measured. Clinically accepted average values for the AC/A ratio with the gradient and heterophoria method are ~3.5 Δ/D and ~5.5 Δ/D respectively in young pre-presbyopic subjects with normal binocular vision. If accommodative convergence was to provide all the vergence needed the average AC/A ratio would have to equal the PD with the heterophoria method.

3.2 *The CA/C ratio*

The convergence accommodation/convergence (CA/C) ratio (Fincham & Walton, 1957; Schor & Narayan, 1982) measures the accommodation produced by a unit change in convergence (D/Δ). Schor and Narayan (1982) described a method, similar to the AC/A gradient method, by which the stimulus CA/C ratio could be measured. With this method prisms are placed in front of one eye and the convergence accommodation induced, with the accommodative system open-looped, is measured. When the accommodation system is open-looped by the use of a 0.2 cpd DOG target (Difference of Gaussian, see Fig. 1) we have found that the average CA/C ratio with this method is 0.112 D/Δ (±0.018 SD) in young pre-presbyopic subjects with normal binocular vision. If vergence accommodation was to provide all the accommodation needed the CA/C ratio would have to be 0.16 D/Δ (i.e. when assuming a PD of 6.0 cm).

4 MEASUREMENTS OF ADAPTATION

4.1 *Accommodative adaptation*

Accommodative adaptation can clinically be measured with a method developed by Tsuetaki & Schor (1987). This method utilizes the 0.2 cpd DOG target which open-loops the accommodative system. With this method the neutral position (i.e., the level of tonic accommodation) is determined with dynamic retinoscopy while fixating the DOG target monocularly (to eliminate convergence accommodation). Accommodation is then stimulated for 30 sec by superimposing letters printed on transparent film on the central white area of the DOG target. After 30 sec the transparent film is removed and the time taken for accommodation to drift back to the tonic position (i.e. when the retinoscopy reflex again becomes neutral) is measured. Tsuetaki & Schor (1987) suggested that if the accommodative after effect (i.e. adaptation) lasted less than 10 sec, the subject had a low level of accommodative adaptation. If the after effect lasted between 10 to 45 sec, the subject had a moderate or normal adaptation, and that any after effect in the order of one minute or more could be classified as being robust. In twenty normal young pre-presbyopic subjects we have found the average duration of the after effect to be 33 ± 8 sec (±1 SD) with this method.

4.2 *Vergence adaptation*

Clinical measurements of vergence or phoria adaptation can be done by the flashed Maddox rod technique described by Henson & North (1980). With this method a phoria is induced by the use of prisms and then the "new" phoria is measured at regular intervals. Between each phoria measurement the subject is allowed binocular vision through the prism. Figure 2 shows the average response of 20 pre-presbyopic subjects with normal binocular vision to both 6Δ BI and 6Δ BO while fixating at 40 cm.

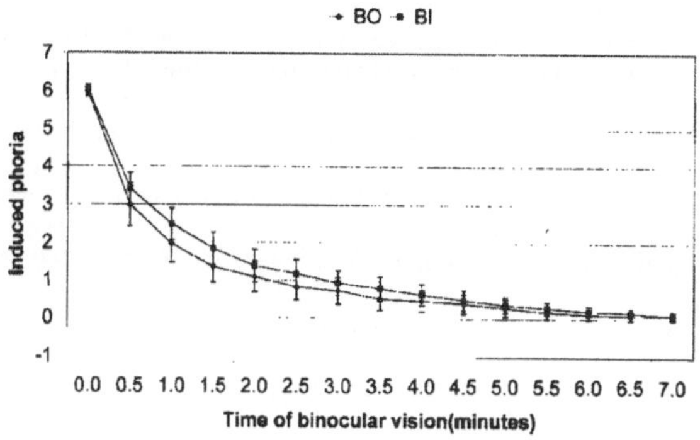

Figure 2. The average (±95% confidence intervals) phoria adaptation response to 6 base-in (BI) and base-out (BO) prism at 40 cm in 20 subjects with normal binocular vision.

5 DISCUSSION

In an attempt to investigate the effect on the vergence system from visual development with a fixed, open-loop accommodative system, we evaluated the binocular status of five subjects binocularly operated for infantile cataract within the first month after birth. At the time of the investigation their average was 17.4 ±2.5 years (±1 SD). All five subjects achieved at least 0.9 of Snellen visual acuity in both eyes monocularly. However, despite all of them being able to see the fly three dimensionally on the Titmus fly stereotest, they all had small exotropias. This raises the interesting question of whether cross-link inputs between accommodation and vergence and/or both accommodative and vergence adaptability are prerequisites for the development of normal binocular vision.

What we do know is that subjects with normal binocular vision poses the ability to vergence adapt to both convergence and divergence demands (see Fig. 2), and to adapt accommodation. In addition, they have AC/A and CA/C ratios that are slightly lower than that needed for one of the systems to provide all the innervation needed to fully drive the other system. This suggests that normal binocular vision is best achieved when both the accommodative and vergence systems have to simultaneously respond in the same direction (i.e. converge while increasing accommodation, and diverge while relaxing accommodation), and not when having to constantly overcome the excess or lack of response of the other system. (i.e. when the cross-links and adaptive abilities are unbalanced).

REFERENCES

Burian, H.M. & von Noorden, G.K. 1974. *Binocular vision and ocular motility.* St Louis: C.V. Mosby Ltd.

Charman, N. 2000. Accommodation and the through-focus changes of the retinal image. In O. Franzén, H. Richter & L. Stark (eds.), *Accommodation and vergence mechanisms in the visual system: 115-127.* Basel: Birkhäuser Verlag.

Culhane, H.M. & Gilmartin, B. 1999. Human dynamic closed-loop accommodation by sympathetic inhibition. *Invest. Ophthalmol. Vis. Sci. 40: 1137-1143.*

Fincham, E.F. & Walton, J. 1957. The reciprocal actions of accommodation and vergence. *J. Physiol 137: 488-508.*

Fry, G.A. 1939. Further experiments on the accommodation convergence relationship. *Am. J. Ophthalmol. 16: 325-336.*

Gilmart, B., Mallen, E.A.H. & Wolffsohn, J.S. 2002. Sympathetic control of accommodation: evidence

for inter-subject variation. *Ophthal. Physiol. Opt. 22: 366-371.*
Heath, G.G. 1956. Components of accommodation. *Am. J. Optom. Arch. Am. Acad. Optom. 33: 569-578.*
Henson, D.B. & North, R. 1980. Adaptation to prism-induced heterophoria. *Am. J. Optom. Physiol. Opt. 57: 129-137.*
Maddox, E. 1886. Investigations on the relationship between convergence and accommodation. *J. Anat. 20: 475-505, 565-584.*
Miles, F.A. 1985. Adaptive regulation in the vergence and accommodation control systems. *Rev. Oculomot. Res. 1: 81-94.*
Rosenfield, M. & Gilmartin, B. 1989. Temporal aspects of accommodative adaptation. *Optom. Vis. Sci. 66: 229-234.*
Saladin, J.J. 1986. Convergence insufficiency, fixation disparity, and control systems analysis. *Am. J. Optom. Physiol. Opt. 63: 645-653.*
Schor, C.M. 1986. Adaptive regulation of accommodative vergence and vergence accommodation. *Am. J. Optom. Physiol. Opt. 63: 587-609.*
Schor, C.M. & Kotulak, J.C. 1986. Dynamic interactions between accommodation and vergence are velocity sensitive. *Vision Res. 26: 927-942.*
Schor, C.M. & Narayan, V. 1982. Graphical analysis of prism adaptation. *Am. J. Optom. Physiol. Opt. 59: 774-784.*
Strak, L. & Takahashi, Y. 1965. Absence of an add-error signal mechanism in human accommodation. *IEEE Trans. BME-1: 138-146.*
Tsuetaki, T.K. & Schor, C.M. 1987. Clinical method for measuring adaptation of tonic accommodation and vergence accommodation. *Am. J. Optom. Physiol. Opt. 64: 437-449.*
Winn, B., Culhane, H.M., Gilmartin, B. & Strang, N.C. 2002. Effect of □-adrenoceptor antagonists on autonomic control of ciliary smooth muscle. *Ophthal. Physiol. Opt. 22: 359-365.*

Transactions 28th Meeting European Strabismological Association, de Faber (ed.)

Etiology of accommodative esotropia – current concepts

Olav H. Haugen
Department of Ophthalmology, Haukeland University Hospital, Bergen, Norway

ABSTRACT: Current understanding of accommodative esotropia holds that uncorrected hypermetropia, abnormal AC/A ratio, and/or a poor motor fusion are three major factors in the etiology of this condition. Usually, accommodative esotropia has been classified as a subgroup of acquired esotropia, that is with an age of onset after six months of age. The strict division between infantile esotropia and accommodative esotropia has been questioned, and the term "early-onset accommodative esotropia" has been used to define a group of children with strabismus onset before six months of age, but with the features of refractive esotropia of normal alignment with optical correction. However, there seems to be some controversy regarding the binocular potential, both in accommodative esotropia in general, and in the early-onset accommodative esotropia group in particular. Hypoaccommodation is probably an import etiological factor in some patients with refractive or non-refractive accommodative esotropia, especially individuals with Down syndrome.

KEYWORDS: accommodative esotropia, etiology, binocular function, hypoaccommodation.

1 INTRODUCTION

In the general discussion on the causes of strabismus, there are basically two main factors: mechanical and innervational factors. One important innervational factor is the refractive state through the near vision complex, namely the connection between accommodation and convergence. This connection is of principal importance in the understanding of accommodative esotropia.

The pioneer work in this field was carried out by Donders (1). Although some of his theories have been modified, the principal understanding of the interplay between accommodation and convergence is still today one of the cornerstones in strabismology.

In accommodative esotropia, uncorrected hypermetropia causes a blurred retinal image. This stimulates the accommodation in order to give a focussed image. Through the near vision complex this leads to an accommodative convergence.

If the motor fusion is insufficient, the result will be a manifest esotropia. However, if the patient have a strong motor fusion, the esotropic stimulus will only cause an esophoria.

Another possibility is that the patient has a low AC/A ratio. In this case there will not be any esodeviation in spite of an uncorrected hypermetropia.

When classifying accommodative esotropia, there are two main subgroups:
refractive and non-refractive. By a refractive esotropia we understand a manifest esodeviation related to hypermetropia, but with a normal AC/A ratio. Clinically, there is an important further subdivision into two classes: pure refractive, where normal alignment of the eyes is completely

restored by optical correction of the hypermetropic refractive error, and partly refractive, where the alignment of the eyes is improved, but not normalised by optical correction.
In non-refractive accommodative esotropia, there is an esodeviation unrelated to the refractive state, but with a high AC/A ratio. Clinically, this gives a significant greater squint angle for near than for distance. Such non-refractive accommodative esotropia may principally be found both in emmetropic, hypermetropic or myopic individuals. However, most of these patients are moderately hypermetropic.

There are some controversies, where clinical experience disturbs our concepts of classification. One of these controversies concerns the time of onset. One of the cornerstones in the classification of strabismus, is the difference between infantile and acquired esotropia, defined according to an age of onset before or after 6 months of age. Classical teaching in strabismology has stated that these are two distinct entities. This concept has been challenged by several authors, who claim that there is a clinical entity of "early-onset accommodative esotropia" (2-5). A study by Havertape et al. (5) defined this condition as an esotropia with onset up till 6 months of age and a refraction of +2.25 or more. They found that among 100 successive children with esotropia with onset before 6 months of age, 15 could be classified as early-onset accommodative esotropia. In this group, there were some with DVD and latent nystagmus, both features which usually are characteristic of infantile esotropia. Among those given glasses initially, 40% were fully corrected with glasses. Unfortunately, the study did not give any information on binocular function.

These studies rise some questions concerning the entity "early-onset accommodative esotropia":
- Is this a separate clinical entity?
- Or: is it merely an infantile esotropia with an accommodative component?
- What is the expected binocular function in this group?

The last question brings us to the next point of controversy: binocular potential.
Classical teaching has claimed that while infantile esotropia has a poor prognosis concerning the binocular outcome, acquired and particularly accommodative esotropia has a normal or near normal potential for binocular function. This clear distinction has also been challenged by a number of studies.
Firstly, there are studies concerning binocular outcome in infantile esotropia, claiming that early surgically alignment is associated with better binocular outcome. However, this topic will not be discussed further in this paper.
Secondly, there are also studies questioning the concept of a normal binocular potential in accommodative esotropia. Two recent studies on refractive accommodative esotropia agree that normal binocularity and stereopsis not always are achieved (6-7). In twenty patients with fully refractive esotropia, Tomac (6) found no patient with more than gross stereopsis (positive Wirth House Fly test). This study, however, did not give data on the time span between the onset of manifest strabismus and full alignment. In a study on 111 patients with fully refractive accommodative esotropia, Fawcett et al. (7) found that a short time (less than 4 months) of constant misalignment before full alignment with glasses was significantly correlated with an outcome of fine random dot stereopsis. On the contrary, longer time of misalignment before optical correction was associated with a poorer outcome.

There seems to exist a hypoaccommodative type of accommodative esotropia, described both by Costenbader (8) and Mühlendyck (9). In these patients there is a poor accommodative ability, and therefore an increased accommodative effort in order to bring a blurred retinal image into focus. This increased accommodative effort leads to an increased convergence response, and, probably in association with a poor motor fusion, this gives a manifest esotropia. This mechanism is probably of importance to certain groups of patients, for instance Down syndrome, whose accommodation in the majority of cases is poor (10). The treatment in these cases is parallel to non-refractive accommodative esotropia, namely bifocal or progressive glasses, but it is important to underline that the mechanism is principally different.

2 CONCLUSION

The present understanding of accommodative esotropia mainly points out uncorrected hypermetropia and poor motor fusion as the main etiological factors in a child that we believe has a normal (or near normal) sensoric potential for binocularity. However, we are challenged by the fact that there is a group of children that seems to be somewhere in the middle between infantile esotropia and accommodative esotropia. How this should be interpreted, especially in terms of binocular potential, is presently a matter of controversy.

REFERENCES

Donders FC. On the anomalies of accommodation and refraction of the eye. London 1864. New Sydenham Society.

Pollard ZF. Accommodative esotropia during the first year of life. Arch Ophthalmol 1976;94:1912.

Baker JD, Parks MM. Early onset accommodative esotropia. Am J Ophthalmol 1980;90:11.

Coats DK, Avilla CW, Paysse EA, Sprunger D, Steinkuller PG, Somayia M. Early onset refractive accommodative esotropia. J AAPOS 1998;2:275-278.

Havertape SA, Whitfill CR, Cruz, OA. Early-onset accommodative esotropia. J Pediatr Ophthalmol Strabismus 1999;36:69-73.

Tomac S. Binocularity in refractive accommodative esotropia. J Pediatr Ophthalmol Strabismus. 2002 Jul-Aug;39(4):226-230.

Fawcett S, Leffler J, Birch EE. Factors influencing stereoacuity in accommodative esotropia. J AAPOS 2000;4:15-20.

Costenbader FD. Management of convergent strabismus. In: Allen JH (editor): Strabismus ophthalmic symposium I. St.Louis 1950 Mosby Year Book:339.

Mühlendyck H. Symptoms and treatment in hypoaccommodation cases. In: International Symposium on Strabismus and amblyopia. Tel Aviv 1985 CERES:25.

Haugen OH, Høvding G. Strabismus and binocular function in children with Down syndrome. A population-based, longitudinal study. Acta Ophthalmol Scand 2001 Apr;79(2):133-139.

Transactions 28th Meeting European Strabismological Association, de Faber (ed.)
© 2004 European Strabismological Association, ISBN 90 265 1965 6

The role of bifocals in the management of accommodative esotropia

G. Holmström
Department of Ophthalmology, University Hospital, Uppsala, Sweden

ABSTRACT: Bifocals have been regarded as a tool of eliminating or reducing the near deviation in patients with accommodative esotropia with a high AC/A ratio since at least 1956, when it was described by Burian. Evaluations of the long-term efficacy of bifocals are described in the literature. They point to the conclusion, that bifocals still have a role to play in the management of esotropia.

KEYWORDS: Accommodative esotropia - bifocals

Bifocals have been used in the treatment of accommodative esotropia with a high AC/A – ratio since at least half a century (Burian – 56). Their role is to eliminate a residual esotropia for near and to achieve binocular vision.

Bifocals should be used in patients who are ortophoric for distance, or have a minimal residual esotropia after full cycloplegic correction, and who still have an esotropia for near, which is converted into esophoria with the help of additional plus lenses. In case of amblyopia, or a residual esotropia, in spite of additional plus lenses, bifocals are contraindicated. The smallest additional plus lens that converts the esotropia for near to an esophoria, should be prescribed. It is, however, noteworthy that the bifocal segment is placed properly and high enough to facilitate the child to use it for near work. Although small bifocal segments and progressive glasses are cosmetically attractive, they do not always achieve this goal. Finally, children with bifocal glasses must repeatedly be refracted in cycloplegia and the near addition should gradually be weaned off.

The long-term efficacy of bifocals has been evaluated in the literature (von Noorden, Morris, Edelman –78, Pratt-Johnson & Tillson – 85, Ludwig, Parks, Getson – 89, Eckstein, Fisher, Esser –97). Von Noorden et al (-78) found that bifocals were successful in 37 % of their patients and 46 % remained dependant of their bifocals. In spite of bifocals, 17 % slowly deteriorated and needed surgery to restore binocular vision. Ludwig et al (-89) found that 62 % of their patients could discontinue bifocals and that a significant reduction of the AC/A – ratio over time was a prognostically good sign. Eckstein et al (-97) reported that near addition could be weaned off in 44 % of patients with bifocals. Poor binocularity and large phoric component for distance and near were prognostically unfavourable signs. In contrary to the previous authors, Pratt-Johnson & Tillson (-85) did not find any significant difference in the final sensory results in children with or without bifocals. However, they conclude that bifocals are a harmless form of treatment, although they could not find enough evidence that they were beneficial.
Based on personal experience in selected cases (a few are presented) and on previous reports in the literature, see above, we feel that bifocals do have a role to play in the management of ac-

commodative isotropic with a high AC/A-ratio. If the child, however, is loosing fusion for near or if the bifocal segment cannot be weaned out in the teens, surgery is the alternative.

REFERENCES

Burian , H.M. 1956. Use of bifocal spectacles in the treatment of accommodative esotropia. Brit. Orthoptic J. 13, 3.

Eckstein, A.K., Fisher, M., Esser, J. 1997. Normakkommodativer Konvergenzexzess – langzeitverlauf bei konservativer therapie mit bifokalbrille. Klin Monatsbl Augenheilk 212: 218-225.

Ludwig, I.H., Parks, M.M., Getson, P.R. 1989. Long-term results of bifocal therapy for accommodative esotropia. J Ped Ophthalmol Strab. November/December 264-270.

Pratt-Johnson, J.A., Tillson, G. 1985. The management of esotropia with high AC/A ratio (convergence excess). J Ped Ophthalmol Strab 238-242.

Von Noorden, G.K., Morris, J., Edelman, P. 1978. Efficacy of bifocals in the treatment of accommodative esotropia. Am J Ophthalmol 85: 830-834.

Transactions 28th Meeting European Strabismological Association, de Faber (ed.)
 ISBN 90 265 1965 6

Outcome of treatment in accommodative esotropia – how often do we restore binocular vision?

L.Lindberg, MD, PhD
Helsinki University Hospital, Helsinki, Finland

ABSTRACT: An overview of the literature concerning different treatment possibilities in accommodative esotropia and the outcome of them is presented. Emphasis is placed on the knowledge of the outcome of restoring binocularity in accommodative esotropia. The published results in the papers are not all together comparable since several different methods were used but the literature cited substantiates the kind of expectations we can have on the outcome of treatment.

KEYWORDS: accommodative esotropia , treatment outcome, binocularity

1 INTRODUCTION

Accommodative esodeviation is an acquired form with association with the activation of the accommodational reflex. If the deviation is within the patient's fusional divergence amplitude, only a latent deviation, that is, esophoria will result. If the deviation is beyond the scope of fusion, a manifest deviation will occur. The onset of accommodative ET is between 6 months and seven years, on average between 2,5 and 4 years of age. It is usually intermittent at onset, becoming constant, often hereditary, sometimes precipitated by trauma or illness. Amblyopia is frequent. The three main forms of accommodative esodeviation are: 1) refractive with high hypermetropia with equal distance and near deviation, that is no more than 10 PrD in difference, 2) non-refractive = high AC/A-ratio with a greater esodeviation at near fixation than at distance fixation or 3) mixed with partially accommodative esodeviation and partially basic esodeviation .

2. "THE NATURAL HISTORY"

The main characteristics of the clinical course of accommodative esotropia despite treatment is that it may continue well into adolescence or early adulthood. Decompensation of a fully accommodative esotropia may occur even in the presence of apparently good binocular vision, and developing of consecutive exotropia in fully refractive accommodative esotropia has been described. Noteworthy is that the anticipated reduction in hyperopia with age that occurs in non-strabismic children does not entirely apply in children with accommodative esotropia and thus giving hope of removing the optical correction has to be well considered. Amblyopia can persist or deteriorate.

3.TREATMENT ALTERNATIVES

Pure refractive accommodative ET is commonly successfully treated with full correction of the hypermetropia. For patients with fusional ability and a small deviation, incorporated base out prisms in the least strength necessary for binocular single vision can be used. The role of bifocals is worth consideration in nonrefractive accommodative esotropia (see presentation by Gerd Holmström, MD for details). Although bifocals may be successfully discontinued in a majority of patients within a few years, a significant percentage require long-term wear. Medical management is hardly ever the only method. Tropicamide, cyclopentolate, homatropine and atropine are among the popular drugs used when the diagnosis and measurement of an accommodative ET is being done. They are also used as a "medical patch" or as an important part of penalisation-process in the treatment of associated amblyopia.

Miotics can be used as supplementing glasses or bifocals or, as mentioned in some articles, they may be effective in reducing the esodeviation to a suitable fusion range postoperatively in uncorrected esotropia. Miotics alone are never more effective than glasses. It has been mentioned that miotics should never be used unless some degree of binocularity can be achieved. However, many authors emphasise that miotics are not better than, and more often, are not as good as glasses correcting the deviation and enhancing binocularity. It also has been suggested that the presence of amblyopia in accommodative esotropia is a contraindication to miotic therapy. Miotics should never be the sole means of determining that an accommodative element is absent. Local and systemic side effects of any medical device are a serious consideration before usage.

3.1 *Surgery for deteriorated / residual accommodative esotropia*

Gradual development of a superimposed nonaccommodative component or a decompensation of a previously fully controlled esotropia are quite often seen. It is generally agreed that extraocular muscle surgery for esotropia is indicated in the correction of nonaccommodative component of mixed esotropia, in the residual deviation of nonrefractive esotropia and in decompensated refractive esotropia. The surgical methods most often used are: Single medial rectus recession (for high AC/A ratio), bimedial rectus recessions with or without augmentation, bimedial rectus recessions with or without posterior fixation suture, posterior fixation suture (= Faden) alone (for high AC/A ratio), and hang-back recessions on medial recti or bilateral rectus resection (used in mixed form accommodative esotropia).

Some use distance deviations the base of grading surgery amounts, some augment that measurement with certain amount by taking into account the near deviation or rely only on the near deviation measurements. Hyperopic correction is always paid attention to when planning surgery. Arnoldi & Tychsen (1996) concluded that surgery may be more effective than bifocals in restoring normal stereopsis and binocular fusion in patients with high AC/A ratio. They also mentioned that more than two thirds of the children in their study had an AC/A ratio within the normal range postoperatively. They prefer bilateral medial rectus recessions performed for the greatest deviation measured at near fixation through the full distance hyperopic correction. Their goals were to eliminate the need for bifocals by substantially reducing the esodeviation at near fixation, restoring a more normal pattern of accommodative vergence and improving the grade of binocularity.

4.OUTCOME OF TREATMENT

4.1. *In refractive accommodative esotropia*

Binocular function in 3 % - 89 %
Monofixation/periferial fusion in 45 % - 76 %
Amblyopia of some degree in 4 % - 48 %
Need for surgery in 10 % - 50 %

Stable refraction
Good esthetics

These above mentioned results are collected from several papers and the large dispersion in the results is due to different treatment modalities used. This shows how heterogeneous this group of patients and the outcome of treatments can be. Binocular vision was tested with several different stereo acuity tests. Testing for fusion or suppression was mainly done with Bagolini lenses. The presence of binocular single vision with fusion contributes to maintaining alignment. In many of the articles the final stereopsis was compared with age of presentation and age in which motor alignment was achieved and it was found that higher grade binocular vision is associated with late presentation. With monofixation one does not mean the Primary monofixaton syndrome. Amblyopia therapy with patching and or penalisation was usually successful. These figures are from the patients last visits, reduction was mentioned to be remarkable in many cases. In Bakers & Parks (1980) paper they noticed that deviations which develop before 12 months of age initially fully corrected later decompensated and needed surgery in approximately 50 % cases. The need for surgery consists of initial or additional operations, some for consecutive exotropia. Dickey's & Scott's (1988) finding that very high rate of deterioration is seen in patients in whom the onset of esodeviation was noted within the first 2 years of age is consistent with the findings of Baker.

4.2. *In non-refractive accommodative esotropia*

Binocular function in 5 % - 96 %
Monofixation/perferial fusion in 28 % - 76 %
Amblyopia of some degree in 4 % - 61 %
Reduction of near angle in 67 % - 96 %
Normalisation of AC/A ratio in 13 % - 69 %
Need for surgery in 13 % - 50 %

Some authors suggested that patients with accommodative ET with high AC/A ratio have a lower incidence of bifoveal fusion and fine stereopsis compared with patients with normal AC/A ratio. In other papers no effect of AC/A ratio on random dot stereoacuity was found. It has been suggested to treat patients with a high AC/A ratio aggressively, providing an optimum lens to correct the near esodeviation in order to save binocularity.

4.3. *Restored binocularity?*

Accommodative esotropia although initially intermittent, tends to progress to a constant deviation if treatment is delayed. Constant esotropia can then lead to permanent loss of central binocular vision. Early effective therapeutic intervention during the intermittent esotropia phase or within a few months of the development of a constant deviation appear therefore necessary if bifixation is to be maintained. Wilson et al (1993) concluded that patients with intermittent esotropia at presentation were nearly three times more likely to remain bifixators over time than patients presenting with constant esotropia. If deterioration of ocular alignment occurs later, or amblyopia is detected, early and aggressive intervention is necessary to prevent loss of bifixation. The following data is from this particular article: Patients with bifixation had stereopsis of 50 seconds of arc or better and central fusion was demonstrated for example with Bagolini glasses. They presented 24 % of the patients with an average follow up time of 89 months. Monofixation patients had stereopsis worse than 60 arc seconds with evidence of peripheral fusion on the Worth four-dot test. A macular scotoma was demonstrated for example with Bagolini striated glasses. They presented 76 % of the patients with an average follow up of 84 months. Primary monofixaton syndrome patients were excluded.

There was no significant difference between the bifixation and monofixation groups for age of onset of strabismus, average hyperopia (5.0 vs 4.10 D) or anisometropia greater that 1.50 D. Patients with bifixation were less likely to have presented with constant esotropia (19 % vs 39%) and were more likely to be aligned within 8 PrD of orthophoria in their first glasses (84% vs 21%). No patient with bifixation had a history of constant esotropia longer than 4 months. In addition, patients with bifixation were less likely to have worn bifocals, undergone esotropia surgery or patching for amblyopia.

Fawcett et al (2000) noted in their study that if the child's age at onset of ET was >25 months, these children tend to have better stereoacuity compared with those with the onset between ages 7 and 17 months of age ($p < .03$). The children who had intermittent ET had better stereo acuity than those with constant ET aligned between 6 and 24 months of age and after age 24 months of age ($p < .001$). Duration of constant misalignment was statistically also very meaningful; those children who had intermittent ET or constant misalignment of < 4 months had better stereo acuity than those with constant ET > 4 months ($p < .001$). The AC/A ratio did not affect random dot stereoacuity outcomes ($p < .10$): with normal and high AC/A ratio the results were not statistically meaningfully different. Fine random dot stereoacuity is strongly associated with a constant misalignment of less than 4 months duration with normal or high AC/A ratio. However, different opinions are published, for example, in a study by Mazow et al (1984) they found no correlation between the age of onset and duration of deviation to the degree of stereopsis achieved.

5. CONCLUSIONS

Restored binocular vision of *some degree* in accommodative esotropia? YES, often in the majority of cases
IF ALIGNMENT IS RESOTRED WITH TREATMENT (GLASSES, BIFOCALS, SURGERY) BEFORE OR SHORTLY AFTER THE ESODEVIATION BECOMES CONSTANT.

Many with accommodative esotropia do not have normal stereopsis even after successful realignment. Recent studies suggest that the duration of misalignment plays a critical role in binocular sensory outcomes in patients with accommodative ET. Patients who achieve orthoposition during the intermittent phase or within a few months of developing a constant misalignment maintain bifixation whereas patients who experience a constant misalignment longer have monofixation. It has been proved that no patient with constant accommodative ET exceeding 12 months´duration maintain or recover any measurable stereopsis.

This entity requires a close follow-up to ensure maintenance of binocularity and appropriate early intervention to modify the course before bifixation is lost.

REFERENCES

Arnoldi K.A. & Tychsen L. 1996. Surgery for esotropia with a high accommodative conver gence/accommodation ratio: effects on accommodative vergence and binocularity. *Ophthalmic Surgery and Lasers* 27:342-348

Baker J.D. & Parks M.M. 1980. Early-onset accommodative esotropia. *American Journal of Ophthalmology* 90:11-18

Bixenman W.W. 1981. Management of nonrefractive accommodative esotropia (correspon dence). *Can J Ophthalmol* (16) July: 163-164

Dickey C.F. & Scott W.E. 1988. The deterioration of accommodative esotropia: frequency, characteristics and predictive factors. *J Pediatr Ophthalmol Strabismus* 25: 172-175

Diorio P.C. 1977 The role of miotics in the management of accommodative esotropia. *Am Orthopt J.* 27: 96-99

Evans B.J.W. 1999. Clinical course of accommodative esotropia (correspondence). *Optom Vis Sci* 76:80

Fawcett S., Leffler J., Birch E.E. 2000. Factors influencing stereoacuity in accommodative eso tropia. *J of AAPOS* 4:15-20

Gökyigit B., Köse B., Kadioglu E., Manzakoglu U. 1997 Binocularity in accommodative eso tropia. In *Transactions of the 24th meeting of European Strabismological Association* Aeolus Press The Netherlands

Havertape S.A., Whitfill C.R., Cruz O.A. 1999. Early-onset accommodative esotropia. *J Pediatr Ophthalmol Strabismus* 36:69-73

Hiatt R.L. 1983. Medical management of accommodative esotropia. *J Pediatr Ophthalmol Stra bismus* 20:199-201
Knapp P. 1967. The clinical management of accommodative esotropia. *Am Orthopt J.* 17:8-13
Kushner B.J. 2001. Fifteen-year outcome of surgery for the near angle in patients with accom modative esotropia and a high accommodative convergence to accommodation ratio. *Arch Ophthalmol* 119:1150-1153
Kushner B.J., Preslan M.W., Morton G.V. 1987. Treatment of partly accommodative esotropia with high accommodative convergence-accommodation ratio. *Arch Ophthalmol*105:815-818
Leitch R.J., Burke J.P., Strachan I.M. 1990. Convergence excess esotropia treated surgically with fadenoperation and medial rectus muscle recessions. *Br. J. Ophthalmol 74:278-279*
Lucas E., Bentley C.R., Aclimandos W.A. 1994. The effect of surgery on the AC/A ratio. *Eye* 8:109-114
Mazow M.L., Kaldis L.C., Prager T.C. 1984. An evaluation of accommodative esotropia. In: Reinecke RD: *Strabismus II.* Grune and Stratton 189-192
Mulvihill A., MacCann A., Flitcroft I., O'Keefe M. 2000. Outcome in refractive accommodative esotropia. *Br. J. Ophthalmol* 84: 746-749
Ohtsuki H., Hazebe S., Kobashi R., Okano M., Fususe T. 1994. Critical period for restoration of normal stereoacuity in acute-onset comitant esotropia. *Am J. Ophthalmology* 118:502-508
Pollard Z.F. 1976. Accommodative esotropia during the first year of life. *Arch Ophthalmol* 94:1912-1913
Pratt-Johnson J.A. & Tillson G. 1985. Management of esotropia with high AC/A ratio (conver gence excess). *J Pediatr Ophthalmol Strabismus* 22:238-242
Preslan M.W. & Beauchamp G.R. 1987. Accommodative esotropia: review of current practices and controversies. *Ophthalmic Surgery* 18: 68-72
Raab E.L. 1984. Hypermetropia in accommodative esodeviation. *J Pediatr Ophthalmol Stra bismus* 21:64-68
Raab E.L. 1991. The accommodative portion of mixed esotropia. *J Pediatr Ophthalmol Stra bismus* 28:73-76
Raab E.L., & Spierer A. 1986. Persisting accommodative esotropia. *Arch Ophthalmol* 104:1777-1779
Rutstein R.P. & Marsh-Tootle W.1998. Clinical course of accommodative esotropia. *Optom Vis Sci* 75:97-102
Shippman S., Weseley A.C., Cohen K.R. 1993. Accommodative esotropia in adults. *J Pediatr Ophthalmol Strabismus* 30:368-371
Swan K.C. 1983. Accommodative esotropia long range follow-up.*Ophthalmology* 90:1141-1145
Watanabe-Numata K., Hayasaka S., Watanabe K., Hayasaka Y., Kadoi C. 2000. Changes in de viation following correction of hyperopia in children with fully refractive accommodative esotropia. *Ophthalmologica* 214:309-311
West C.E. & Repka M.X. 1994. A comparison of surgical techniques for the treatment of ac quired esotropia with increased accommodative convergence/accommodation ratio. *J Pediatr Ophthalmol Strabismus* 31:232-237
Williams H.P. 1974. Comparison of the accommodative effects of Carbachol and Pilocarpine with reference to accommodative esotropia. *Br. J. Ophthalmol* 58:668-673
Wilson M.E., Bluestein E.C., Parks M.M. 1993. Binocularity in accommodative esotropia. *J Pediatr Ophthalmol Strabismus* 30:233-236
Zak T.A. 1986. Results of large single medial rectus recession. *J Pediatr Ophthalmol Strabis mus* 23:17-21

Session 5
Vergence problems/Refractive surgery/ Strabismus and cataract

Transactions 28th Meeting European Strabismological Association, de Faber (ed.)
© 2004 European Strabismological Association, ISBN 90 265 1965 6

A Study on the Treatment of Convergence Insufficiency

F.F. Naqui, A. Bruce & J.A. Bradbury
Bradford Hospitals NHS Trust, Bradford, West Yorkshire, UK

ABSTRACT: A retrospective study to investigate the treatment and outcome of patients with Convergence Insufficiency was undertaken. 94% of patients who completed their orthoptic treatment plan were symptom free. Patients completing treatment were found to have a mean age of 31yrs, greater than the mean age of those who failed to complete 15.5 yrs ($p=<0.05$). Patients failing to complete treatment were followed up with a telephone questionnaire. Reasons for non completion included; ineffective exercises, relocating, home treatment, and symptoms resolving. To improve completion rate amongst the younger group the exercise strategy should be reviewed. Better provision of instructions using DVD or video is recommended along with the redesign of the current exercise regime, developing computer based exercise programmes.

KEYWORDS: Convergence Insufficiency, orthoptic treatment, age.

1 INTRODUCTION

Convergence insufficiency (CI) is one of the most common causes of ocular discomfort and is in fact the most common cause of asthenopia (Leeuwen et al 1999). It is also one of the most successful applications in the art of orthoptics. Orthoptic exercises are usually the first choice of treatment and are reported to relieve symptoms in the majority of treated patients (Wicks 1994).

2 DESIGN

A retrospective study was carried out to investigate the treatment and outcome of patients with CI. The cases were identified from our new case data base for 2000-2001. Patients who discontinued their treatment for unknown reasons were then followed up and a telephone questionnaire carried out.

3 METHOD

Criteria for inclusion in the study included:

- Attendance to the orthoptic department with symptoms suggestive of CI (blurred vision/diplopia/headache)
- No decompensating phoria
- Diagnosis of CI on Orthoptic assessment
- The commencement of Orthoptic treatment (e.g. pen convergence, dot card & stereograms)

The patients who did not complete their treatment were then contacted via phone and asked to complete a questionnaire regarding the effectiveness of their exercises and their reasons for non-attendance/ compliance.

4 RESULTS

31 cases fulfilled the criteria (age range 8-81yrs, mean age 24yrs)
17 completed their treatment (5 male 12 female, mean age 31yrs)
16 became symptom free post orthoptic treatment (94%)
14 did not complete their treatment. (6 male 8 female, mean age 15.5yrs)

4.1 *Questionnaire Results of Patients NOT completing Treatment:*

Moved away	4 (29%)
Patients found exercises ineffective and are still symptomatic.	4 (29%)
Exercises were found to be useful with symptoms improving and are continued at home.	3 (21%)
Symptom free and did not feel need for further treatment	1 (7%)
Unable to attend appointments	2 (14%)

5 DISCUSSION

Those patients who did not complete their treatment were found to be of a significantly younger age ($p=<0.05$) than those who did. This group who discontinued their treatment with no recurrence of symptoms may not have been true "CI patients" although volunteering asthenopic symptoms, perhaps from prolonged close work or exams. There has been a suggestion that CI may be linked to psychological distress, giving rise to asthenopic symptoms. Psychological distress was not evaluated in this study; however a previous study (Massey 2000) found no indication of psychological distress in CI patients.
Motivation in carrying out the exercises may be reduced in the teenage group that failed to complete their treatment. In general teenagers appear to become bored easily and are less tolerant of repetitive exercise.
This younger group will rely on their parents/carers to bring them for appointments, if the parents have work commitments and/or other priorities this may lead to failure to attend.
None of the patients were aware that orthoptic exercises have a good success rate and knowledge of this could improve compliance.

6 CONCLUSIONS

In order to improve the completion rate amongst the teenage group we should review our current exercise strategy. Instructions for patients to take home could be produced in the form of a video/DVD to ensure that the exercises are carried out properly in the home environment.
Many patients like to know the facts and figures of success rates. It could be helpful to ensure that patients know that there is a successful outcome in 94% of cases on completion of treatment.
The types of orthoptic exercises recommended in the treatment of CI have been with us for a number of years. In order to appeal to teenagers it may be time for us to revise these exercises and develop a computer based system that would appeal to this group of patients.

7 REFERENCES

Leeuwen.A.F, Westen.M.J. et al 1999. Gaze-shift dynamics with and without symptoms of CI: Influence of monocular preference and the effect of training. *Vision Research* 39: 3095-3107.

Massey T. 2000 Do patients with Convergence Insufficiency show a profile of significant psychological distress? *Br Orthopt J 57:* 11-14.

Wicks.H.R. 1994 A Report of a clinical Audit on the Management of Convergence Insufficiency. *Br Orthopt J* 51: 35-37.

Transactions 28th Meeting European Strabismological Association, de Faber (ed.)
© 2004 European Strabismological Association, ISBN 90 265 1965 6

Binocular vision problems after refractive surgery

D.J.M. Godts, M.J. Tassignon, L. Gobin
University Hospital Antwerp, Department of Ophthalmology, Edegem, Belgium

ABSTRACT: Five cases of patients presenting binocular vision problems after refractive surgery have been analysed. In one patient, a latent superior oblique palsy decompensated after LASIK of the most myopic eye to achieve monovision. A second patient, operated for a fourth nerve palsy ten years ago, presented a recurrence of his palsy after bilateral LASIK for myopia. The third patient complained of intermittent diplopia caused by aggravation of a pre-existing intermittent esotropia that worsened after LASIK for hypermetropia. The fourth patient had permanent diplopia after LASIK of his highly anisometropic and exotropic eye. Finally, the fifth patient experienced a decrease in fusion and stereopsis at the time he became anisometropic after bilateral PRK and LASIK. These cases clearly illustrated the need of an accurate preoperative orthoptic examination in order to prevent postoperative complaints secondary to changes in binocular vision.

KEYWORDS: Binocular vision problems, refractive surgery, diplopia, orthoptics

1 INTRODUCTION

Patients undergoing refractive surgery may experience binocular vision impairment after surgery. A variety of complaints can be recognized when listening carefully to the patient's history. These may vary from blurred vision to diplopia according to the person's capacity to compensate for these changes in binocular vision induced by surgery. The aim of this paper is to stress the importance of an orthoptic evaluation before refractive surgery and to define risk groups for binocular vision impairment after refractive surgery.

2 MATERIAL AND METHODS

Five patients, referred to our department after refractive surgery, were analysed.
The first patient is a 36-year-old woman with intermittent vertical diplopia after an uneventful LASIK of her most myopic, left eye. She had postponed LASIK treatment of her best, right eye and was looking for a second opinion. The patient had never had binocular vision problems and was never been adapted with contact lenses in the past. Preoperative best-corrected visual acuity was 20/20 in both eyes. The refractive error before surgery was –1.75 (–0.75 _ 145°) in the right eye, and –3.50 (–1.00 _ 25°) in the left eye. Postoperative visual acuity in the left, treated, eye did improve to 20/25 with a small additional correction of –0.75 (–0.25 X 50°). The right eye remained dominant postoperatively. Orthoptic examination showed a right hyperphoria of 3 prism diopters (PD) in primary position increasing at distance (5 PD) and at left gaze (8 PD). Ocular motility evaluation showed a V pattern, an underaction of the right superior oblique muscle and a positive Bielschowsky head-tilt-test. The Lancaster test was suggestive for a right superior oblique palsy (fig. 1). Vertical fusion amplitude was increased up to 7 degrees. Accommodation measured with the RAF-ruler was 10 D for the

right eye but was reduced to 5 D for the left eye. Convergence was normal. No cyclotorsion was found but fundus examination showed a bilateral tilted disc and extorsion of both maculae, more pronounced in the left eye.

Fig. 1: Lancaster patient I

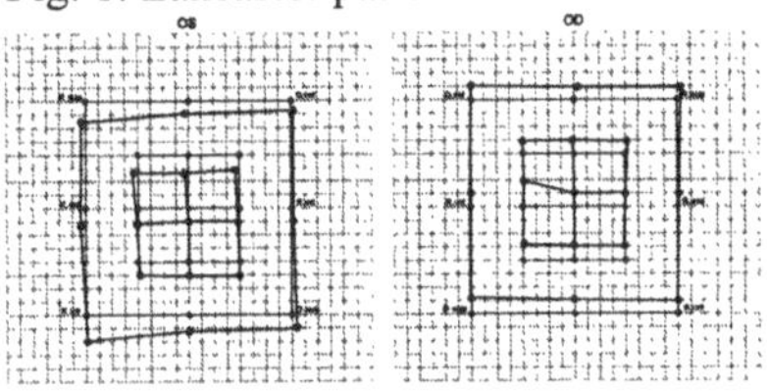

The second patient was a 42-year-old man with complaints of intermittent diplopia after having had an uneventful LASIK for myopia of both eyes simultaneously. The patient underwent strabismus surgery on both eyes in 1990 for a congenital right fourth nerve palsy. Preoperative best-corrected visual acuity was 20/20 in both eyes. The refractive error before surgery was –5.25 in the right eye and –5.00 in the left eye. Postoperative uncorrected visual acuity was 20/40 in the right eye and 20/32 in the left eye. Postoperative best-corrected visual acuity at distance was 20/25 in the right eye and 20/20 in the left eye. The right eye needed an additional correction of –1.00 (–0.25 X 20°) and the left eye an additional correction of –0.50 (–0.25 X 170°). Uncorrected visual acuity at near was 20/40 in the right eye and 20/25 in the left eye. Orthoptic examination showed a right hyperphoria of 3 PD at near and 2 PD at distance, slightly increasing in down and left gaze. The right eye was dominant. Ocular motility evaluation showed a V pattern, an underaction of the right superior oblique muscle (fig. 2) and a positive Bielschowsky head-tilt-test. Vertical fusion amplitude was increased to 6° on synoptophore. Excyclotorsion of 1° was measured in both eyes. On fundus examination the left eye had an important torsion of the macula compared to the right eye. The diagnosis of a recurrent right fourth nerve palsy was made.

Fig. 2: Lancaster patient II

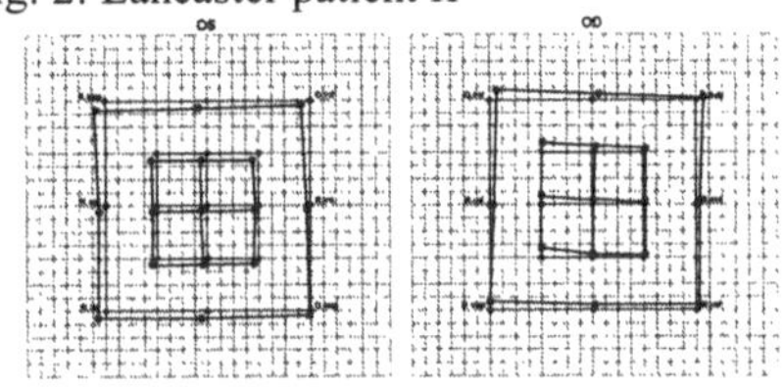

The third patient is a 40-year-old woman complaining of intermittent diplopia after LASIK for hyperopia of her left eye. She reported a history of intermittent esotropia since childhood. Postoperative best-corrected visual acuity was 20/20 in the right eye with +1.50 and 20/63 in the left eye with +1.25 (–3.50 X 150°) in the left eye. With the prism cover test, performed with glasses, an esotropia of 18 PD was found at near vision and of 10 PD at distance vision. Without glasses the esodeviation increased up to 25 PD at near and to 18 PD at distance. The diagnosis of partial accommodative esotropia was made. Ocular motility showed a V pattern with over action of the left inferior oblique muscle. The objective angle of strabismus was +7° and the subjective angle was –1° measured with the synoptophore. These results are suggestive for an abnormal retinal correspondence with peripheral fusion on the subjective angle of strabismus. Suppression of the left eye was present in free space. Accommodation measured with the RAF test was 5D in both eyes, which is low but acceptable considering patient's age. Fundus examination showed an extreme extorsion of both maculae. Bielschowsky head-tilt-test was negative.

The fourth patient is a healthy 39-year-old man who had manifest diplopia after having had an uneventful LASIK of his myopic right eye. The patient was anisometropic since years. The left eye was almost emmetropic. He presented an important exotropia of his right myopic eye. Preoperative best-corrected visual acuity was 20/25 in the right eye with correction of –9.50 (–0.75 X 80°) and 20/20 in the left eye with correction of –0,5 (–0.75 X 15°). Spectacle correction was –5.25 for his right eye and (–0.25 X 85°) for his left eye but was seldom used. He was never advised to try out contact lenses before performing refractive surgery. Postoperative uncorrected visual acuity was 20/25 in the right eye and 20/40 in the left eye. Orthoptic examination revealed a right exotropia of 50 PD and a right hypertropia of 14 PD for distance and for near. Ocular motility evaluation showed an over action of the right inferior oblique muscle, a V pattern and absence of convergence. The Bielschowsky head-tilt-test was negative. No fusion or suppression could be demonstrated. Fundus examination showed a peripapillar staphyloma in the right myopic eye and was without particularity in the left eye.

The fifth patient is a healthy 25-year-old young student was referred to our department for severe difficulties to read for a prolonged time and because of glare at night after having had multiple sessions of refractive surgery procedures to correct his myopia. He first had a bilateral PRK to correct –6.50D on the right eye and –7.00D on the left eye. One year later his right eye was re-treated with LASIK for residual myopia and another year later the left eye was re-treated for residual myopia with PRK and mitomycine. The patient's orthoptic history was negative. Best-corrected postoperative visual acuity was 20/25 in the right eye with –0.75 and 20/32 in the left eye with +1.50. Uncorrected visual acuity at near was 20/20 in the right eye and 20/100 in the left eye. The left eye could be improved up to 20/50 with +2.00. Orthoptic examination showed an esophoria of 16PD at near and 4 PD at distance, with normal ocular motility. Horizontal fusion was in the normal range but stereopsis, measured with the Titmus stereo test, was reduced (200 seconds of arc). Accommodation was 5D in both eyes, which is poor considering the young age of the patient. These measurements explain the complaints of the patient in sustained reading conditions. Fundus examination was without particularity in both eyes. The patient was equipped with a contact lens on the left eye to correct his hyperopia. Although this resulted in a subjective improvement in binocular vision the patient did not well tolerate the contact lens, which was soon abandoned. A conservative approach consisting in a spectacle correction with additional prismatic correction to support convergence at reading distance was refused.

3 DISCUSSION

Increasing reports on binocular vision impairment and diplopia after refractive surgery are found in the literature (Marmer et al. 1987; Mandava et al. 1996; Chaduteau et al 1998; Schuler et al. 1999; Holland et al 2000; Yap & Kowal 2001; Kushner & Kowal 2003). Recently also positive reports of treating binocular vision problems and strabismus by refractive surgery are described (Nemet et al. 2002; Stidham et al. 2002). In this paper we emphasise the importance of a detailed anamnestic and orthoptic examination prior to refractive surgery to avoid dominance problems, diplopia and binocular vision problems.

Dominance problems can occur when the dominant eye is undercorrected after surgery (Jain et al 1996), what happened in all our patients. Disturbing the ocular dominance in this way resulted in a decompensation of the heterophoria in patient I and II. In patient I even the non-dominant eye was treated instead of the dominant eye for monovision.

Diplopia occurred after decompensation of a hyperphoria (patient I and II), after loss of suppression (patient IV) and after changing the eye position and disturbing in this way the abnormal retinal correspondence (patient III). Also a change in the prismatic effect of the spectacles on binocular vision can result in diplopia (Pedrotti 1998). The prismatic effect is zero in emmetropic patients or patients with equal ametropia in both eyes but will be substantial in anisometropic patients. This so called anisoprism[10] effect can by calculated by the following formula:

$$P_{prism}\,(PD) = 100\,\tan\left\{\frac{40}{c} - \sqrt{\left(\frac{40}{c}\right)^2 - 1}\right\} \qquad \text{(Pedrotti 1998)}$$

where c is the glass correction in diopters (D) and assuming the index of refraction of the glass to be 1.5. The patient's spectacle vertical prismatic effect, expressed in prism diopter (PD = _), has been calculated before and after refractive surgery for all cases examined (table 1). In patients with anisometropia, muscular effort is needed both to maintain binocular single vision and to compensate the anisoprism effect of the spectacle correction.

Table 1. Vertical anisoprism before and after excimer laser expressed in prism diopters (PD = _).

Case	Power	Preoperative			Postoperative			Induced change in RE–LE balance
		RE	LE	Balance	RE	LE	Balance	
I	spherical equivalent (D)	−2.25	−4.00	+1.75	−2.25	−0.75	−1.50	−3.25
	prism diopter (_)	−2.80	−5.00	+2.20	−2.80	−0.94	−1.86	−4.06
II	spherical equivalent (D)	−5.25	−5.00	−0.25	−1.00	−0.50	−0.50	−0.25
	prism diopter (_)	−6.55	−6.25	−0.30	−1.24	−0.62	−0.62	−0.32
III	spherical equivalent (D)	?	?	?	−1.50	−0.50	+2.00	2.00
	prism diopter (_)	?	?	?	−1.87	−0.62	+2.49	2.49
IV	spherical equivalent (D)	−10.00	−0.75	−9.25	0.00	−0.75	−0.75	10.00
	prism diopter (_)	−12.40	−0.94	−11.46	0.00	−0.94	−0.94	12.40
V	spherical equivalent (D)	−6.50	−7.00	−0.50	−0.75	+1.50	−2.25	−2.75
	prism diopter (_)	−8.10	−8.50	−0.40	−0.74	+1.90	−2.64	−3.04

Patient I is very illustrative to demonstrate the vertical anisoprism influence of the spectacles on patient's binocular vision. Preoperatively, this patient presented an anisometropia of 1.75 D inducing a vertical anisoprism of 2.2 _ (table 1). She also presented a right hyperphoria of 3 PD. After LASIK of her most myopic, left eye an anisometropia in the opposite direction was induced. The total postoperative change in prismatic vertical balance between right and left eye was 4.06 _. As a result, the preoperative latent hyperphoria became manifest postoperatively.

Binocular vision problems and also reading problems occur when accommodation is reduced what happened in one eye in patient I and in both eyes in patient II. Reduced stereopsis was seen in patient V due to the postoperative anisometropia. Decreased stereopsis after monovision and anisometropia has been described before (Bagolini et al. 1991; Brooks et al. 1996; Wright et al. 1999).

Risk groups for postoperative binocular vision impairment and minimal screening techniques were suggested earlier (Kowal 2000; De Faber & Tjon-Fo-Sang 2001). We agree with these authors and like to make the following recommendations:

- The patient's history of precious strabismological or amblyopia therapy should urge the surgeon to ask for an orthoptic examination.
- Patients with anisometropia, who have never been adapted with contact lenses before, should be picked out for an orthoptic examination to rule out the presence of a hyperphoria.
- Patients who feel more comfortable with spectacles than with contact lenses should be oriented for an orthoptic examination to rule out the compensation of a heterophoria by the prismatic effect of their spectacles (anisometropic, decentered, overcorrected or under-corrected spectacles).
- Dominancy is important to determine since it is not wise to undercorrect a dominant eye.
- Monovision can only be proposed in patients with equal visual acuity, normal binocular vision and good fusion capacity, correcting the dominant eye for distance. In case of doubts, simulation with contact lenses should always be tried out.

Patients who normally should have no risk for binocular vision problems after refractive surgery are patients with:

- Low/moderate myopia
- No strabismus or diplopia
- No prisms or decentered glasses
- No hyperphoria
- Small esophoria or exophoria
- Maximum of 0.5 D difference between the glasses and the cycloplegic refraction

Patients with a moderate risk for binocular vision problems after refractive surgery are patients with:

- Intended monovision
- Overcorrected myopia
- Prism glasses
- Hypermetropia
- Ex-strabismus
- Hyperphoria

Patients with a high risk for binocular vision problems after refractive surgery are patients with:

- Manifest strabismus
- Hypermetropia with poor fusion
- Intermittent diplopia
- Anisometropia
- Amblyopia

REFERENCES

Bagolini, B., Dickmann, A,. Savino, G., Muci, A. 1991. Evaluation orthoptique dans la chirurgie réfractive. *Journal Français d'Orthoptique* 23: 131-134.

Brooks, S.E., Johnson, D., Fischer, N. 1996. Anisometropia and binocularity. *Ophthalmology* 103: 1139-1143.

Chaduteau, G.C. & Kohanc, B. 1998. De la nécessité du bilan orthoptique avant chirurgie réfractive. *Journal Français d'Orthoptique* 30: 106-108.

De Faber, J.T.H.N. & Tjon-Fo-Sang, M. 2001. Strabismologic advice for the refractive surgeon. In de Faber, J.T.H.N. (ed.) *Transactions, 26th meeting European Strabismological Association*: 41-43. Lisse: Swets Zeitlinger.

Holland, D., Amm, M., de Decker, W. 2000. Persisting diplopia after bilateral laser in situ keratomileusis. *J. Cataract Refract. Surg.* 26: 1556-1557.

Jain, S., Arora, I., Azar, D.T. 1996. Success of monovision in presbyopes: review of the literature and potential applications to refractive surgery. *Survey of ophthalmology* 40: 491-499.

Kowal, L. 2000. Refractive surgery and diplopia. *Clinical and experimental Ophthalmology* 28: 344-346.

Kushner, B.J. & Kowal, L. 2003. Diplopia after refractive surgery. *Arch ophthalmol* 121: 315-321.

Mandava, N., Donnenfeld, D.E., Owens, P.L., Kelly, S.E., Haight, D.H. 1996. Ocular deviation following excimer laser photorefractive keratectomy. *J. Catararct Refract. Surg.* 22: 504-505.

Marmer, R.H. 1987. Ocular deviation induced by radial keratotomy. *Ann.Ophthalmol*: 451-452.

Nemet, P., Levinger, S., Nemet, A., 2002. Refractive surgery for refractive errors which cause strabismus. *BinocularVision & Strabismus Quarterly.* 17 (3): 187-190.

Pedrotti, L.S. & Pedrotti, F.L. 1998. Optics and Vision, Prentice hall, *Optical Instrumentation*: 157-169.

Schuler, E., Silverberg, M., Beade, P., Madel, K. 1999. Decompensated strabismus after laser in situ keratomileusis. *J. Cataract Refract. Surg.* 25: 1552-1553.

Stidham, D.B., Borissova, O., Borrissov, V., Prager, T.C. 2002. Effect of hyperopic laser in situ keratomileusis on ocular alignment and stereopsis in patients with accommodative esotropia. *Ophthalmology* 109 (6): 1148-1153

Wright, K.W. Guemes, A. Kapadia, M.S. Wilson, S.E. 1999. Binocular function and patient satisfaction after monovision induced by myopic potorefractive keratectomy. *J. Cataract Refract. Surg*. 25: 177-182.

Yap, E.Y. & Kowal, L. 2001. Diplopia as a complication of laser in situ keratomileusis surgery. *Clinical and Experimental Ophthalmology* 29: 268-271.

Transactions 28th Meeting European Strabismological Association, de Faber (ed.)
© 2004 European Strabismological Association, ISBN 90 265 1965 6

Refractive Surgery and Binocularity

A. Dickmann, P. Valente, M.T. Rebecchi , G. Savino , A. Salerni , L. Buzzonetti
Department of Ophthalmology, Catholic University of Sacred Hearth – Rome – Italy

ABSTRACT: Aim of this study is to evaluate pre and post operative sensorial and motor balance in myopic anisometropic patients performing laser in situ keratomileusis (LASIK), in order to detect the cases that may actually benefit from refractive surgery and those in which LASIK could be useless or even harmful.

Ten patients with high myopic anisometropia (>4.5 D) were enrolled in this study. A complete orthoptic examination was always performed pre- and post-operatively (six months). Eight patients performed uncomplicated LASIK. Two patients showing risk to develop a postoperative diplopia were left off surgery.

To prevent post-operative diplopia and/or angle deviation increase, a complete pre-operative orthoptic evaluation with contact lenses is recommended to simulate post-operative refractive changes. The importance of Red Glass Bar in evaluating the strength and the depth of binocular cooperation (normal or anomalous) or suppression is stressed

KEYWORDS: Refractive surgery, myopic anisometropia, diplopia, Red Glass Bar.

1 INTRODUCTION

Refractive surgery may induce problems in the binocular condition of some patients (Bagolini et Al. 1991, Kowal et Al 2002, Sugar et Al. 2002). Laser in situ keratomileusis (LASIK) has become a standard procedure for the correction of moderate or severe myopia (Sugar et Al. 2002).

In patients with myopic anisometropia motor and sensorial outcomes after LASIK are especially depending on the pre-operative binocular condition. In fact, in some subjects an intractable diplopia may arise (Holland et Al. 2000, Kowal et Al. 2000, Kushner et Al. 2003, Valente et Al. 2003, Yap et Al. 2001), while in other ones this kind of surgery may result ineffective concerning a possible binocular cooperation improvement.

In this study we performed a complete pre- and post-operative orthoptic evaluation to assess binocular vision state and eye motor balance. Our aim was to detect the subjects whose binocularity actually improved and those in whom refractive surgery proved to be useless or even harmful about binocular cooperation.

2 METHODS

Ten consecutive patients with high myopic anisometropia (>4.5D), three males and seven females, mean age 38,7 years (range 29 to 49 years) were enclosed in this study.

A complete ophthalmological (UCVA and BSCVA, manifest and cycloplegic refraction, fundus examination, IOP, slit-lamp examination, corneal topography, ultrasonic pachymetry) and orthoptic examination (4-PD Base-Out Prism Test, TNO Test, Bagolini's Striated Glasses, Worth's Test, Red Glass Bar, Prismatic Cover Test, Fusional Amplitudes when possible) was always performed, with glasses and contact lenses preoperatively and postoperatively.

Two patients, showing a risk to develop a postoperative diplopia, were not treated. Eight patients (fourteen eyes) performed uncomplicated LASIK (Bausch & Lomb Technolas 217C excimer laser; Hansatome microkeratome). We planned monocular LASIK (the second eye treated two weeks after the first one).

Operated patients were evaluated at one day, seven days, and one, three, six and twelve months.

3 RESULTS

Preoperative conditions and postoperative results are summarized in Table 1. Postoperative findings in the Table are obtained at six months from refractive surgery. Data of refraction are shown as spherical equivalent.

In our sample two subjects showed NBV (Normal Binocular Vision), seven ARC (Anomalous Retinal Correspondence, four subjects showing an Anomalous Binocular Vision), one Suppression of the more ametropic eye. Patients 4 and 10 were rejected from surgery for a high risk of postoperative diplopia due to the very low results obtained at RGB. The other patients, showing diplopia with red glasses bar test at values higher than 4 or 5, could safely perform LASIK.

Two comments should be made. In case 5 firstly has been treated the suppressed eye and LASIK induced a transitory diplopia due to the switch of fixation to the more ametropic eye (Kushner et Al. 2003); double vision disappeared when the better eye was operated on and became again the fixing one. About case 1, it may be important to remark that at the first visit time very low values at RGB were observed (that is the patient showed signs of a very weak NBV); for this reason we decided to submit him to exercises of fusional amplitude while he wearing contact lenses. In one month good values of fusional amplitudes were achieved and RGB test exhibited an improvement as shown in Table 1.

4 CONCLUSIONS

Laser in situ keratomileusis is commonly performed in myopic anisometropia. About binocular cooperation, refractive surgery in patients with myopic anisometropia may be useful, useless or even harmful inducing diplopia (Bagolini et Al. 1991, Holland et Al. 2000, Kowal et Al. 2000, Kushner et Al. 2003, Valente et Al. 2003, Yap et Al. 2001).

In this study we performed a complete pre- and post-operative orthoptic evaluation to assess the binocular vision condition, in the attempt to detect, first of all, criteria of ruling out surgery patients with high probability to develop post-operative diplopia.

Another aim of our study was to identify, if possible, both the subjects in which binocularity has, in some way, improved (useful) and those who could obtain no advantages concerning their binocular cooperation (useless).

Regarding preoperative binocularity condition, in our sample three types of situation are represented: NBV (Normal Binocular Vision), Suppression of the more ametropic eye and ARC (Anomalous Retinal Correspondence) which in some cases supports an ABV (Anomalous Binocular Vision).

Concerning our post-operative findings some considerations can be made:

1. In our patients never developed a post-operative permanent diplopia (see text above for case 5);
2. we observed an increase of stereoacuity only in one subject (case 1);
3. about Bagolini's striated glasses, only one case showed an improvement from suppression to fusion (preoperatively NRC was present) (case 8);
4. Worth test exhibited a response from suppression to fusion only in one case (case 3) with ARC;
5. in four subjects RGB demonstrated a variation (cases 1, 3, 8 and 9).

It is possible to note that in five cases refractive surgery proved useless about opportunity of improvement of the binocular conditions (ARC in four cases, Suppression in one case).

Slight improvements in binocular cooperation (useful refractive surgery) have been observed in three subjects independently from the type of preoperative sensorial condition.

Refractive surgery has never been harmful (untractable postoperative diplopia) in our subjects, but we rejected two patients from surgery because the RGB preoperative results (cases 4 and 10).

The possibility of a refractive surgery proving to be unsafe seems to be related not to the type of binocular condition but to its depth, that is to its ability to oppose resistance to the dissociation power of the new refractive condition. In this study RGB proved to be an useful and easy tool to measure the strength of sensorial condition. In all patients submitting to surgery we never observed diplopia with filters lesser than n.8.

Furthermore, RGB provides suitable information about a possible subclinic perturbation of the postoperative sensorial conditions; in fact subjects 8 and 9 showed a slight worsening of the responses, even if they do not display any symptom.

Concerning a possible increase in angle deviation we have not observed significant variations (in case 5 a temporary increase of exodeviation after treatment of the non fixing eye could be found); however, in cases 2 and 3 a slight improvement at Prismatic Cover Test has been noticed.

Our study suggests to perform a careful ocular and orthoptic evaluation on all high myopic anisometropic patients undergoing LASIK. In particular we recommend a pre-operative examination with contact lenses to simulate post-operative refractive results.

To prevent post-operative diplopia Red Glass Bar test is very useful to evaluate the depth and the strength of sensorial situation.

In case 5 we observed that diplopia occurred when firstly has been treated the suppressed eye, therefore we suggest to perform LASIK beginning from less ametropic eye.

Finally, to obtain a strong and comfortable binocular vision, a training of fusional amplitudes in particular cases (NBV) may be useful (case 1).

5 REFERENCES

Bagolini, B., Dickmann, A., Savino, G., and Muci, A. 1991. Orthoptic work-up of patients being considered for refractive surgery. In *Advances in amblyopia and Strabismus. Trans. Of the VIIth International Orthoptic Congress, Nurnberg, Germany, 2-6 June,* p.194-196.

Holland, D., Amm, M., and de Decker, W. 2000. Persisting diplopia after bilateral laser in situ keratomileusis. *J. Cataract Refract Surg* 26: 1555-1557

Kowal, L. 2000. Refractive surgery and diplopia. *Clinical and Experimental Ophthalmology* 28: 344-346

Kowal, L., De Faber, J., Calcutt, C., and Fawcett, S. 2002. Refractive surgery and strabismus: workshop. In J T de Faber (ed.), *9th meeting of the international Strabismological Association Sydney, Australia 17-20 April.*

Kushner, B.J., and Kowal, L. 2003. Diplopia after refractive surgery. *Arch Ophthalmol.* 121: 313-321.

Sugar, A., Rapuano, C.J., and Culberston, W.W., 2002. Laser in situ Keratomileusis for myopia and astigmatism: safety and efficacy, a report by American Academy of Ophthalmology. *Ophthalmology* 109: 175-187

Valente, P., Dickmann, A., Buzzonetti, L., Rebecchi, M.T., and Scullica, L. 2003. Orthoptic evaluation in high myopic anisometropia patients undergoing to LASIK. In *VII Congress ESCRS, Rome, February 7-9* (Poster accepted).

Yap, E.Y., and Kowal, L. 2001. Diplopia as complication of laser in situ keratomileusis surgery. *Clinical and Experimental Ophthalmology* 29: 268-271.

Table 1:

	Pat.s	Sens. state	P CT	Manifest Refraction	BSCVA	WORTH	Striated Glasses	TNO	RGB
1	Pre	NBV	D: X N: X'	OD: -9.00 OS: -1.75	OD:20/32 OS: 20/20	Fusion	NRC	480	D 10 OO N no dipl
	Post	NBV	D: X N: X'	OD: -1.00 OS: -0.25	OD:20/32 OS: 20/20	Fusion	NRC	240	D no dipl N 16OD 9OS
2	Pre	ARC	D:14 XT 8 LHT N:10 XT' 8 LHT'	OD: -12.50 OS: -3.50	OD:20/50 OS: 20/25	OD suppr.	ARC	0	D no dipl N no dipl
	Post	ARC	D:6 XT 16 LHT N:6 XT' 8 LHT'	OD: -0.25 OS: +0.50	OD:20/50 OS: 20/25	OD suppr.	ARC	0	D no dipl N no dipl
3	Pre	ARC	D: ortho N: 16 XT'	OD: -0.75 OS: -5.50	OD: 20/32 OS: 20/20	OD suppr	ARC	480	D 8 OD 12 OS N 13 OO
	Post	ARC	D: ortho N: 2 XT'	OD: 0 OS: -0.50	OD: 20/20 OS: 20/20	Fusion	ARC	480	D no dipl N no dipl
4	Pre	ARC	D: 8 XT N: 8 XT'	OD: 0 OS: -15.75	OD: 20/20 OS: 20/40	Fusion	ARC	0	D 4 OD 9 OS N 3 OD 4 OS
5	Pre	ARC	D: ortho N: 2 XT'	OD: -13.50 OS: - 6.50	OD: 20/25 OS: 20/20	Fusion	ARC	0	D 13 OO N 13 OO
	Post	ARC	D: ortho N: 2 XT'	OD: -0.50 OS: -0.75	OD: 20/25 OS: 20/20	Fusion	ARC	0	D 13 OO N 13 OO
6	Pre	ARC	D: ortho N: ortho	OD: -6.25 OS: -1.25	OD: 20/50 OS: 20/50	Fusion	ARC	480	D no dipl N no dipl
	Post	ARC	D: ortho N: ortho	OD: -0.50 OS: -1.00	OD: 20/50 OS: 20/50	Fusion	ARC	480	D no dipl N no dipl
7	Pre	ARC	D:2 XT N:2 XT'	OD: -3.50 OS: -10.00	OD: 20/25 OS: 20/32	Fusion	ARC	480	D no dipl N no dipl
	Post	ARC	D: 2 XT N: 2 XT'	OD: -0.25 OS: -0.25	OD: 20/20 OS: 20/25	Fusion	ARC	480	D no dipl N no dipl
8	Pre	NBV	D: ortho.N: X'	OD: -3.25 OS: -11.25	OD: 20/20 OS: 20/25	Fusion	D suppr.NCRN	120	D no dipl N no dipl
	Post	NBV	D: ortho N: X'	OD: -3.25 OS: -2.25	OD: 20/20 OS: 20/20	Fusion	NRC	120	D OD14 OS8 N OD10 OS9
9	Pre	Suppr.	D: 30 XT N:35XT'	OD: -2.00 OS: -7.00	OD: 20/20 OS: 20/25	OS supp.	OS suppr.	0	D no dipl N no dipl
	Post	Suppr.	D: 30 XT N: 35 XT'	OD: -2.00 OS: 0.00	OD: 20/20 OS: 20/20	OS supp.	OS suppr.	0	D N OD no dipl. OS 11
10	Pre	ARC	D:2 XT N:2 XT'	OD: -5.50 OS: -0.25	OD: 20/32 OS: 20/20	Fusion	ARC	0	D OD 3 OS 4 N OD 3 OS 4

P CT: Prismatic cover test; BSCVA: measured in Snellen; D: distance; N: near; X: exophoria; XT: exotropia; LHT: left eye hypertropia

Transactions 28th Meeting European Strabismological Association, de Faber (ed.)
© 2004 European Strabismological Association, ISBN 90 265 1965 6

Strabismus after treatment of unilateral congenital cataracts. A clinical model for strabismus physiopathogenesis?

D. Thouvenin, S.Nogue, L. Fontes, O. Norbert
Clinique Saint Nicolas. Toulouse, France.

ABSTRACT: Unilateral cataracts in children provoke an interruption of binocular vision development at a more or less sensible stage function of the age of occurrence. We report 75 cases of unilateral cataracts in children followed more than 3 years after surgery (mean 6.5 years). Visual results are reported. We focused on binocular and oculomotor state. When opacification occurs before age 1, 60% of cases present a typical but "acquired" infantile strabismus syndrome. It may, in itself, limit VA of the sound eye, because of its specific fixation anomalies (MLN, Fixation in Adduction...). Unilateral congenital cataracts may then have binocular consequences and lead to bilateral low vision. This last comment should represent another motivation for real treatment of these deep amblyopias. Neutralisation is the most common binocular scar found in cases opacified later. 70% of these last case present only microtropias. KEYWORDS: Unilateral congenital cataracts. Visual results. Binocular vision. Infantile strabismus.

1 INTRODUCTION

Unilateral congenital cataracts have many sensorial consequences : interruption of monocular visual development which leads to deprivation amblyopia and interruption of binocular visual development with sensorial and motor disorders.

On a monocular aspect, the brain plasticity period spread over the first decade. The more precocious, intense and extended the deprivation period, the deeper and more difficult to treat the amblyopia. This is the usual point of discussion when talking of unilateral cataracts in children.

On a binocular aspect, the major period of development is limited to the six first months of life. Early unilateral deprivation disrupts binocular vision (BV) maturation process. The consequences should be similar to infantile strabismus syndrome. Secondary unilateral deprivation occurs as BV has already matured. Its deterioration should be all the more light since cataract appears late in the first decade.

2 GOAL OF THE STUDY

Verification of binocular consequences of unilateral cataracts in children on a retrospective study and clinical confirmation of theoretical neurophysiological data.

3 PATIENTS AND METHODS

75 cases of unilateral cataracts in children, last exam realised at least 3 years after cataract surgery (med 6.8 years).

We separated the cases in 5 age groups function of age at surgery :

0 to 6 months : 16 cases = group 1
6 months to 1 year : 12 cases = group 2
1 to 2 years : 8 cases = group 3
2 to 4 years : 14 cases = group 4
4 to 8 years : 25 cases = group 5

Surgical procedure, treatment of aphakia and patching procedure are usual and have been discussed elsewhere, with monocular visual results [Thouvenin: 1995, 2003]. We although report monocular visual results to be more complete on cases description.

We focused the study essentially on binocular state : oculomotricity, state of BV (Normal or abnormal Retino Cortical Correspondence (nrcc or arcc), neutralisation) and stereoscopy (Lang stereotest and TNO).

4 RESULTS

4.1 *Monocular visual acuity*

In group 1 and 2 (surgery before age 1), 40% of the cases gained over 0.4, 40% gained between 0.1 and 0.4, and 20% stayed below 0.1. The proportions are even a little better if we focus on children operated on before age 3 months (11 cases), classically with the worst prognosis.

After age 1, 66.8% gained over 0.4, 26.6% gained between 0.1 and 0.4 and 6.6% stayed below 0.1.

These results are obtained after more than 3 years of amblyopia therapy, medium 6,8 years, and are discussed elsewhere [Thouvenin, 2003].

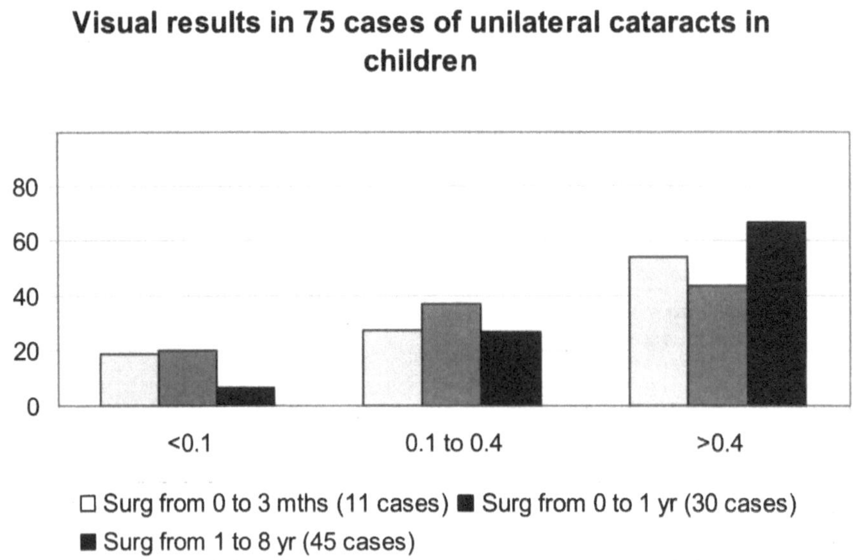

4.2 *Binocular vision*

4.2.1 *Some clinical signs are really specific of infantile strabismus syndrome, the most primitive state of BV*

Manifest Latent Nystagmus
Fixation in adduction.
Dissociated Vertical Deviation
Asymmetry of OptoKinetic Nystagmus

Three of these signs are found together in more than 75% of cases in group 1, and 60% of cases in group 1 + 2. None of these three signs are found in 84 % of cases of group 3, 4 and 5, as seen bellow:

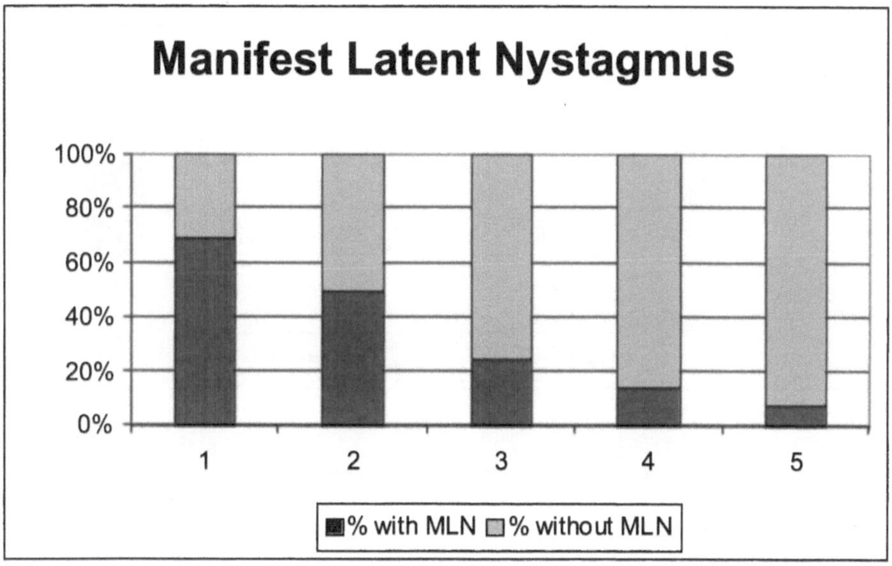

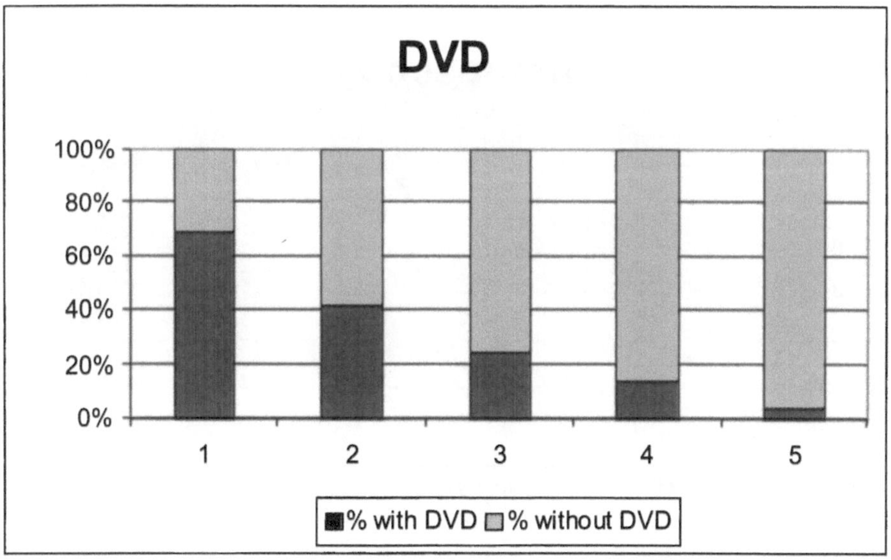

4.2.2 *Some signs testify more or less altered BV :*

4.2.2.1 State of BV = RCC and neutralisation :

48 cases present neutralisation (masking evaluation of RCC), distributed in all groups.

15 cases present proved ARCC, almost all in groups 1 and 2

12 cases present documented NRCC, 80% in group 5.

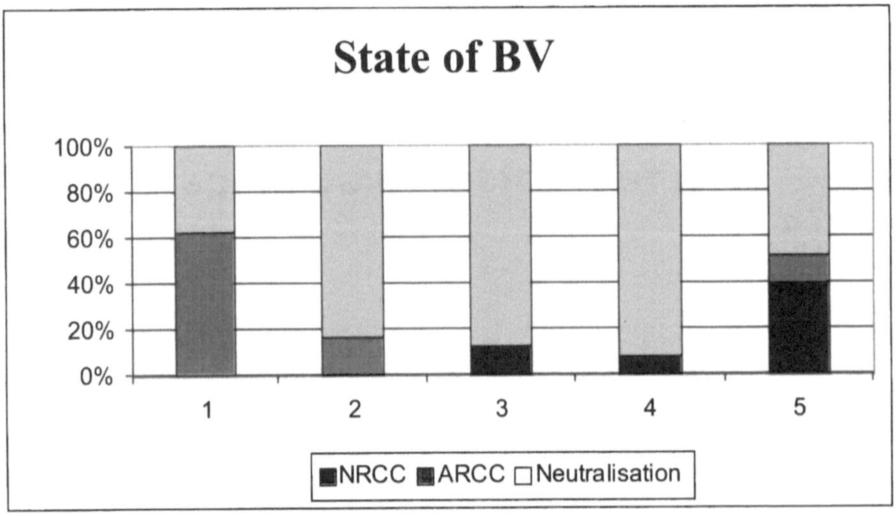

4.2.2.2 Stereoscopy improves markedly with age of surgery

No real stereoscopy can be identified on Lang test (and eventually TNO) in groups 1, 2 and 3. Gross stereoscopy (Lang 500" and TNO > 120") is found in 3 cases in group 4 and 8 cases in group 5, and fine stereoscopy in 1 case in group 5 (TNO 60").

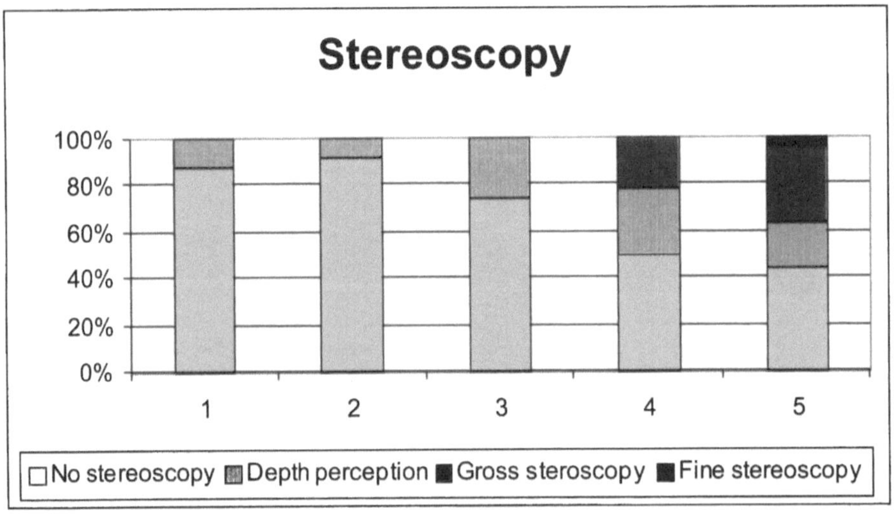

4.2.3 *The type of horizontal deviation presents no specificity :*
Microtropia is found in 40% of group 1, 2 &3 and 70% of group 4 & 5. The frequency of esodeviation seems to lessen with age of surgery : 40% in group 1 & 2, 15% over age 1. Exotropia is found in all age groups around 15%.

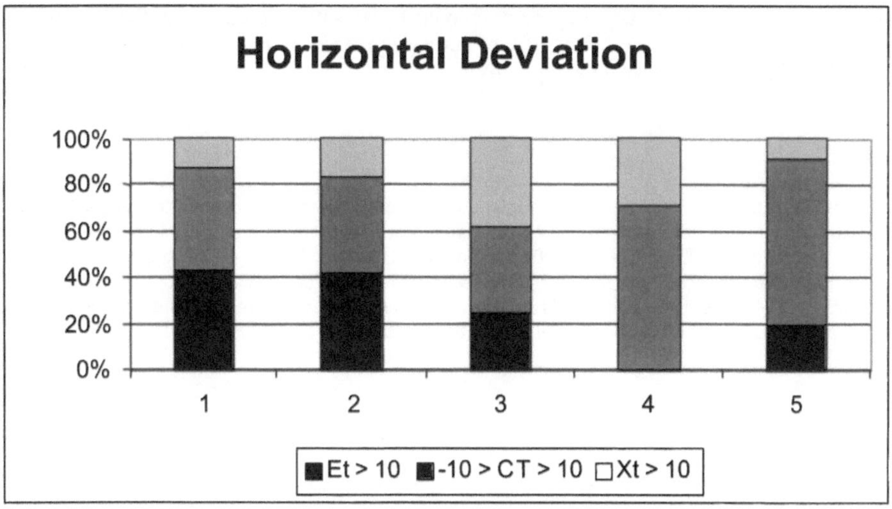

5 DISCUSSION

We can separate two groups with totally different binocularity :

5.1 *Opacification before age 1 (groups 1 & 2)*

We observe a specific binocular anomaly. Binocularity cannot develop itself and definitive sensorial signs are observed : ARCC, no real stereoscopy. Infantile strabismus syndrome is observed in 80% of cases in group 1, and 60% in group 1+2. 40% present esotropia, 42% present microtropia and 18% exotropia. This infantile strabismus syndrome is peculiar. It is often called "congenital monophtalm syndrome" also observed in other cases of congenital monocular blindness. It is spontaneously non alternating because of amblyopia but may become alternating in the specific case of treated monocular congenital cataracts with amblyopia treatment. It may, in itself limit VA of the sound eye, because of fixation anomalies (MLN, Fix in Add...) [Thouvenin: 2000]. This last point represents a major reason to cure these amblyopias. It is possible that vision recovery of the operated eye as tenuous as it may be, lessen motor anomalies of the sound eye, by balancing visual inputs when fixating in binocular status

5.2 *Opacification after age 1 (groups 3 to 6)*

Initial development of binocularity is normal. The later the lens opacification, the better the underlying BV quality. Sensorial scars may be limited to neutralisation, eventually with normal underlying binocularity. 70% of groups 4 and 5 have micro or orthotropia, essentially associated with good monocular visual results. These last cases developed the highest grades of stereoscopy. « Sensorial strabismus » may appear if deprivation is extended, 10% present esotropia and 20% exotropia.

6 CONCLUSION

Infantile unilateral cataracts lead to a peculiar infantile strabismus syndrome, spontaneously non alternating that maybe threatful for the vision of the sound eye. This reason must motivate full treatment of these cataracts. It is an example of « acquired » infantile strabismus, and a clinical proof that post natal conditions may also lead to this situation.

Later opacified unilateral cataracts appear on a more or less developed BV. Neutralisation is the most common scar. Normal BV may be recovered in late juvenile cataracts. Strabismus is related to the interruption of fusion, but 70% of our case present micro or orthotropia. Exotropia is found in less than 20% of cases in all age groups.

REFERENCES

Thouvenin D., Lesueur L., Arne J.L. 1995 - Intercapsular lens implantation in pediatric aphakia : study of 87 cases compared to 88 cases without lens implantation..- J. Fr. Ophtalmol., ,18, 11, 678-687.

Thouvenin D., Taurines E., Noblet P. 2000 - Oculomotor Status in Treated Monocular Congenital Cataracts. - De Faber, ed. Trans 26th meeting ESA. Swets and Zeitlinger. Lisse. ; 44-50.

Thouvenin D., S. Nogue, L. Fontes, JL Arne 2003. Long term functional results of the treatment of unilateral congenital cataracts with early surgery. About 20 cases. J. Fr. Ophtalmol,

Transactions 28th Meeting European Strabismological Association, de Faber (ed.)
© 2004 European Strabismological Association, ISBN 90 265 1965 6

Strabismus in pediatric cataract

J.T.H.N. de Faber, M.J. Tjon-Fo-Sang
Pediatric Ophthalmology and Strabismus Service
The Rotterdam Eye Hospital, The Netherlands

ABSTRACT: From 1990-2000, lens extraction was performed in 200 eyes with pediatric cataract. This study is a retrospective analysis of the frequency of strabismus in this cohort. After lens extraction, there were twice as many new cases of strabismus in bilateral aphakic patients compared to bilateral pseudophakic patients. In the patients with unilateral cataract ,both apakic and pseudophakic, the frequency of post lens extraction strabismus was comparable.Fifty-seven percent of the children with bilateral cataract had a best corrected visual acuity (BCVA) higher than 0.8. Only 23% of the patients with unilateral cataract had a BCVA higher than 0.5. Pediatric pseudophakia may rapidly achieve visual rehabilitation.

KEYWORDS: congenital cataract, strabismus, pseudophakia

1. INTRODUCTION

Strabismus is a common disorder in patients with congenital cataract and can be noted either pre- or postoperatively to lens extraction. France[1] reported an incidence of 43% of strabismus preoperatively in patients with congenital cataracts. Postoperatively, this number increased to 71%. In addition, ocular misalignment was noted to occur more frequently in patients with unilateral than in those with bilateral cataract.[1 2] In the study of France et al.[1] however, the children were aphakic after cataract surgery.

IOL implantation has been reported to reduce the incidence of strabismus in aphakic children.[3] In a study by Awner et al.,[4] strabismus was found preoperatively in 6 cases (29%) with unilateral cataract. Postoperatively, with IOL implantation, 3(15%) additional cases developed strabismus.

We performed a retrospective analysis of the results of lens extraction of pediatric cataract in our clinic. In this study we focused mainly on the occurrence of ocular misalignment.

2. MATERIAL AND METHOD

From 1990-2000, 351 patients were treated for congenital or pediatric cataract in our clinic. We excluded all patients operated after the age of 10, and patients operated for traumatic cataract, secondary cataract (juvenile rheumatoid arthritis, buphthalmus, atopic cataract, use of corticosteroids) and cataracts associated with PHPV, Marfan's syndrome, or Peter's anomaly. In this study, we included the results of lens extraction in 128 patients (65 male, 63 female; 200 eyes). The cases were divided in 4 subgroups: eyes with bilateral cataract and IOL implantation (bilIOL, N=99; 57 patients); eyes with bilateral cataract and aphakic (bilAPH, N=58; 32 patients); eyes with unilateral cataract with IOL implantation (uniIOL, N=25; 25 patients) and eyes with unilateral cataract and aphakic (uniAPH, N=18; 18 patients).

3. RESULTS

The median age of surgery was 595 days (approximately 1 year and 8 months), and the mean time of follow-up was 4 years and 2 months (range 22 days to 12 years).

The children with IOL implantation tended to be older, which is demonstrated in the mean age of the children at surgery: bilIOL 4.7 yrs, bilAPH 4.8 months, uniIOL 3.2 yrs, and uniAPH 3.6 months.

Strabismus- In the bilIOL group, 5 (9%) patients had strabismus pre-operatively; 2 were eso- and 3 exotropic. Postoperatively, 8 (14%) additional cases of strabismus were recorded. Of these, 4 had esotropia, 3 exotropia and 1 only had dissociated vertical deviation. In the bilAPH patients, the same percentage of patients, i.e. 9% (3 patients (1 esotropic, 2 exotropic)) had an ocular misalignment before cataract surgery. Postoperatively however, quite a few more patients, i.e. 9 (28%) developed strabismus (6 esotropic, 3 exotropic). Patients with unilateral cataract also tended to show a higher frequency of ocular misalignment post-operatively. In the uniIOL group, 7 (28%) cases developed strabismus; 3 esotropia and 4 exotropia. In the uniAPH group, 6 (33%; 3 esotropic, 3 exotropic) cases developed strabismus after surgery. Before cataract surgery, 5(20%) patients had strabismus pre-operatively (4 esotropic, 1 exotropic) in the uniIOL group, whereas in the uniAPH group, only 1 (5.5%) patient had esotropia.

Best Corrected Visual Acuity (BCVA) – The frequencies for the BCVA, as measured in Snellen visual acuity has been stated in the table for each of the subgroups. In a number of patients the visual acuity could not be measured, because the patients were still in their preverbal phase. When these cases were excluded, 57.1% of the children with bilateral cataract had a BCVA of 0.8 or higher in their best eye. In the patients with unilateral cataract, only 23% of the patients had a BCVA higher than 0.5.

	<0.25	0.3 – 0.5	0.6 – 0.7	0.8 – >1.0	preverbal
bilIOL	6	14	7	54	19
bilAPH	19	16	3	16	47
uniIOL	40	24	16	8	12
uniAPH	39	39	6	11	6

Table. The percentage of patients with the best corrected visual acuity as measured in Snellen (<0.25, 0.3-0.5, 0.6-0.7, 0.8->1.0). Patients were divided in 4 groups: those with bilateral cataract and IOL implantation (bilIOL) or aphakic (bilAPH), and those with unilateral cataract and IOL implantation (uniIOL) or aphakic (uniAPH). The last column reflects the percentage of patients who were still preverbal at the last follow-up and therefore had no measurement of visual acuity.

Nystagmus – In the bilIOL group, 10% of patients demonstrated nystagmus, whereas in the aphakic patients with bilateral cataract, this number was much higher: 41.7%. In the patients with unilateral cataract, the frequency of nystagmus was quite similar in the implant and aphakic patients: 8 and 5.6% respectively.

Amblyopia treatment– As would be expected, amblyopia treatment was far more often required in patients with unilateral cataract. In the uniIOL group 72% received amblyopia treatment and in the uniAPH group this number was even 77.8%. By contrast, 17.4% of the bilIOL patients received amblyopia treatment. The bilAPH patients required slightly more amblyopia treatments: 28.3%.

4. DISCUSSION

In this study, there was a higher incidence of postoperative strabismus in the bilateral aphakic patients compared to the patients with bilateral lens implantations. It may be that pseudophakia, and therefore faster and better visual rehabilitation, reduces the incidence of strabismus, as reported by Awner et al.[4] On the other hand, in our study, the patients who had a lens implantation were older. Apparently, the deprivation amblyopia had not been to the extent that surgery was warranted at an earlier age. It could well be that in these cases, binocular vision developed more or less before lens extraction was performed.

Except for the cases with bilateral lens implantation, we found an approximately twice as high rate of postoperative new strabismus compared to the study by Awner et al.[4] The patients in his study however, were somewhat younger (mean age 26 months) and all received intraocular lens implantation. Our patients who had a lens implantation were on average 3.2 years. It could be postulated that earlier surgery is beneficiary to the development of the binocular vision, and therefore prevented the development of strabismus.

We found the highest rate of preoperative strabismus in the older patients with unilateral cataract. Strabismus has been reported to be more common in children with unilateral than bilateral cataract.[2] Again, these children were older and deprivation amblyopia must have played a key factor in the occurrence of strabismus.

Overall there was a fairly even spread between eso- and exotropia in the various subgroups, before and after cataract surgery, with or without lens implantation.

More than half of the patients with bilateral cataract had a visual acuity of 0.8 and higher. In the patients with unilateral cataract, only 23% had a visual acuity >0.5.

5. CONCLUSION

In this study, only half as many of the children with bilateral lens implantation develop strabismus postoperatively when compared to the bilateral aphakic children. Pediatric pseudophakia may rapidly achieve visual rehabilitation.

REFERENCES

France TD, Frank JW. The association of strabismus and aphakia in children. J Ped Ophthalmol Strab 1984; 21(6): 223-6.

Hiles DA, Sheridan SJ. Strabismus associated with infantile cataracts. Int Ophthalmol Clin 1977; 17: 193-202.

Ben Ezra D. Cataract surgery and intraocular lens implantation in children. Am J Ophthalmol 1996; 121: 224-5.

Awner S, Buckley EG, DeVaro JM, Seaber JH. Unilateral pseudophakia in children under 4 years. J Pediatr Ophthalmol Strab 1996; 33: 230-6.

Transactions 28th Meeting European Strabismological Association, de Faber (ed.)

Combined strabismus and cataract surgery in adults

N.G. Ziakas, K. Boboridis & N.S. Georgiadis
Department of Ophthalmology, AristotleUniversity of Thessaloniki, Greece

ABSTRACT: *Introduction*: To present our experience with combined strabismus and cataract surgery in adult patients.

Design: Prospective noncomparative interventional case series study.

Methods: Three cases of combined strabismus and cataract surgery are described in 3 adults. Two had longstanding traumatic cataract with secondary strabismus and the other senile cataract and pre-existing strabismus for which she already had surgery with unsatisfactory outcome.

Results: Visual acuity improved in all 3 patients. Satisfactory ocular alignment was achieved with good cosmetic outcome in all cases.

Conclusions: Combined strabismus and cataract surgery in adults is a safe procedure that can optimise visual alignment and improve visual acuity in a single operation.
KEYWORDS: Strabismus, cataract, combined, adults

1 INTRODUCTION

Cataract and strabismus are amongst the commonest pathologies that are encountered by ophthalmologists. However, whilst the potential benefits of combined surgery for cataract and glaucoma,[1] and cataract and vitreoretinal pathologies[2] are well documented, there are very few reports of cataract and strabismus surgery being performed as a combined procedure.[3-6]

We describe three cases of combined strabismus surgery with adjustable sutures and phacoemulsification with intraocular lens (IOL) implantation. All three procedures were done in adult patients with longstanding strabismus. We outline each case and discuss the role that combined surgery may have in the management of such selected patients with symptomatic cataract and strabismus.

2 CASE REPORTS

2.1 *Case 1*

A 43-year-old woman with a history of a penetrating left eye (LE) injury at the age of 5 years treated with iris excision and cornea suturing. She then progressively developed a dense cataract and a convergent LE squint. She attended the eye department concerned mainly for her cosmesis. On examination, her visual acuity (VA) was 6/6 in the right eye (RE) unaided, and light perception (LP) in the LE. She had full range of extraocular movements, and a LE esotropia which measured 40Δ at 6 meters (m) and 45Δ at 1/3m with the Krimsky prism bar reflexion test. In the LE there was a dense white cataract with distorted pupil and multiple anterior and posterior synechiae. Ultrasonography did not revealed any posterior segment abnormalities and there was no afferent pupillary defect. Cycloplegic refraction did not show any refractive error in the RE, and couldn't be performed in the LE.

She underwent a LE medial rectus recession of 9mm on adjustable suture, and a lateral rectus resection of 7mm combined with phacoemulsification with IOL implantation under general anaesthesia (GA). Postoperatively, she was overcorrected and the medial rectus was re-advanced by approximately 2mm. She was discharged home with a VA of 6/60 and a remaining esotropia of 5Δ both for near and distance. On her last visit, 9 months postoperatively, her deviation remains 5Δ for near and distance and her VA 6/60 due to amblyopia and to some pigmentary macular changes, presumably from her old trauma. The final outcome of her combined strabismus and cataract procedure was improved VA and excellent cosmesis.

2.2 *Case 2*

A 75-year- old woman with a history of LE esotropia and amblyopia as a child. She had surgery at the age of 5 years and then she progressively developed a LE divergent squint. Over the last 5 years she noticed a gradual reduction of her LE vision and her divergent squint got worse. On examination, her VA was 6/6 in the RE with –1sphere (sph), and 6/60 in the LE with –5sph. She had full range of extraocular movements, and a LE exotropia which measured 65Δ at 6m and 55Δ at 1/3m with the Krimsky prism bar reflexion test. Slit lamp examination showed a dense nuclear sclerotic cataract in the LE. There was no afferent pupillary defect and dilated fundoscopy did not reveal any abnormalities. Cycloplegic refraction showed a refractive error of –1sph in the RE, and –6.5sph in the LE.

She underwent an exploration of the LE medial rectus which was found at 11mm from the limbus and was re-advanced to 5mm from the limbus. She also underwent a 7mm recession of the lateral rectus on adjustable suture, and phacoemulsification with IOL implantation GA. Postoperatively, she did not require any adjustment and and her VA was 6/24 with –1sph. She was discharged home with a remaining exotropia of 5Δ for near and 10Δ for distance with her spectacles on. On her last visit, 9 months postoperatively, her deviation is 10Δ for near and 15Δ for distance and her VA remains 6/24 due to amblyopia. The final outcome of her combined procedure was improved VA and cosmetically acceptable squint.

2.3 *Case 3*

A 55-year-old man with a history of penetrating RE injury at the age of 12 years. The injury was probably caused by a thorn and was managed conservatively at the time. He then progressively developed a RE divergent squint and a dense cataract. On examination, his VA was hand movements in the RE, and 6/6 unaided in the LE. He had full range of extraocular movements, and a RE exotropia which measured 60Δ at 6m and 50Δ at 1/3m with the Krimsky prism bar reflexion test. Slit lamp examination showed a dense white cataract in the RE. Ultrasonography did not revealed any posterior segment abnormalities and there was no afferent pupillary defect. Cycloplegic refraction showed a refractive error of +0.5sph in the LE, and could not be performed in the RE.

He underwent a RE lateral rectus recession of 10mm on adjustable suture, and a medial rectus resection of 6mm combined with phacoemulsification and IOL implantation under GA. Post-operatively, he was overcorrected and the lateral rectus was re-advanced by approximately 3mm. He was discharged home with a VA of 6/24 with -1sph and a remaining exotropia of 5Δ both for near and distance. On his last visit, 9 months postoperatively, his deviation is 2Δ for near and 5Δ for distance with his spectacles on, and his VA 6/12. The final outcome of his combined strabismus and cataract procedure was improved VA and excellent cosmesis.

3 DISCUSSION

Combined cataract and strabismus surgery was first described by Maltzman *et al* in 1986.[3] They reported a series of ten patients with large angle concomitant exotropia and cataract or aphakia who underwent combined horizontal strabismus and extracapsular cataract surgery or insertion of an anterior chamber IOL. They reported no complications and no long term complaints of diplopia or cosmetic dissatisfaction with an average follow-up of 15 months. There is another case report of combined surgery in an adult involving surgery in only one horizontal muscle,[4] and a report of combined surgery in a series of paediatric cases.[5] Recently, Squirrell *et al* reported a series of three patients undergoing combined strabismus and phacoemulsification with IOL implantation.[6] They had restrictive or paralytic strabismus with intactable diplopia pre-operatively and senile cataracts. They reported no complications, and good results regarding the VA and the post-operative alignment with resolution of the symptomatic diplopia.

We report a series of combined cataract and strabismus surgery in three adult patients with cataract and strabismus of different aetiologies. In all cases strabismus surgery was performed first with the use of adjustable suture technique, and cataract surgery next with phacoemulsification. Visual acuity of the operated eye improved in all cases, and satisfactory post-operative ocular alignment achieved and retained in all 3 patients. No complications were encountered, and all patients noticed a marked cosmetic improvement, while none had long term complaints of diplopia. Ours is the first report of the use of adjustable suture technique for strabismus surgery combined with cataract surgery. We also are the second ones to use modern phacoemulsification cataract surgery for this type of combined procedures. According to our findings combined strabismus and cataract surgery in adults is a safe procedure that can optimise visual alignment and improve visual acuity in a single operation in selected cases.

4 REFERENCES

1. Shields MB. Another reevaluation of combined cataract and glaucoma surgery. *Am J Ophthalmol* 1993;115:806-11.

2. Senn P, Schipper I, Perren B. Combined pars plana vitrectomy, phacoemulsification, and intraocular lens implantation in the capsular bag: a comparison to vitrectomy and subsequent cataract surgery as a two step procedure. *Ophthalmic Surg Lasers* 1995;26:420-8.
3. Maltzman BA, Caputo AR, Cinotti DJ. Combined intraocular lens and strabismus surgery. *J Cataract Refr Surg* 1986;12:65-9.
4. Gayton JL, Ledford JK. Combined cataract and strabismus surgery. *Ann Ophthalmol* 1993;25:295-7.
5. Zwaan J, Al-Sadhan Y. Combined intraocular and strabismus surgery. *Ophthalmic Surg Lasers* 1998;29:456-61.
6. Squirrell D, Edwards M, Burke J. Combined strabismus and phacoemulsification cataract surgery: a useful option in selected patients. *Eye* 2001;15:736-8.

Session 6
Strabismus surgery

Transactions 28th Meeting European Strabismological Association, de Faber (ed.)
© 2004 European Strabismological Association, ISBN 90 265 1965 6

The Early vs. Late Infantile Strabismus Surgery Study:

First Results

Kristina Unnebrink[a], Carmen Bauer[a], Gerold H. Kolling[b], Huib J. Simonsz[c],

For the Early vs. Late Infantile Strabismus Surgery Study Group

[a]Coordination Centre for Clinical Trials, [b]Department. of Ophthalmology,

University of Heidelberg, D-69120 Heidelberg, Germany,

[c]Department of Ophthalmology, University Hospital, NL-3015 Rotterdam, The Netherlands

1. INTRODUCTION

The Early vs. Late Infantile Strabismus Surgery Study Group is a group of strabismologists and orthoptists from 58 clinics in 11 European countries. We investigated whether early or late surgery is preferable in infantile strabismus, in a non-randomised, prospective, multi-centre clinical trial.

2. METHODS

Infants between 6 and 18 months of age received a standardised entry examination[1] and were then operated either before their second anniversary ('early'), or between their 32nd and 60th month of age ('late'). Each of the participating centres had decided to treat all eligible children either early or late, at the beginning of the trial. The children were evaluated at age six. In order to minimise possible assessment bias at the final examinations in this non-randomised study, an external observer was present at every final examination.

3. RESULTS

Recruitment ran from May 1993 until October 1996. Fifty-eight clinics have entered a total of 532 patients (231 early surgery group, 301 late surgery group). We reported before that the two groups were almost similar at entry examination regarding (1) refraction, (2) degree of amblyopia, (3) angle of strabismus and (4) limitation of adduction[2]. The dropout rate of about 25% has been relatively low, considering the very long follow-up period.

On conclusion of the final examinations of the last children in March 2003 the database was closed. The first results were presented at the ESA meeting in June.

Early surgery leads to better stereopsis and higher amount of simultaneous perception than late surgery (p=0.001). This seems to be mainly due to fewer patients in the early treatment group who have no binocular vision at all (32.4% Bagolini negative in the early treatment group, 47.4% in the late one). Only 1% of both groups had positive stereopsis using randomised tests. The classified angle of squint at the final examination does not differ between the two treatment groups (p=0.97). The rate of patients who did not require surgery was higher in the late treatment group (20%) than in the early one (8%).

The quotient of visual acuities is larger in the early treatment group than in the late treatment group (p=0.023), i.e. the degree of amblyopia is slightly less in the early group.

CONCLUSIONS

Normal stereopsis is a rare condition in our study. Convergent angle of squint and amblyopia can be treated successfully in both groups. It is unknown whether the slightly better binocularity in the early group will succeed in a more stable alignment for the next years.

REFERENCES

The Early vs. Late Infantile Strabismus Surgery Study Group (1993): The protocol for the Early vs. Late Infantile Strabismus Surgery Study. *Strabismus* 1, 135-157

Meyer K, Breitschwerdt H, Kolling GH, Simonsz HJ (1998): The Early vs. Late Infantile Strabismus Surgery Study: Do sources for bias exist in this non-randomized trial? *Br J Ophthalmol* 82, 934-938

Unnebrink K, Bauer C, Kolling G, Simonsz HJ (2001): The Early vs. Late Infantile Strabismus Surgery Study: State of the Final Examinations and Some Preliminary Findings. in: Transactions 26th Meeting European Strabismological Association, Barcelona, Spain, September 2000. de Faber JT (Ed.), Swets&Zeitlinger Publishers, Lisse, Abingdon, Extorn (PA), Tokyo, 57-60

ACKNOWLEDGEMENTS

This work was supported by the Deutsche Forschungsgemeinschaft, Bonn, Germany, Ko 1295-1.

Transactions 28th Meeting European Strabismological Association, de Faber (ed.)
© 2004 European Strabismological Association, ISBN 90 265 1965 6

Hardly any difference between bilateral recession (BR) and unilateral recession resection (RR): Results of a controlled, prospective, randomized multicentre study.

J. R. Polling 1 ,M. J. C. Eijkemans 2 ,J. Esser 3 ,B. Lieb 4 ,G. H. Kolling 5 ,E. Schulz 6 ,B. Lorenz 7 , P. Roggenkämper 8 ,V. Herzau 9 ,A. Zubcov 10 ,M. P. M. ten Tusscher 11 ,D. Wittebol-Post 12 ,G. C. Gusek 13 ,H. J. Simonsz 1
Department of ophthalmology 1 &public health 2 ,Erasmus Medical Center Rotterdam,and depart- ment of ophthalmology of the university clinics in Essen 3 ,Freiburg 4 ,Heidelberg 5 ,Hamburg 6 , Regensburg 7 ,Bonn 8 ,Tübingen 9 ,Frankfurt 10 ,Maastricht 11 ,Utrecht 12 and Erlangen 13

Introduction:The choice of BR or RR is not based on evidence and arguments for and against have never been substantiated in a prospective,randomised study. A randomised study with strictly defined inclusion and exclusion criteria was performed among children with infantile esotropia. We analysed differences between the effect of a RR and a BR on the postoperative latent distance angles and the convergence excess.

Methods:From 1998 to 2001, nine German and five Dutch clinics recruited 122 three-to eight- year-old patients with an infantile esotropia,with normal development and in good health. They had never been operated for strabismus before. The exclusion criteria were:binocular vision (Bagolini positive),distance angle >24 °or <10 °,near-angle /distance-angle ratio >3/2,more than 1 line interocular acuity difference,hypermetropia >6D or myopia <-3D,substantial up-or downshoot >8 ° hypertropia in 25 °adduction,V-or A-pattern >8 °or large manifest hypertropia >4 °. All clinics used a consensus,standardised orthoptic examination and surgical techniques. The millimetres of recession and/or resection to operate were calculated by dividing the latent angle at dis- tance fixation (degrees)by 1. 6,the day before surgery. After that the child was randomised to have either BR or RR surgery the following day. The children were seen twice before surgery and twice after surgery,the last visit being three months postoperatively.

Results:Because of strict inclusion criteria 122 patients were included. Hardly any difference bet- ween both techniques was found for either the postoperative latent angle or the postoperative ma- nifest angle. Reduction of convergence excess was slightly greater with the BR,although this was not statistically significant. One third of the patients had postoperative binocular vision and a better alignment. Note,however,that the Bagolini may have become positive because of better alignment, or vice versa.

Transactions 28th Meeting European Strabismological Association, de Faber (ed.)
© 2004 European Strabismological Association, ISBN 90 265 1965 6

The effect of seprafilm on adhesions in strabismus surgery – an experimental study

Seyhan B. Özkan, Erkin Kır,
Adnan Menderes University Medical School Department of Ophthalmology, Aydın, Turkey
Nil Culhacı,
Adnan Menderes University Medical School Department of Pathology, Aydın, Turkey
Volkan Dayanır
Adnan Menderes University Medical School Department of Ophthalmology, Aydın, Turkey

ABSTRACT: The purpose of this study is to histopathologically evaluate the influence of seprafilm on postoperative adhesions. Seven adult rabbits were used for the study. The superior rectus (SR) muscle was resected and limbal conjunctival dissection was done inferonasally in both eyes. Seprafilm was inserted between the conjunctiva and SR, and under the dissected inferonasal conjunctiva of one eye. The fellow eyes served as controls. Histopathological sections were obtained on 6th postoperative week. There was no significant difference between the seprafilm inserted and control eyes with regard to inflammation, neither at the area of SR resection nor at the area of conjunctival dissection. Fibrosis was significantly less in the surgical areas where seprafilm was used as compared to the control groups. It is concluded that application of seprafilm may prove useful in strabismus surgery especially where adhesion formation may influence the outcome, and in cases where recurrent conjunctival dissection may be needed.
KEY WORDS: Adhesion, seprafilm, strabismus surgery.

1. INTRODUCTION

One of the major problems in strabismus surgery is the development of postoperative adhesions particularly in patients who require multiple surgeries. The adhesions may involve conjunctiva, Tenon's capsule, intermuscular membrane, orbital fat, sclera and extraocular muscle. The formation of such a scar tissue may affect the function of extraocular muscles and may result in motility problems that may alter the outcome of surgery.

In an attempt to decrease surgical adhesions, various materials and medicines are used such as supramide (Supramide Extra; S.Jackson Inc., Alexandra, Va), silicone sleeve, vicryl mesh, polypeptide sleeve, oxidized regenerated cellulose sleeve (Interceed; Johnson and Johnson Medical, Arlington, Texas), sodium hyaluronate, mitomycin C and 5 fluorouracil (1-11). None of these modalities carry the properties of an ideal material convenient for routine strabismus surgery. Seprafilm (Seprafilm ™, Genzyme Corp., Cambridge, MA) is a bioabsorbable membrane composed of sodium hyaluronate and carboxymethylcellulose and it has been used to decrease adhesions mainly in abdominal surgery. In a series of four patients Assaf (12) reported that seprafilm is tolerated well by ocular tissues in patients with previous adhesions. In that report only the tolerance of seprafilm was evaluated and it was suggested that seprafilm might be a potentially useful material to be used in strabismus surgery. To the best of our knowledge there is no report about the histopathological effect of seprafilm in ocular surgery.

The purpose of this study is to evaluate the effect of seprafilm on postoperative scar and adhesion formation histopathologically in an experimental model.

2. MATERIALS AND METHODS

This study was performed after the approval of Animal Ethics Committee of Adnan Menderes University. Seven adult male New Zealand albino rabbits weighing about 3kg were used. Xalazin hydrochloride (5mg/kg) and ketamine hydrochloride (3.5mg/kg) were used for anaesthesia. Limbal conjunctiva was incised at the superior quadrant. Superior rectus was isolated and secured with a muscle hook. Two knots with 6/0 vicryl (Ethicon Inc., Sommerville, NJ) suture were placed on the sides 3mm from the muscle insertion. Following resection, it was resutured to the original insertion. Seprafilm, measuring 9x7mm, was placed between the resected muscle and conjunctiva (Group 1). The fellow eye served as control and the same procedure was repeated without the insertion of seprafilm (Group 2). Conjunctiva was closed with 7/0 Vicryl (Ethicon Inc., Sommerville, NJ) sutures. In the inferonasal region, a fornix based limbal conjunctival dissection was performed where seprafilm, measuring 7x5mm, was placed (Group 3) under the conjunctiva before closure with 7/0 vicryl suture while the fellow eye served as the control (Group 4). The dissection is performed in a large area to promote more tissue reaction. Rabbits were sacrificed with intravenous pentobarbital 6 weeks after the surgery and both eyes were enucleated.

All specimens were examined by one pathologist in a masked fashion. The eyes were fixed in buffered formalin and serial cuts were taken through the superior rectus, and inferonasal conjunctival region. They were then embedded in paraffin. Serial sections 4µm in thickness were taken from each block and stained with hematoxylin-eosin for histopathological examination of inflammation. The specimens were also stained with Masson trichrome to demonstrate collagen fibers, and were graded for the amount of scar tissue formation. Inflammation and fibrosis were graded on a scale of 0-4 (2,6).

The inflammatory reaction is composed of lymphocytes, plasma cells, histiocyres, and polymorphonuclear leukocytes. The grades were: 0, no inflammation; 1, a few lymphocyte and plasma cell beneath the epithelium; 2, mild inflammatory infiltrate composed of lymphocytes, plasma cells and polymorphonuclear leukocytes beneath the epithelium and congestion; 3, grade 2 plus neutrophils in the epithelium; 4, high concentrations (collections) of lymphocytes, plasma cells, polymorphonuclear leukocytes, and histiocytes both intraepithelial and subepithelial and ulceration.

A scale of 0 to 4 for fibrosis was based on the amount of collagen formation. 0: no fibrosis, 1: mild perimusculer fibrotic reaction (stained collagen was detectable only in thin bands immediately adjacent to muscle), 2: easily detected thick bands, 3: well developed, dense bands of collagen, 4: a severe fibrotic response replacing large areas.

Statistical analysis was performed with "Wilcoxon signed ranks test".

3. RESULTS

Table 1 demonstrates the mean values of inflammation and fibrosis in the 4 groups. There were no signs of muscle necrosis in any cases. Neither the resected superior rectus region nor the dissected inferonasal conjunctival region where seprafilm was used, differed statistically from the control group with regard to inflammation (p=0.655 and p=0.157 respectively). However, both regions showed significantly less fibrosis than the control groups; p=0.046 for the superior rectus and p=0.015 for the inferonasal regions (Table 1).

Table 1. Histopathologic evaluation of inflammation and fibrosis

	Area Of Superior Rectus Resection			Area of Inferonasal conjunctiva dissection		
	Group 1	Group 2	P*	Group 3	Group 4	P*
Inflammation	0.71±0.95	0.85±0.37	0.655	1.85±0.37	2.42±0.53	0.157
Fibrosis	0.57±0.71	1.14±0.37	0.046	0.71±0.48	2.14±0.37	0.015

*Wilcoxon signed ranks test

4. DISCUSSION

Predictability of the outcome of strabismus surgery has always been a problem even in uncomplicated cases. The variability of the dose response relation is a well known entity in strabismus surgery and thus reoperations may be inevitable in particular cases. Reoperation represents a complicated procedure for the strabismus surgeon since such cases carry the risk of conversion of a concomitant deviation into a restrictive type. Restriction develops related to the fibrous tissue and adhesion formation involving conjunctiva, Tenon's capsule, extraocular muscle, intermuscular membrane and sometimes orbital fat tissue. Such adhesions may prevent the normal functional effect of contraction of an extraocular muscle and prove a strabismus surgery ineffective. Once the adhesions develop, it is very difficult to reverse its effect. Control of haemorrhage, gentle surgical technique, and prevention of excess cautery are also necessary measures to reduce postoperative adhesions. Inflammatory reaction related to postoperative infection or suture reaction may also lead to formation of adhesions. Despite all measures multiple operations create a cumulative effect for development of adhesions (6). Various materials and pharmaceutics have been tried to lessen postoperative adhesion and scar formation. Supramid plastic sleeve (1) and silicone sleeve (5) are nonabsorbable materials that act by forming a mechanical barrier. They are currently not in use, and are known to lead to infection and foreign body reaction. Absorbable materials as Interceed, vicryl mesh and polypeptide sleeve are also not recognized as decreasing adhesion formation (7,8,10). The results on the effect of sodium hyaluronate, which is absorbable are contradictory. Fulga et al. (13) reported sodium hyaluronate as ineffective in prevention of adhesion formation in a rabbit model; whereas Searl et al.(6) and Yaacobi et al. (8) reported a favourable result. Experimental studies utilizing antimetabolites mitomycin C and 5-fluorouracil had positive results in decreasing adhesion formation (2,9). However these agents have the potential risk of serious side effects. Antimetabolites are known to cause severe corneal and scleral complications in their use in glaucoma and pterygium surgery (14-16). They are known to decrease vascularity and are also thought to increase the risk of anterior segment ischemia in patients who have undergone multiple strabismus surgeries (2,11,17).

Seprafilm is an absorbable membrane composed of sodium hyaluronate and carboxymethylcellulose both of which are anionic polysaccharides. Hyaluronate is ubiquitously present in soft tissues, synovial fluid, umbilical cord and vitreous. Carboxymethylcellulose has widespread application in the pharmaceutical and chemical industries.

In our experience, once seprafilm is in contact with the tissue it is more difficult to reposition it and following hydration of the material it glides easily and may lose its location. The surgeon must be careful during first positioning and additional sutures may be required especially at the limbal area to prevent slippage of seprafilm through the corneal surface.

Seprafilm is produced in a large size to be used in large surgical areas and the cost of the material unnecessarily increases for ophthalmic use. We suggest that seprafilm in a convenient size for ophthalmic use may decrease the cost of the material and facilitate its use in routine strabismus surgery without significant additional cost.

Seprafilm has been observed to separate tissues by forming a temporary barrier and hence decrease adhesions (18). Adhesions have been histopathologically shown to decrease when seprafilm is used in gynecological and intraabdominal surgeries (19,20). Current literature has no histopathologic data evaluating the effect of seprafilm use on adhesions in ophthalmic surgery.

This study shows that fibrosis which is a sign of adhesion, is significantly less in the seprafilm utilized surgical areas as compared to control. Seprafilm significantly decreases postoperative adhesion formation between the conjunctiva and muscle in muscle surgery group and between the conjunctiva and sclera in conjunctival surgery group. The placement of such a material may be useful in other ophthalmic surgeries such as retinal detachment surgery where adhesion formation may create serious additional problems. The results of our study demonstrated that seprafilm may be useful in strabismus surgery especially where adhesion formation may be expected to influence the outcome, and in cases where recurrent conjunctival dissection may be needed.

REFERENCES

Dunlap EA. Surgery of muscle adhesions and effects of multiple operations. Br J Ophthalmol 1974;58:307-12.

Mora JS, Sprunger DT, Helvesten EM, Evan AP. Intraoperative sponge 5-fluorouracil to reduce postoperative scarring in strabismus surgery. J AAPOS 1997;1:92-7.

Beck DE. The role of seprafilm bioresorbable membran in adhesion prevention. Eur J Surg Suppl 1997;577: 49-55.

Urban RC, Kaufman LM. Mitomycin in the treatment of hypertrophic conjunctival scars after strabismus surgery. J Pediatr Ophthalmol Strabismus 1994;31(2):96-8.

Morales AG, Polack FM, Arata AF. Silicone implant to extraocular muscles. Br J Ophthalmol 1966; 50: 235-44.

Searl SS, Metz HS, Lindahl KJ. The use of sodium hyalorunate as a biologic sleeve in strabismus surgery. Ann Ophthalmol 1987;19:259-68.

Elsas FJ, Gowda DC, Urry DW. Synthetic polypeptide for strabismus surgery. J Pediatr Ophthalmol Strabismus 1992;29(5):284-6.

Yaacobi Y, Hamed LM, Kaul KS, Fanous MM. Reduction of postoperative adhesions secondary to strabismus surgery in rabbits. Ophthalmic Surg 1992;23(2):123-8.

Cruz OA, Matkovich L. Effects of intraoperative topical mitomycin C on strabismus surgery in the rabbit: a preliminary study. Ophthalmic Surg 1995;26:237-40.

Sondhi N, Ellis FD, Hamed LM, Helveston EM. Evaluation of an absorbable muscle sleeve to limit postoperative adhesions in strabismus surgery. Ophthalmic Surg 1987;18:441-3.

Cruz OA, Evaluation of mitomycin to limit postoperative adhesions in strabismus surgery. J Pediatr Ophthalmol Strabismus 1996;33:89-92.

Assaf AA. Seprafilm in repeated strabismus surgery to reduce surgical scarring. Advances in Strabismology: G. Lennerstrand (ed.) pp.377-80.

Fulga V, Koren R, Ezov N, Gal R, Nimrod A, Savir H. Sodium hyaluronate as a tool in strabismus surgery in rabbits. Ophthalmic Surg Lasers 1996;27(3):228-33.

Dougherty PJ, Hardten DR, Lindstrom RL. Corneoscleral melt after pterygium surgery using a single intraoperative application of mitomycin- C. Cornea 1996;15(5):537-40.

Manche EE, Afshari MA, Singh K. Delayed corneal epitheliopathy after antimetabolite augmented trabeculectomy. J Glaucoma 1998;7(4):237-9.

Knapp A, Heuer DK, Stern GA, Driebe WT Jr. Serious corneal complications of glaucoma filtering surgery with postoperative 5-flourouracil. Am J Ophthalmol 1987;103(2):183-7.

Smith S, D'Amore PA, Dreyer EB. Comparative toxicity of mitomycin C and 5-fluorouracil in vitro. Am J Ophthalmol 1994;118(3):332-7.

Skinner KC, Colt MJ, Carver RC, Burns JW. The evaluation of HAL-F bioabsorbable membrane for the prevention of postsurgical adhesion formation in two animal models. Proceedings of the 2nd International Symposium on Post Surgical Adhesions and Gynecologic Surgery, Palm Beach FL, 1992.

Vrijland WW, Tseng LN, Eijkman HJ, Hop WC, Jakimowicz JJ, Leguit P, Stassen LP, Swank DJ, Haverlag R, Bonjer HJ, Jeekel H. Fewer intraperitoneal adhesions with use of hyaluronic acid-carboxymethylcellulose membrane: a randomized clinical trial. Ann Surg 2002;235(2):193-9.

Tsapanos VS, Stathopoulou LP, Papathanassopoulou VS, Tzingounis VA. The role of Seprafilm bioresorbable membrane in the prevention and therapy of endometrial synechiae. J Biomed Mater Res 2002;63(1):10-4.

Transactions 28th Meeting European Strabismological Association, de Faber (ed.)

Antinomic deviations: Esodevation associated with exodevation

Alain C SPIELMANN, Annette SPIELMANN
Nancy - FRANCE

ABSTRACT
Introduction : Antinomic deviations are defined as a basic exoposition of the eyes associated with innervational convergence excess leading to esoposition.
Material and Methods : 34 patients with both Exodeviation (X) and Esodeviation (E) were studied. Surgery consisted in Lateral Recti (LR) recess with Fadenoperation on the Medial Recti (MR).
Results : Four types of antinomic deviations were found :
- Primitive X with excess of physiological accommodative vergences.
- Consecutive X due to surgical overcorrection of an accommodative esotropia.
- Infantile X with fixation in adduction, DHD ± convergence excess.
- Consecutive infantile X: overcorrection of a congenital esotropia
Conclusion : Although Fadenoperation on MR may seem paradoxical in exodeviations, it is the most logical procedure to deal with convergence excess and fixation in adduction prevalence.

KEYWORDS : Antinomic deviation, Convergence excess, Esotropia, Exotropia, Fixation in adduction, Surgery.

1. INTRODUCTION

The term ''antinomic'' seems very appropriate to define strabismus associating a basic exodeviation with convergence excess or fixation in adduction prevalence leading to esodeviation. A retrospective study was carried out to evaluate the clinical features of these strabismus and the surgical results of LR recess associated with MR posterior fixation suture.

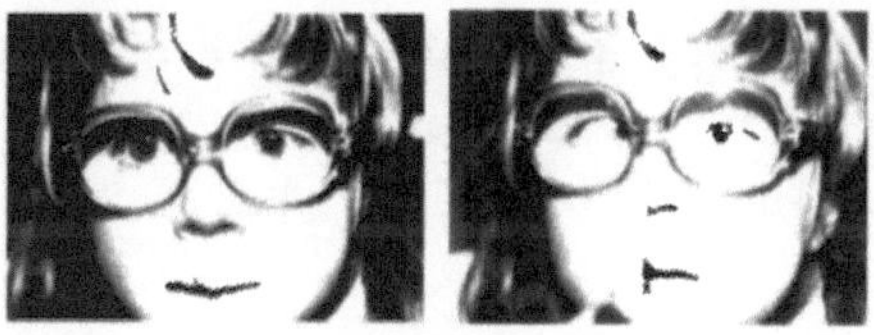

Fig 1 : typical antinomic deviation patient with fully corrected hyperopia

X at distance fixation
E at near fixation

2. MATERIAL AND METHODS

34 files of patients operated on by LR recess and MR Fadenoperation from 1995 to 2002 were studied. Some of them were infantile X with abnormal innervations such as fixation in adduction and DHD. In these cases, one eye is in a position of adduction when fixing, but is in exoposition when fixation is shifted to the other eye or under occlusion (= monocular eso / exodeviations). The range of deviation was studied pre- and post-operatively : from the maximal X with full optical correction to the maximal E at near fixation with or without glasses (in some cases, it was a minimal X but with fixation in adduction prevalence). The surgical

procedure was : 1) for the maximal X : unilateral (11 cases) or bilateral (23 cases) LR recess (adjustable suture in 20 cases). 2) for the convergence excess and the fixation in adduction : Fadenoperation on both MR.

Results (fig. 2 to 5, graphs I and II)
Four clinical types of antinomic deviations have been identified :
1 : Primitive antinomic exotropia : exoposition with excess of physiological accommodative vergences (fig 2)

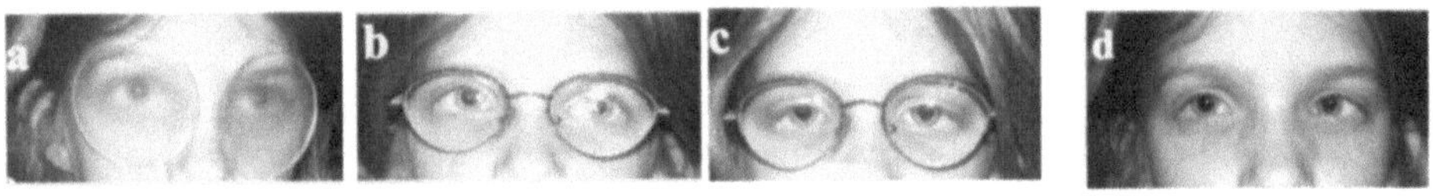

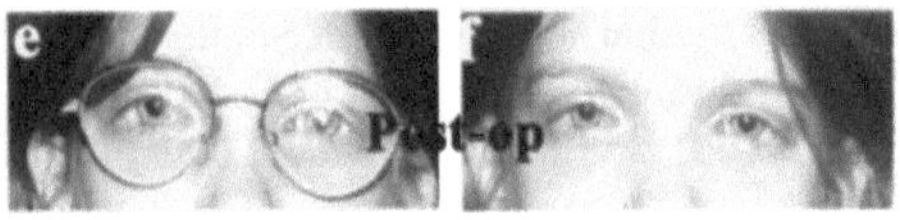

*Fig. 2 :a) X without fixation, b) X with glasses, c) E at near fixation, diplopia,
d) E without glasses, e) postop.orthophoria with glasses f)) postop.orthophoria without glasses*

2 : Consecutive antinomic exotropia : surgical overcorrection of the basic position of an accommodative esotropia with undercorrection of the innervationnal deviation.

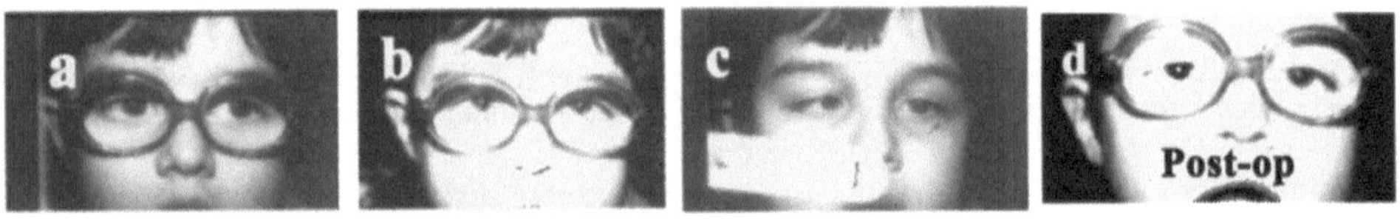

Fig. 3 : a) usual expositon at distance fixation, b) small eotropia at distance fixation, c) esotropia at near fixation without glasses, d) postoperative orthophoria

GRAPH 1 Group 1 and group 2
1- Antinomic EXO 6 cases *2- Antinomic Consecutive EXO 8 cases*

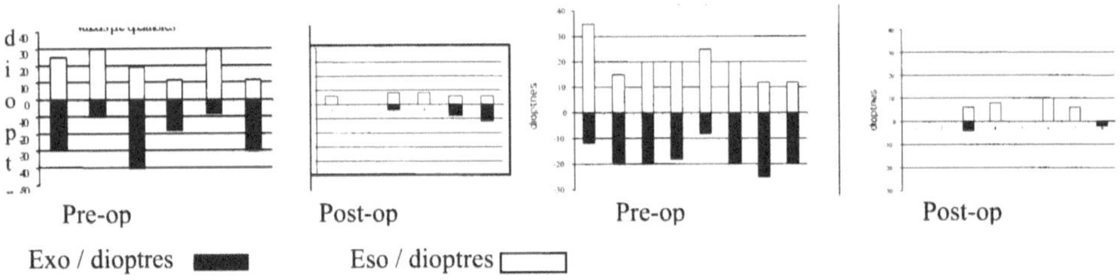

3 : Infantile antinomic exotropia : basic exoposition with abnormal innervations : fixation in adduction (+/- MLN), DHD ± accommodative deviations
3a) with 'binocular' esodeviation
3b) with monocular esodeviation (fixation in adduction prevalence)

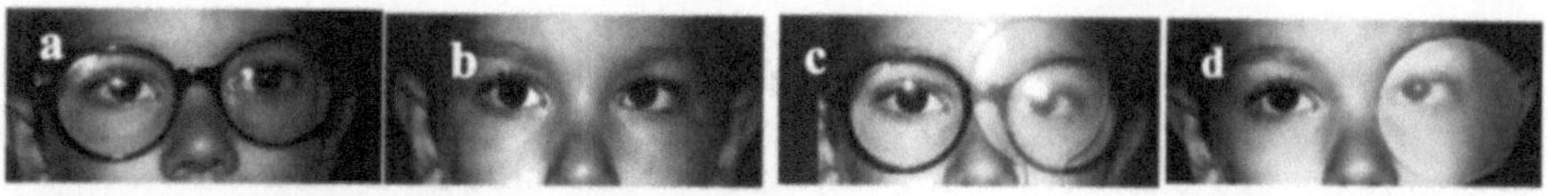

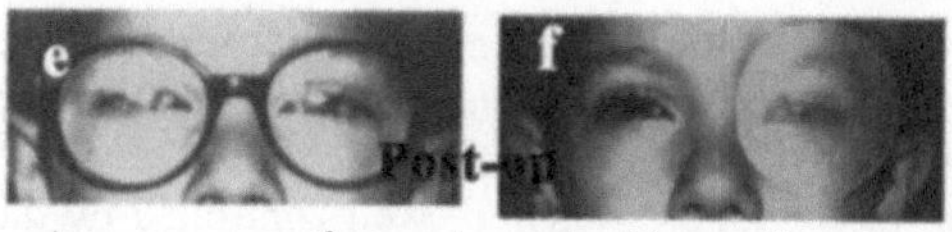

Fig. 4 : a) X with full optical correction b) E without glasses c) E under occlusion DHD d) convergence excess without glasses DHD and DVD e) post-op : orthotropia.with glasses f) orthotropia, without glasses no occlusion eso

4 : Consecutive infantile antinomic exotropia : overcorrection of an infantile esotropia with abnormal innervations ± accommodative deviations

4a) with 'binocular' esodeviation

4b) with monocular esodeviation (fixation in adduction prevalence)

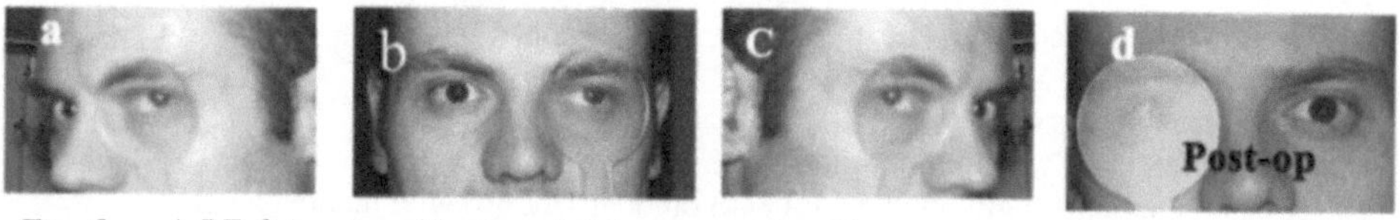

Fig. 5 : a) RE fixing in adduction, LE in exoposition b) exoposition c)LE fixing in adduction, RE in exoposition. d) postoperative result : orthotropia, no head posture.

GRAPH II Group 3 and group 4

Antinomic primitive infantile exotropia 12 cases | *Antinomic consecutive infantile exotropia 9cases*

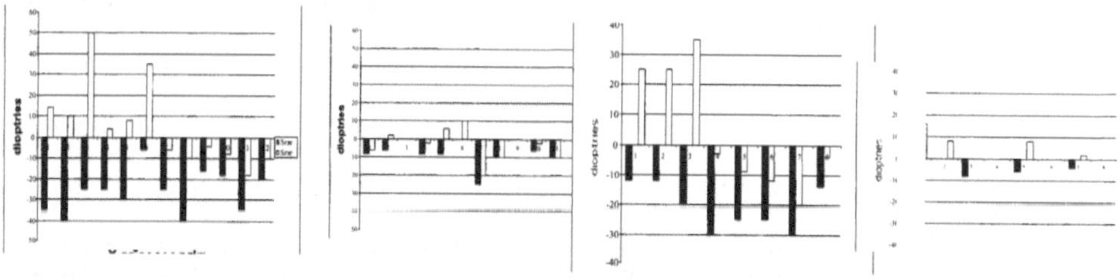

3. DISCUSSION

Intermittent exotropias with convergence excess have been studied for a long time (1, 2, 3, 4, 5). The possibility that the convergence excess could lead to a genuine esodeviation was already known but a study of these rare cases had never been carried out. We named these cases antinomic deviations. The convergence excess can come not only from accommodative innervations (refractive error or high AC/A ratio) but also from abnormal innervations in cases of infantile strabismus. Antinomic deviations are different from intermittent exotropia since the diminution of the angle is not due to fusional vergences : they lead to esotropia but not to orthophoria. Antinomic deviations are different from antipodean deviations due to anisometropia when the angle of deviation is different according to the fixing eye (6).

Many cases had already been operated on. Consecutive exotropias were the results of large recess of the MR without Fadenoperation. Some cases were linked to hyperopia without full optical correction. Conversely, many other cases had already undergone surgery with undercorrection as a result (surgeon frightened by the major convergence excess ?).

Our surgical results are good in all our groups of antinomic deviations. The outcome may be less predictable in the group of infantile X (younger age with no adjustable surgery, lack of binocular vision and intensity of abnormal innervations).
The convergence excess, as well as the fixation in adduction, was very well controlled by the fadenoperation, despite the LR recess. The mean remaining distance/near differences were inferior to 10 dioptres in all our groups.

4. CONCLUSION

Antinomic X, association of an exodeviation with an esodeviation, are characterised by a basic exoposition with major convergence excess and/or fixation in adduction prevalence. A classification is proposed :
1 : Primitive antinomic X
2 : Consecutive antinomic X
3 : Infantile antinomic X : 3a) with binocular E, 3b) with monocular E
4 : Consecutive infantile antinomic X :4a) with binocular E, 4b) with monocular E
Although the use of a Fadenoperation on the MR may seem paradoxical in an exodeviation, this is the most rational procedure to deal with the convergence excess. LR adjustable recessions appear safer and more predictable in these difficult cases.

REFERENCES

1 - Brodsky MC, Fray KJ – Surgical management of intermittent exotropia with high AC/A ratio. *J.AAPOS*. 2 : 330-332, 1998.
2 - Kushner BJ _ Selective surgery for intermittent exotropia based on distance/near differencies. *Arch Ophthalmol.*. 116 : 324-328, 1998.
3 - Kushner BJ – Diagnosis and treatment of exotropia with high accommodation ratio. *Arch Ophthalmol.* 177 : 221-224, 1999.
4 - Kushner BJ, Morton GV – Distance/near differences in intermittent exotropia. *Arch. Ophthalmol.* 116: 478-486, 1998.
5 - Roth A, Rossillion B, Delarue L, Huguenin F – Intermittent exotropia with convergence excess. In : JT de Faber ed. : Transaction of the XXVII ESA-meeting, Florence. pp.93-96. Swets & Zeitlinger Pub. 2001.
6 - Shippman S, Hermann JS : Antipodean squint. *J Pediatr Ophyhalomol Strabismus.* 15 : 210, 1978.

Transactions 28th Meeting European Strabismological Association, de Faber (ed.)

Comparison of modified anchored "hang-back technique" (HBT) with conventional HBT in bi-medial rectus recession (BMR)

Andrew K K Chung, Shafiq U Rehman, John A Bradbury
Ophthalmology Department, Bradford Royal Infirmary, Bradford, West Yorkshire, United Kingdom.

Objective: A prospective study to establish whether BMR using modified HBT is comparable to conventional HBT.

Methods: Consecutive patients under the age of 16 underwent BMR during 1999 and 2000 with at least 6 months post-operative follow-up period were included.In 1999, all patients had operations performed with conventional HBT whereas those in 2000 were carried out with modified HBT. Angles of strabismus were measured pre-operatively and at 2 weeks, 2 months and 6 months post-operatively.

Results: 39 and 43 patients underwent BMR using conventional and modified HBT respectively. Pre-operative angles for near and distance were 43.6D vs 43.5D and 36.4D vs 36.8D. At 6 months post-op, the mean angles for near and distance were 6.4D (range:35D Eso – 40D Exo)and 5.4D (range:35D Eso – 35D Exo))in the conventional group:8.1D (range:35D Eso – 20 Exo)and 6.3D (range:35D Eso-25D Exo)in the modified group. The overall success rate (alignment to within 10D of orthotropia for distance and near)was similar between the two groups (conventional HBT:69.2%vs modified HBT:67.4%, p=0.352).However, modified HBT was found to be associated with significantly lower consecutive exotropia rate at 6 months post-op (4.7%vs 20.5%, p=0.031)

Conclusion: BMR using modified HBT is as effective as conventional HBT but with significantly lower rate of consecutive exotropia.

Transactions 28th Meeting European Strabismological Association, de Faber (ed.)
© 2004 European Strabismological Association, ISBN 90 265 1965 6

Parameters to calculate the amount of conventional eye muscle surgery

André Roth, MD
Medical School, University of Geneva (CH)

ABSTRACT: Conventional surgery is calculated on the basis of the waking-state angle. In order to reduce the variance of the results, passive force imbalance in the horizontal rectus pair should be taken into account. *Patients and method*: In 80 children with infantile esotropia the angle under anaesthesia and the differential of muscle extensibility were assessed. Bilateral posterior fixation and uni or bilateral medial rectus recessions, adjusted if necessary during surgery according to the intra-operative data, were carried out. *Results*: The postoperative minimum angle was most often between –4° and + 4° in the cases where adjustment was carried out. *Discussion and conclusion*: The results 1) demonstrate the validity of intra-operative data as additional parameters, 2) suggest that by taking these into account variance in results is reduced.
KEYWORDS: Conventional eye muscle surgery, amount of recession, eye position under anaesthesia, muscle stretch test, differential of passive muscles forces.

The squint angle in infantile esotropia is variable, with basic components such as the imbalance of tonic vergence and the anatomized part of the deviation and variable components, including Bielschowsky's compensatory movements (insignificant in infantile esotropia) and accommodation or non accommodation-dependent convergence excess. The basic components, corresponding to the minimum angle, will be corrected by conventional surgery, the variable by posterior fixation sutures.

For the conventional surgery, calculations are usually based on one parameter only, the waking-state angle, with the amount of surgery calculated to best correct the minimum angle. We know, however, that the greater the number of parameters taken into account, the smaller the variance in results will be. The purpose of this study is to confirm that intra-operative data can be valid additional parameters from both the theoretical and clinical point of view.

PATIENTS AND METHOD

A series of 80 children underwent surgery for infantile esotropia, with ages ranging from 11 to 100 months (median 44 months) from 1994 to 1998.

Bilateral medial rectus posterior fixation sutures combined with uni or bilateral recession were carried out in all cases. The global amount of recession was calculated on the basis of the minimum angle in the waking state, this ranging from 0° to 17° (figure 1). The mean recession effectiveness on the minimum angle is given as 1.5°/mm in the case of two-muscle surgery of medium value [1]. This amount has, however, to be reduced by 1/3 when recession if combined with posterior fixation sutures, leading to a value of 0.45 mm per 1° of minimal angle. The global amount was then distributed between the two medial recti and adjusted if necessary during surgery according to intra-operative data. The present study, still in progress, is confined to the effect on the postoperative minimum angle.

Intra-operative data were recorded prospectively and assessed under deep and stable anaesthesia with over 90% muscle relaxation, this latter being obtained by non-depolarizing curarization, according to the method already described [2].

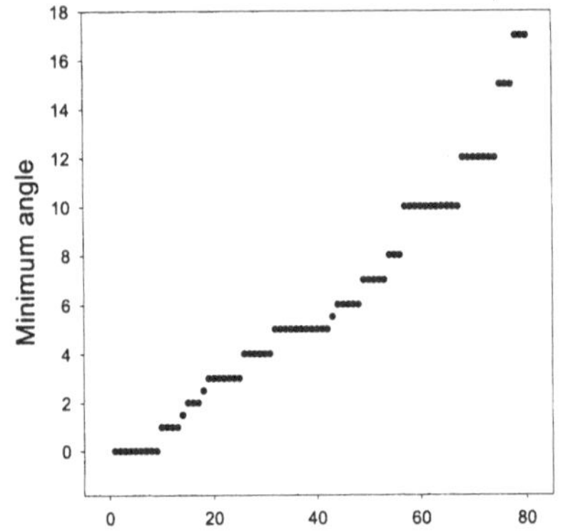

Fig.1 : The preoperative minimum angle in waking state in 80 children with infantile esotropia (ranging from 0° to 17°) in order of increasing angle size.

First intra-operative parameter: angle under anaesthesia

Eye- position under general anaesthesia was assessed by Hirschberg's corneal reflections using a spotlight centred vertically 1 m above and between the patient's eyes (taking into account a parallactic error of 3° per eye) [2]. The horizontal angle under anaesthesia results from passive tension exerted by the medial and lateral recti and their musculo-fibro-elastic situation.

Second intra-operative parameter: differential of muscle extensibility

The imbalance of passive muscle tension in an antagonistic horizontal muscle pair can be better evaluated by measuring its inverse function, muscle extensibility. This latter was measured by the muscle stretch test using the Rapp-Roth myometer on all four horizontal recti (using a small buttonhole incision through the conjunctiva and Tenon's capsule for the lateral rectus).

This is essential because, "considered in isolation, the extensibility of a muscle cannot be interpreted by itself alone; its significance (and the imbalance in an antagonistic muscle pair) depends equally on the extensibility of the ipsilateral antagonist"; moreover there was "no correlation between the values measured in a muscle pair" [2] ($r^2 = 0.004$) (figure 2). A differential of extensibility (or gradient) can, on the other hand, be calculated [3]:

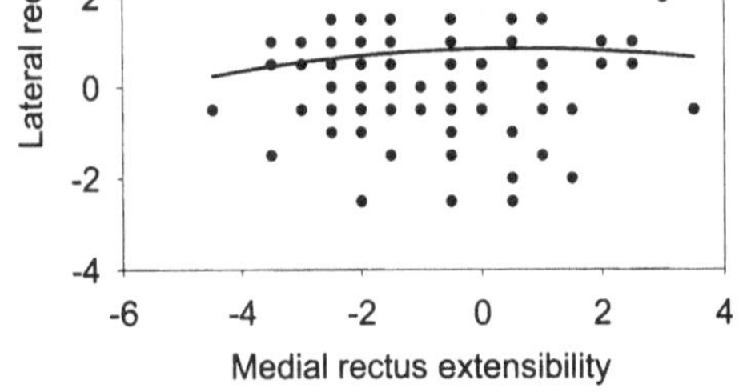

Fig. 2 : Extensibility of lateral rectus versus extensibility of medial rectus in 160 eyes (80 patients): there was no correlation (several symbols represent more than one eye). N = 160, $r^2 = 0.004$

differential = extensibility of lateral rectus minus extensibility of medial rectus.

The differential expresses the balance or imbalance between the two muscles; "it may be zero, or positive indicating a imbalance towards convergence, or negative indicating an imbalance towards divergence" [2].

RESULTS

Validity of the intra-operative data as additional parameters
In our series the angle under general anaesthesia ranged from –16° to + 20° and showed significant correlation with the minimum angle ($p < 0.001$) (figure 3a). The coefficient r^2 was 0.29, indicating that the two parameters are nonetheless partially independent.

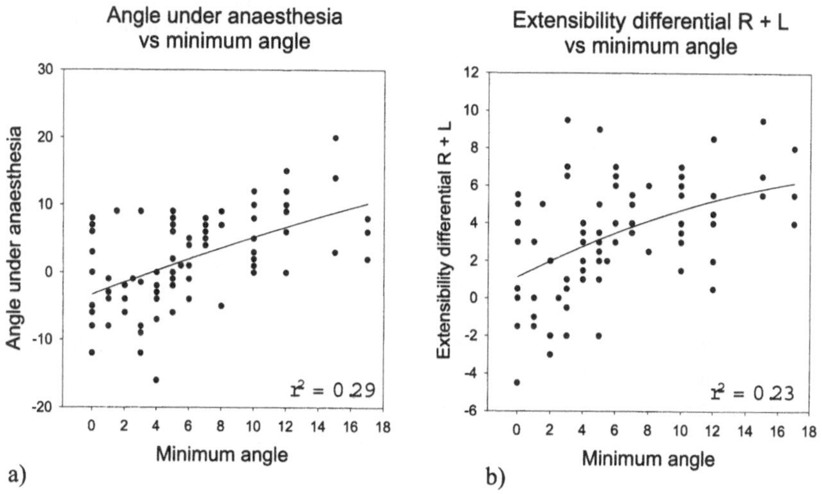

Fig. 3 : Correlation between
a) angle under anaesthesia and minimum angle (N = 0.80)
b) sum of the differential of extensibility of both eyes and minimum angle (N = 0.80)

The correlation of the sum of the differential of the two eyes was equally good both with the minimum angle ($p < 0.001$, $r^2 = 0.23$) and the angle under anaesthesia ($p < 0.001$, $r^2 = 0.36$), shown in graphs 3b and 3c (figures 3b and c). The second order regression curve on graph 3c, (deleting 2 outlayers indicated by open circles) is almost linear with $r^2 = 0.36$ (0.32 including the 2 deleted cases).

Surgical outcome on the minimum angle
49 children were followed up over two to seven years. After two years the results remained stable. Figure 4 shows that, as a general rule, the amount of recession was increased for small angles and decreased for large angles.

Table I: Postoperative results according to the adjustment carried out (see text)

Amount / minimum angle ratio	< 0.4	0.4 – 0.5	> 0.5	Total (N = 49)
Microtropia -2° to +4°	8	14	15	37 (75.5%)
Exotropia -7° to –18°	3		1	4
Esotropia 5° to 10°	1	6	1	8

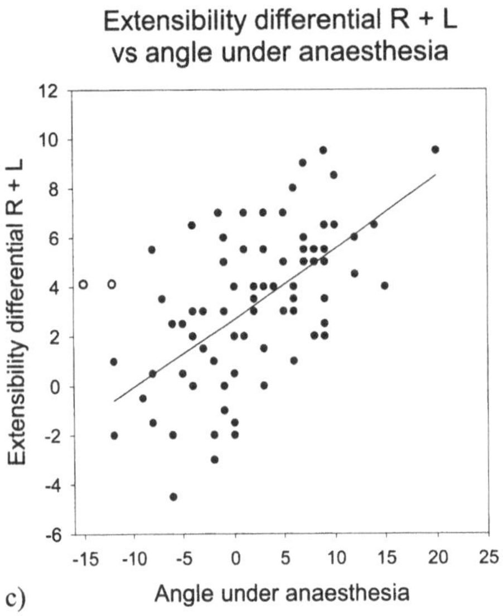

c)

Fig.3: c) sum of the differential of extensibility of both eyes and angle under anaesthesia, two outlayers being deleted (open circles). N = 78, $r^2 = 0.36$

The results, summarized in Table I, show that the expected values were obtained without any intra-operative adjustment in 20 cases (ratio of global recession carried out to that calculated between 0.4 and 0.5), and with adjustment in 29 cases (in 12 cases the amount was reduced [ratio <0.4], in 17 cases increased [ratio > 0.5]). Microtropia (-4° to +4°) was obtained in 37 cases (75.5%), 14 of these without, and 23 with, adjustment. In 12 cases, however, the results were outside the expected value, 6 without any adjustment and 6 despite adjustment.

DISCUSSION

Intra-operative data show significant correlation with the minimum angle in the waking state and between themselves but remain, nevertheless, partially independent. The angle under anaesthesia and the extensibility differential can therefore be considered as additional parameters for the calculation of the amount of recession.

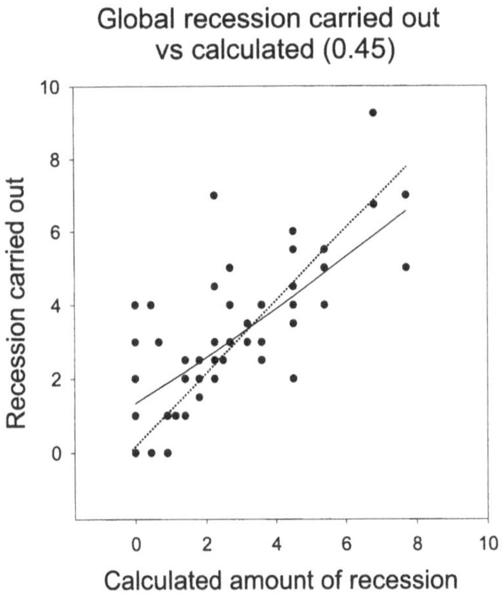

Fig. 4 : Global amount of recession carried out (unbroken line) versus calculated (dotted line 0.45/1° minimum angle)

At the beginning of the study we adjusted, as was our custom, the amount of global recession according to the extensibility of the medial rectus only, reducing it if the extensibility was reduced and conversely. It soon became clear, however, that this strategy was not entirely satisfactory. We decided to make adjustments according to the differential of extensibility, i.e. to increase the amount of recession in the case of imbalance towards convergence and to reduce or even renounce it in the case of imbalance towards divergence, as indicated in Table II.

Table II : guidelines for intra-operative adjustment

E.P.A. / E.D.	Convergent	Straight	Divergent
≥ + *1*	recession up to 4-5 mm max.*	recession up to 2-3 mm max.*	according to min. angle
0 to < +1	recession up to 2-3 mm max.*	according to min. angle	no recession
< *0*	according to min. angle	no recession	plication

EPA eye position under anaesthesia, ED extensibility differential
* on each medial rectus

A good result was obtained in14 out of 20 cases (70%) without adjustment, and in 23 out of 29 (79%) with adjustment. The confidence interval is too small, however, for the difference to be significant. Of the 12 unsatisfactory results, however, no or too little adjustment was made in 4 cases, inverse in 5 (see above). For the remainder, intra-operative data were contradictory on two occasions (one of the outlayer, figure 3c) and in one case misleading (intra-operative data indicating a trend towards convergence but an overcorrection of –7°, despite a low coefficient of 0.29) (figure 5).

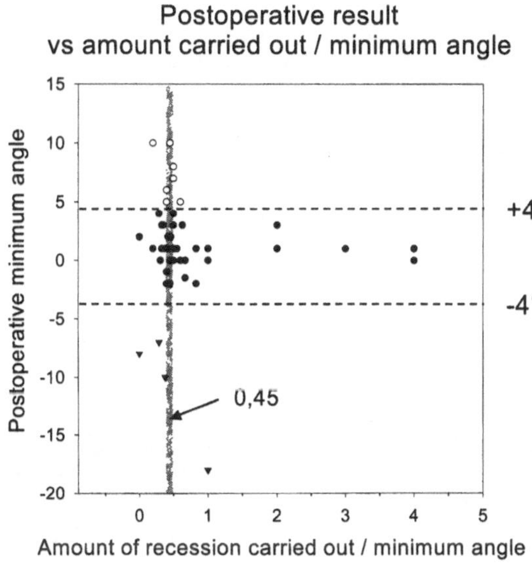

Fig. 5 : Results as a function of the ratio between the amount carried out and the minimum angle

CONCLUSION: Calculation of the amount of conventional muscle surgery is a matter for parametric calculation. Our study shows that intra-operative data are useful additional parameters that, when taken into account, significantly reduce the variance of results.

REFERENCES

1. KAUFMANN H. – *Strabismus.* F. Enke, Stuttgart, 2nd ed., 1995.

2. ROTH A., SPEEG-SCHATZ Cl. – *Eye muscle surgery.* Swetz & Zeitlinger, publ., Lisse, NL, 2001.

3. ROTH A:, SANSONETTI-FERRARIO A., DRAME S. – The gradient of passive muscle forces measured during eye-muscle surgery for concomitant strabismus. In: SPIRITUS M., ed.: Trans. 24th ESA Meeting 1997, Aelous Press, NL, 1998: pp. 45-48.

Transactions 28th Meeting European Strabismological Association, de Faber (ed.)
© 2004 European Strabismological Association, ISBN 90 265 1965 6

Early onset strabismus, DVD and A pattern : efficacy of the superior rectus recession

V.Paris
Liège University, Belgium

ABSTRACT: Eight consecutive patients presenting an A pattern (range:10-45PD) , DVD and different kind of horizontal deviations undergone a weakening of the superior rectus (SR) alone to treat their alphabetic syndrome. The recession of the SR never exceed 6mm and was unilateral in 3 cases. In all patients but two this procedure was efficient to collapse the A pattern. In one case (with the highest incomitance) a weakening of both superior obliques was necessary. In one additional case a slight incomitance was only present from 10° on downgaze. We never obtained overcorrection. The follow up is from 1 to 9 years. Our results suggest that this procedure can be effective to treat up to 30 D of vertical incomitance.. Ours results are compared with the literature. These findings seem to demonstrate the efficacy of the SR weakening on the baseline incyclotorsion associated with DVD.

KEYWORDS : DVD, A pattern, Early Onset Strabismus

1 INTRODUCTION

There is a close association between DVD and torsion. Cyclomovements were systematically observed at the fundus in patients with DVD (Inoue 1993) and a high frequence of alphabetic pattern (72%) was described in untreated patients (Calcutt 1994) .
Based on the observations of Guyton and Weiss, it was proposed that the baseline cyclodeviation , resulting from dynamic torsion in DVD, can be associated with an A pattern in case of a baseline incyclotorsion and a V pattern in case of a baseline excyclotorion (Brodsky 1999).
For treating alphabetic syndromes associated with DVD it is therefore logical to weak the inferior oblique (IO) in case of V pattern and SR in case of A pattern. The aim of this study is to demonstrate the efficacy of the SR weakening alone in that latter situation.
This association was first described long time ago (Helveston 1969) . A single recession of the SR was proposed in these cases and led to the resolution of an apparent superior oblique overaction and of the A pattern in some cases (Coats et al. 1994) .
The first quantified description of this procedure was published four years later and confirmed that SR recession with neither oblique surgery or vertical displacement of horizontal muscle can collapse an A pattern(Melek, Mendoza & Ciancia 1998).
However , in both studies the percentage of overcorrections (A pattern transformed in V pattern) was significant (respectively : 40% and 66%).

2 METHOD

We have retrospectively studied eight consecutive patients aged from 3 to 31 years (mean : 14,6 years), presenting an A pattern with a size of incomitance from 10 to 45 PD (mean:20 PD) They had not undergone prior surgery on the oblique muscles .
Five cases had never been operated before . Symmetric or asymmetric recessions of the SR were performed with a range of 4 to 5.5 mm (scleral attachment) . Except in the microtropic patient (case n°5) , all cases underwent a simultaneous surgery on horizontal rectus muscles.

Table 1. Preoperative description

case	Age (years)	Horizontal Deviation (PD)	Vertical Incomitance (PD)	DVD (PD)
1	3	Et 30	12	R : 5 variable hypo L : 16
2	3	Et 50	45	R : 16 L : 16
3	4	Xt 60	25	R : 10 L : 15
4	23	Xt 40	15	R : 14 L : 12
5	23	Microet	10	R : 0 L : 16
6	25	Secondary Xt 16	30	R : 6 L : 12
7	31	Secondary Xt 50	15	R : 5 variable hypo L: 25
8	4	Recurrence Et 30	10	R : 14 L : 0

In case n°3 and n°4 the DVD was so asymmetric that it provoked a variable hypotropia on the other eye. In case n°5 and in case n°8 the DVD was considered as unilateral.

3 RESULTS

In five cases , the SR weakening was sufficient to eliminate the A pattern with only one procedure.
In case n°2 (with the highest preoperative incomitance) a secondary bilateral recession of the superior oblique (SO) was necessary to achieve a good result.
In that case however and the case n°3 , a small incomitance (respectively 8 and 6 PD) persisted from 10° on downgaze.

Table 2. Postoperative Alphabetic Pattern

Case	Surgery 1	Result	Surgery 2	Result	F up
1	R3 L5	A0			6
2	R5 L5	A30	Bilat recess SO	A8 (inversed Y)	9
3	R6 L6	A6 (inversed Y)			2
4	R5.5 L5	A0			1.5
5	R5	A0			1
6	R4.5 L5	A0			1
7	R4	A0			1
8	R4	A0			7

R and L in table 2 mean respectively that the right and the left superior rectus were recessed .
The number indicates the amount of surgery (in mm).
The follow up is expressed in years.
In case n° 5,7,8 the DVD was so asymmetric that an unilateral procedure was performed.

Table 3. Postoperative DVD

Case	Surgery 1	Result	Surgery 2	Result	F up
1	R3 L5	5/5			6
2	R5 L5	0/6			9
3	R6 L6	3/3			2
4	R5.5 L5	5/3			1.5
5	R5	0/0			1
6	R4.5 L5	4/6			1
7	R4	4/8			1
8	R4	16/5	RIO transp. LIO rec.	4/0	7

The results which are indicated in table 3 show the residual DVD respectively on the right and on the left eye expressed in PD.
All these deviations were latent but the last one (case n°8).
Interestingly, this uncorrected DVD didn't affect the result on the alphabetic pattern which remained controlled. It was treated , six months later by an anterotransposition of the right IO and a recession of the left IO (surgery 2 in table 3) and led to a good long term result.

Table 4. Postoperative Horizontal Deviation

Case	Age	Intial horizontal deviation	Final horizontal deviation
1	3	Et 30	Micro Et
2	3	Et 50	Micro Et
3	4	Xt 60	Micro Et
4	23	Xt 40	Intermittent Xt 15
5	23	Micro Et	Micro Et
6	25	Secondary Xt 16	Micro Et
7	31	Secondary Xt 50	Micro Et
8	4	Recurrence Et 30	Et 12

The horizontal results were also good as we can see in table 4.

4 DISCUSSION

We have shown that a SR weakening alone can collapse an A pattern until 30 PD of incomitance and that the same result can be obtained from a primary or a secondary surgery.
Our findings do not confirm the observations of Coats et al. who observed a major difference between a primary and a secondary surgery with regard to the surgical response (results were much better in the secondary group). These authors didn't mention any quantified analysis of their results but were surprised by the efficacy of the SRR in resolving an A pattern and an apparent SO overaction. In 40% of their cases, they even observed the development of IO overaction. However, we share the same findings when considering that an unilateral procedure can be efficient and that a good result in resolving an A pattern do not preclude a proportional control of the DVD . That could mean that the SR weakening per se is efficient in treating what we consider as a baseline incyclotorsion.

To our knowledge it is only the second time in the literature that a quantified study of A pattern treated with only SRR is proposed. Melek et al. were the first . They selected the same number of patients but didn't mention their age.
Nevertheless, the sizes of A patterns were less important than ours (mean: 10 PD, range: 5-15 PD), their SRR were more important (mean:9mm) and symmetric in all the cases.

These procedures led only to 3 elimination of the A pattern ; 5 were overcorrected (switch into V pattern). They share with other authors (Mc Call & Rosenbaum 1991) the view that it is necessary to add a SO weakening in case of a size of A pattern superior to 15 PD.
Our study shows that good results can be obtained until 30 PD of incomitance with only moderate SRR even unilaterally and even in rather young patients.

More than ten years ago , two authors (Spielmann 1989, Wilson 1991) proposed the best clinical analysis of the early onset strabismus, considering this difficult pathology as a dissociated complex with three components (horizontal, vertical and torsional). Any of them can have significant variations or may predominate in a given patient.

One can ask : why choosing a symmetric or an asymmetric procedure ?
We have presented our results compared with others.
An other original approach was published last year (Gamio 2002) . Based on the Guyton's theory regarding the ethiopathogenesis of DVD (DVD would be secondary to cyclotorsion , mediated primarily by the oblique muscles), she performed bilateral and symmetrical weakening of the four obliques and presented good results both for DVD and for alphabetic patterns associated with DVD in most of her cases. We know that equal innervation does not imply equal eye movement. So , is the four obliques surgery the treatment of the cause and the superior rectus surgery the treatment of the consequence of the initial innervational disorder provoquing the DVD and its torsional consequences ?

5 CONCLUSION

Our results are consistent with the dissociated strabismus complex , believing that early onset strabismus obey to a complicate and individual equilibrium between its three components.

The high efficacy of the SR weakening on the baseline incyclotorsion is demonstrated by its efficacy to treat A patterns and even by the frequency of cycloovercorrections. Therefore , in case of DVD and V pattern it is not surprising to obtain good results by weakening the IO but we advocate to take care of the simultaneous recession of the SR if necessary to treat DVD in that particular cases.

REFERENCES

BRODSKY M.C. : "Dissociated Torsional Deviation" in correspondence , 1999, Binocular Vision & Strabismus, first quarter, vol.14,N°1,6

CALCUTT C.L., MURRAY A.D.N.: 'A' and 'V' Patterns in Untreated Infantile Esotropia and Their Association With DVD; 1994; Proceedings of the Joint ISA and AAPOS meeting; Vancouver; Lennerstrand Ed; 355-358.

COATS D.K., PAYSEE E.A.,SATO M., HELVESTON E.M.: "A Pattern Horizontal Strabismus, DVD and Superior Oblique Overaction ; 1994; Proceeding of the Joint ISA and AAPOS meeting ; Vancouver, Lennerstrand Ed; 381-384.

GAMIO S.: A Surgical Alternative for Dissociated Vertical Deviation Based on New Pathologic Concepts: Weakening All Four Obliques Eye Muscles. Outcome and Results in 9 cases; 2002; Binocular Vision & Strabismus, first quarter, vol.17,N°1,15-24.

INOUE M., et al : Cyclomovements in Dissociated Vertical Deviation (DVD); 1993; First international symposium Ophthalmology; Bordeaux; Book of abstracts; 315.

Mc CALL L., ROSENBAUM A.: Incomitant Dissociated Vertical Deviation and Superior Oblique Overaction; 1991; Ophtalmology; 98; 911-918.

MELEK N.B., MENDOZA T., CIANCIA A.O.: Bilateral Recession of Superior Rectus Muscles: its Influence on A and V Pattern Strabismus; 1998; Journal of AAPOS, vol 2; 6; 333-3.

SPIELMANN A.: Les Déviations d'Occlusion: Esodéviations, Hyperdéviations, Cyclodéviations – Les Déviations Dissociées du Strabisme Précoce Opposées aux Hétérophories ; 1989 ; J. Fr. Orthopt. ; 21 ; 121-138.

WILSON E., SAUNDERS R.A., BERLAND J.E. : Dissociated Horizontal Deviation and Accommodative Esotropia : Treatment Options When Eso and Exo-Deviation Coexist; 1994; Proceedings of the Joint ISA and AAPOS meeting; Vancouver; Lennerstrand Ed; 370-373.

Session 7
Botulinum toxin/EMG

Transactions 28th Meeting European Strabismological Association, de Faber (ed.)

Does Botulinum Toxin have a role in the treatment of small angle esotropia ?

E.L.M Dawson, V.Geh, J.P.Lee
Moorfields Eye Hospital, London, England.

ABSTRACT: A retrospective review of the Toxin Clinic database was carried out over an 18 year period, identifying patients with esotropia under 20 prism dioptres. Sixty eight patients with esotropia of 20 prism dioptres or less were treated with Botulinum Toxin. There 47 females and 21 males, with a mean age of 34 years (range 11-78). Thirty two (47%) patients had residual esotropia, 20 (29%) had primary esotropia, 11 (16%) had consecutive esotropia, 4 (6%) had secondary esotropia and 1 (1.5%) had a decompensating esophoria. The mean pre toxin angle was 16 prism dioptres (range 6-20). Four hundred and thirty four injections were given, with an average of 6 per patient (range 1-36). Forty five (66%) patients underwent continued toxin treatment with an interval of 3 to 31 months. Thirteen (19%) patients achieved long term benefit from only one injection. Seven were unable to demonstrate binocular vision pre injection but demonstrated it post injection. Following an initial injection 9 (13%) patients proceeded to surgery. Botulinum Toxin is a successful treatment for these patients.

KEYWORDS: Botulinum Toxin Esotropia

1 INTRODUCTION

For some time now it has been our practice in patients presenting in adolescence or adulthood with a small angle esotropia to recommend treatment with Botulinum Toxin to the ipsilateral medial rectus. The rationale for this is based on our impression that these patients, when surgically corrected, have a strong tendency to develop consecutive exotropia. This experience was supported by Ciancia in his Knapp Lecture given at AAPOS (2001), where in his personal series of infantile esotropia patients who had undergone surgery, an increasing proportion developed exotropia on long term follow up.

2 METHODS

A retrospective review of the Toxin Clinic database was carried out over an 18 year period, identifying patients presenting with esotropia under 20 prism dioptres.

2.1 *PATIENT DATA*

Sixty eight patients with esotropia of 20 prism dioptres and under were treated with Botulinum Toxin. All patients were treated with 2.5 units of Botulinum Toxin A, under local anaethesia, as an out-patient procedure, under EMG guidance. There were 47 females and 21 males, with a mean age at presentation of 34 years. There was a wide range from 11 to 78 years old.
Thirty two (47%) patients had residual esotropia, 20 (29%) had primary esotropia, 11 (16%) had consecutive esotropia, 4 (6%) had secondary esotropia and 1 (1.5%) had a decompensating esophoria. Preceeding treatment included surgery in 45 cases, ranging from 1 to 5 operations. Eight patients had tried fresnel prisms and 3 had been prescribed exercises.

3 RESULTS

The mean pre-toxin angle was 16 prism dioptres, with a range of 6 to 20 prism dioptres. Four hundred and thirty four injections were given. There was an average of 6 per patient and a range of 1 to 36 injections (Figure 1). Thirty one (46%) patients underwent continued toxin treatment with an interval of 3 to 31 months. In 8 (18%) of these patients the interval between injections increased with time. Twenty four (35%) patients achieved long term reduction of angle of deviation. Three patients failed to attend after one injection. Seven (10%) patients were unable to demonstrate any binocular vision pre-injection but demonstrated fusion and stereopsis post injection, of up to 60 seconds of arc. Two of these required no further treatment. Following treatment, 10 (15%) patients proceeded to surgery. Of these 5 were in the group with unexpected post injection binocularity. Two patients had weak binocular vision pre-injection but good binocular vision post injection. Three patients who had a positive prismatic post-operative diplopia test proceeded to surgery post injection as no diplopia was experienced after the toxin treatment. These 3 patients did not want to continue with toxin treatment, as no diplopia was experienced after the toxin treatment. These 3 patients did not want to continue with toxin treatment, as they had only 3 month intervals between injections. Twenty (29%) patients of the total group were discharged after a minimum of 9 months follow up.

Figure 1: Number of injections per patient

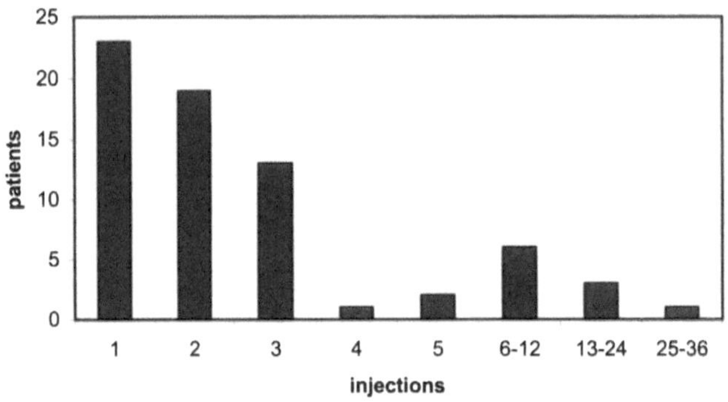

4 CONCLUSION

Botulinum Toxin is a successful treatment for these patients and was tolerated, with no side effects. It appears to have a definite role in the treatment of small angle esotropia.

REFERENCES

Ciancia AO. 2001. Evolution of Surgically Corrected Infantile Esotropia: Factors in Overcorrection. Knapp Lecture, AAPOS.

Transactions 28th Meeting European Strabismological Association, de Faber (ed.)
© 2004 European Strabismological Association, ISBN 90 265 1965 6

Esotropia in paediatric aphakic patients:

the role of botulinum toxin

V. Hauviller, S. Gamio
Hospital de Niños, Buenos Aires, Argentina

ABSTRACT: The frequency of heterotropia in paediatric aphakic patients is variable: 10 -70%. The variability of the angle produces often a risk for overcorrection and makes difficult to take the surgical decision . Our purpose is to assess the results of the injection of botulinum toxin in both medial recti in strabismic aphakic patients.
10 consecutive paediatric patients with strabismus post aphakia were included.
7 were bilateral. Average age was 63 months. All of them were injected in both medial recti with botulinum toxin type A. Average follow up was 31 months after the last injection. Global success rate was 70%(average 1,55 treatments per patient. Successful outcome was considered ortho plus 10 PD. In our group of patients the injection of botulinum toxin seems to be a good alternative treatment for orthotropic outcome
KEYWORDS: botulinum toxin, aphakic, paediatric, esotropia

INTRODUCTION: Heterotropia occurs quite frequently in paediatric aphakic patients with a prevalence that varies between the series (France et al, 1984) (Anaya et al, 1990) (Awner et al, 1996) (DeVaro et al,1997). It can interfere with the postoperative anti-amblyopia therapy necessary in this group. It is thought to be due to sensory factors that disrupt binocular vision both before and after cataract surgery.
When using high plus spectacle lenses, spherical aberration at the lens margin optically reduces vision in the deviated eye. Or a large angle of deviation can make contact lenses fitting difficult. Because of the variability of the angle, the strabismic surgery is frequently postponed until reliable measures are available. Consecutive exotropia is not unusual in these cases and amblyopia is exacerbated by the sensory deficit imposed by aphakia.
We report here the findings of our study, in which we injected botulinum toxin into both medial recti in esotropic aphakic patients.

PATIENTS:It included 10 consecutive paediatric patients who were operated on for congenital cataract and developed esotropia. The average age at the time of injection was 63,3 months (range from 9 to 121). The average initial angle was 28 PD (range from 20 to 40). The average follow up was 31 months after the last injection (range from 10 54). 7 were bilateral and 3 unilateral. The unilateral cases and 2 bilateral cases were fitted with contact lenses. 5 bilateral cases wear glasses.

Of the 8 co-operative children severe amblyopia was found in 2 bilateral cases. In the unilateral cases, visual acuity in the affected eye ranged from count fingers to 1/20.
All of them were injected in both medial recti with 2.5-3.75 U of botulinum toxin type A. EMG feedback was utilised where possible. The non co-operative patients were injected under general anaesthesia, at which time biomicroscopy, tonometry, and funduscopy were performed.

RESULTS: Ortho ± 10PD was achieved in 7 patients (70%), 2 undercorrections and 1 over correction (graphic 1).

4 patients received one treatment,1 was injected twice and 2 patients received 3 injections . This works out at an average of 1,55 treatments per patient
Transient palpebral ptosis was observed in 4 cases. Vertical deviation in 2.
Subsequently: dissociated vertical deviation was found in 3 patients and latent nistagmus in one, but there were no cases of oblique muscles dysfunction.

DISCUSSION: There have been several reports on Botulinum toxin in adults (Hakin and Lee, 1991) and a small series in children have been published (Hauviller and Gamio,1999).
According to Hakin and Lee, the temporary reduction of the squint by the use of toxin was sufficient to restore fusional control in adult aphakic patients, but orthotropia persisted in 3 patients without fusion potential.
Among the predictors of success : fusion potential (Hakin and Lee, 1991), younger age (Campos et al, 2000), mild amblyopia (Tejedor and Rodriguez, 2001), small angle (Hauviller et al, 2001) only the latter is present in this group of patients.
In our paediatric patients the fusion capability is reduced, especially in the unilateral cases. It is possible that selective structural long-standing changes produced by the toxin on the extraocular muscles are responsible for the permanent effect in some of them, as demonstrated by Spencer et al.

CONCLUSION: Within our group of patients the injection of botulinum toxin appears to be an effective therapy for the deviation, with advantages of safe and easy administration .

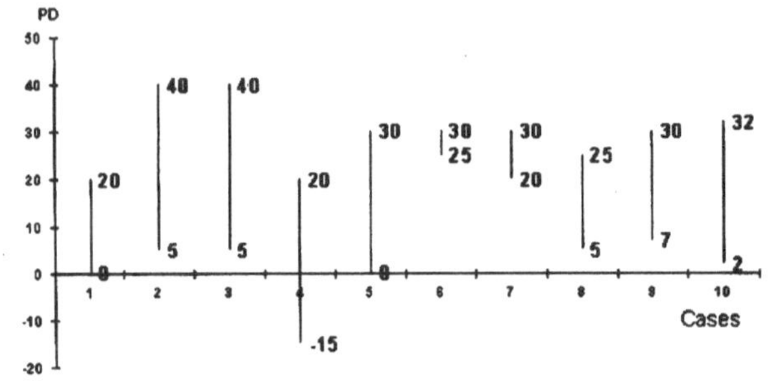

Graphic 1: 10 treated patients. Initial and final angle in PD. 2 undercorrected,1 overcorrecte

REFERENCES

Amaya L, Speedwell L, Taylor D, 1990: Contact lenses for infant aphakia. Br J Ophthalm 74, 150-154.
Campos E., Schiavi C, Bellusci C ,2000: Critical age of botulinum toxin treatment in essential infantile esotropia. J of Ped Opthalm and Strab 37:328-332.
De Varo J, Buckley E, Awner S, Seaber J,1997: Secondary posterior chamber intraocular implantation in pediatric patients. Am J Ophthalm 123,24-30.
France TD, Frank J, 1984: The association of strabismus and aphakia in children J Ped Ophthalm, vol 21 n 6, 221-224.
Hakin KN, Lee JP ,1991 :Binocular diplopia in unilateral aphakia: the role of botulinum toxin. Eye 5,447-450.

Hauviller V, Gamio S,1999: Estrabismo en la afaquia infantil: su tratamiento con toxina botulínica . Congreso Latinoamericano Estrabismo, ed Arroyo Yllanes ,Acapulco , México, 96-97.
Hauviller V,Gamio S,Tartara A , 2001: Botulinum toxin therapy in paediatric esotropia: risk factors for failure. Transactions 27th meeting European Strabismological association, 199-201.
Spencer RF and McNeer KW 1987: Botulinum toxin paralysis of adult monkey extraocular muscle. Structural alterations in orbital , singly innervated muscle fibers, Arch Ophthalmol. 105 ,1703-1711.
Tejedor J, Rodriguez JM 2001: Long-term outcome and predictor variables in the treatment of acquired esotropia with botulinum toxin. Invest Ophthalmol Vis Sci. 42(11):2542-6.

Transactions 28th Meeting European Strabismological Association, de Faber (ed.)
© 2004 European Strabismological Association, ISBN 90 265 1965 6

Levator denervation for upper lid retraction secondary to seventh nerve palsy

K. G. Boboridis, N. G. Ziakas, N. S. Georgiadis
Oculoplastic service, Ophthalmology Department, Aristotle University of Thessaloniki, Greece

ABSTRACT: Botulinum Toxin is used for weakening of the levator complex in the management of upper lid retraction following Facial nerve palsy. Prospective non comparative interventional case series study. Twenty seven consecutive patients with VII nerve palsy, upper lid retraction and symptomatic lagophthalmos (3-8 mm) were included. Botulinum Toxin (37,5 - 75 IU) was administered with a 26 G needle deep into the upper lid sulcus, above the levator muscle. Follow up ranged from 6 to 8 months. Lid position improved within ten days from treatment. Upper lid retraction and lagophthalmos was corrected with lid position above the visual axis. No ocular motility defects observed. Facial nerve function improved spontaneously in eight teen cases, the remaining nine required retreatment in three months time. Botulinum Toxin weakening of levator muscle is an effective management of upper lid retraction following facial nerve palsy especially in temporary nerve palsy.
KEYWORDS: Botulinum toxin, levator, seventh nerve palsy, lagophthalmos, lid retraction

1 INTRODUCTION

Botulinum Toxin type A has been extensively used for the management of blepharospasm, hemifacial spasm, strabismus, involutional lower lid entropion and in cosmetic applications. Chemical denervation of the levator muscle has been reported for correction of disthyroid (Uddin & Davies 2002) upper lid retraction and total ptosis for cornea protection (Adams et al. 1987; Kirkness et al. 1988). Its use in the management of upper lid retraction from seventh nerve palsy has not been extensively documented (Putterman 1990).

Facial squeal from peripheral VII nerve paralysis include brow ptosis, upper lid retraction, paralytic lower lid ectropion and lip angle ptosis. The unopposed levator muscle action from the paralyzed orbicularis muscle results in lid elevation lag on down gaze and incomplete closure. Ophthalmic sequences are lagophthalmos, lacrimal pump failure, corneal exposure, keratitis and corneal ulcer.

Conservative management involves the use of topical lubricating medications, moist chamber and taping the lids closed. Surgical management includes tarsorrhaphy placement of gold weight, levator recession, palpebral springs, lower lid ectropion repair, vascularised muscle flaps and hypoglossal nerve anastomosis.

Our purpose was to investigate the efficacy of Botulinum Toxin in the management of upper lid retraction and symptomatic lagophthalmos secondary to facial nerve palsy by applying the toxin to the levator muscle through the lid skin and retaining free visual axis.

2 METHODS

Our inclusion criteria were VII nerve palsy of sort duration (< 2 months), symptomatic lagophthalmos of more than 3 mm with failure of conservative lubricating medication and normal Bell's phenomenon. We've included 27 consecutive patients (mean age of 64 years, range 47 – 74 years) who suffered from facial nerve palsy with a mean duration of 2,5 months (range 1 – 5 months).

The causative factors included acoustic neuroma (n=16), petri bone fracture (n=3), parotid gland tumour (n=1), middle ear surgery (n=1) and Bell's paralysis (n=6). There was mean lagophthalmos of 5,4 mm (range 3 – 8 mm) and mean upper lid retraction 1,5 mm (range 0 – 4 mm) measured from the unaffected contralateral side upper lid position. In cases with inferior sclera show of more than 1 mm due to paralytic ectropion a lid tightening procedure was also performed.

After obtaining an informed consent our standard method of treatment involved the use of a 27 G needle to inject 37,5 - 75 IU of the commercial toxin preparation Dysport (12,5 IU/0,1 ml dilution) through the middle of upper lid skin, above Whitnall's ligament towards the orbital apex, above the levator muscle belly.

The outcome measures recorded were vertical palpebral aperture, marginal reflex distance for upper and lower lid, levator function, lagophthalmos, the state of corneal epithelium (punctate keratopathy) and patient symptoms. Follow up was performed the following day, in two weeks and every month post treatment.

3 RESULTS

In all cases there was observed reduction of lagophthalmos by mean of 3,2 mm (range 2 – 4 mm) and depression of upper lid position by mean of 3,1 mm (range 2 – 6 mm) compared to the contralateral upper lid, therefore reduction of palpebral aperture (Fig. 1).

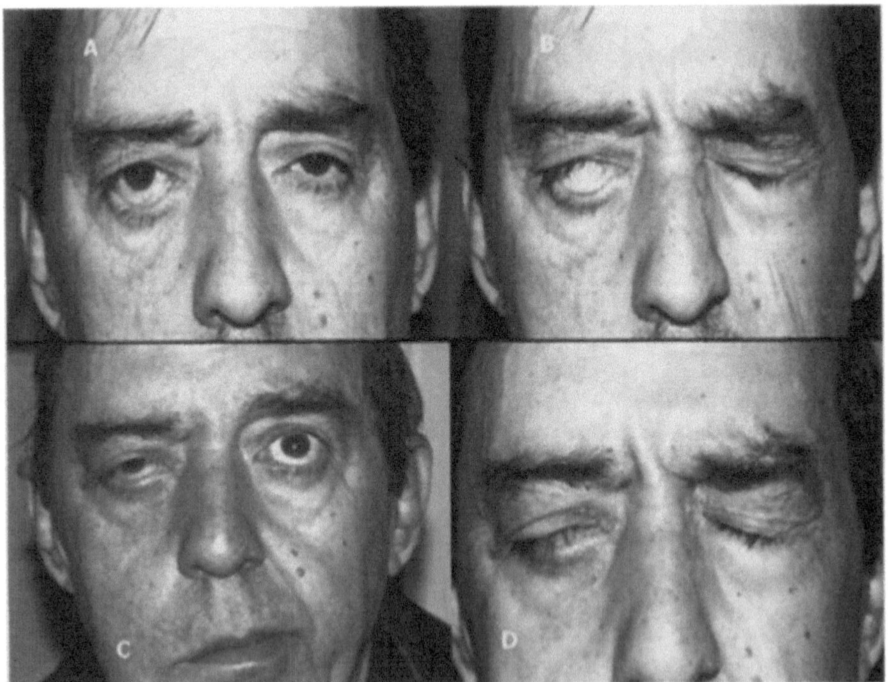

Figure 1. Patient with right seventh nerve palsy. Lid in primary position of gaze (A) and lagophthalmos on lid closure (B) pre treatment. Lower lid level on primary position of gaze (C) and improved lid closure with much reduced lagophthalmos (D) one month following treatment.

The lower lid position was at the level or above the middle of the pupil sparing the visual axis in all cases. There was no significant levator function alteration and the mean duration of the toxin action was 10 weeks, requiring repeated treatment. Punctate keratitis was cured and all patients noticed subjective improvement of symptoms.

There was no ocular motility disturbance and no persistent upper lid ptosis observed as reported in the literature (Heyworth & Lee 1994). No significant complications were recorded with the only minor unwanted side effect the contralateral upper lid retraction due to Herring's law which was well tolerated by all patients (Fig. 2).

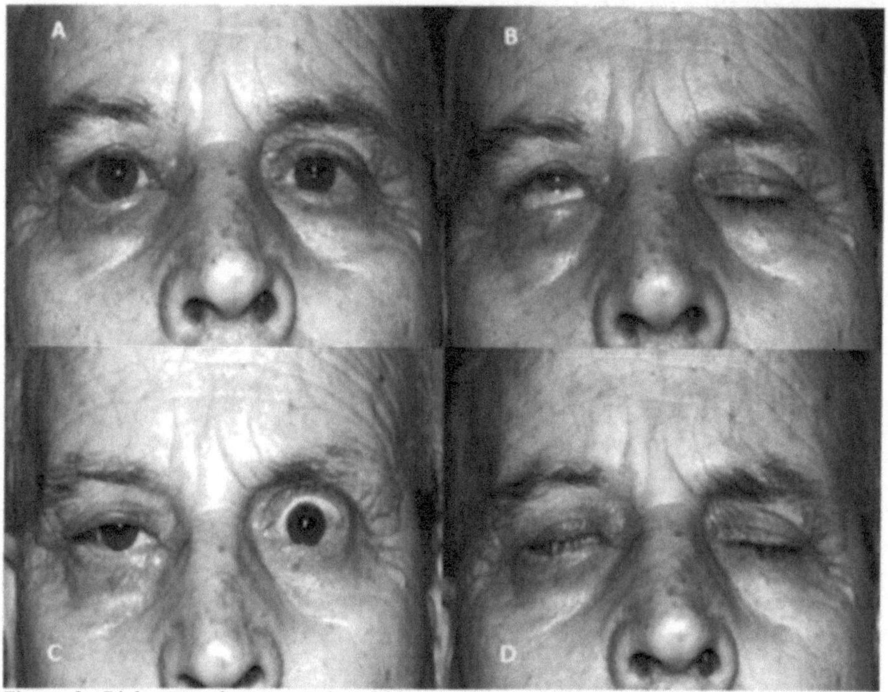

Figure 2. Right seventh nerve palsy. Lid retraction on primary position of gaze (A) and severe lagophthalmos on lid closure (B) pre treatment. Lower lid position on primary gaze with clear visual axis and marked contralateral upper lid retraction (C) one month following botulinum toxin injection. Much improved lid closure with only 1 mm of lagophthalmos (D).

4 CONCLUSIONS

In our experience the use of Botulinum toxin type A for chemical denervation of the levator muscle is an effective option for the temporary management of upper lid retraction secondary to seventh nerve palsy until a permanent surgical correction can be performed six to eight months from onset.

Adequate cornea protection is maintained with lower lid position and lagophthalmos reduction. Patient satisfaction is high with subjective improvement, reduction of intensive conservative management and a minimally invasive procedure.

The only concern may be the low reproducibility of the technique, high cost of the medication and the need for repeated treatment every three months.

REFERENCE

Adams, G. G., C. M. Kirkness, et al. (1987). "Botulinum toxin A induced protective ptosis." Eye (London, England) 1 (Pt 5): 603-8.
Heyworth, P. L. and J. P. Lee (1994). "Persisting hypotropias following protective ptosis induced by botulinum neurotoxin." Eye (London, England) 8 (Pt 5): 511-5.
Kirkness, C. M., G. G. Adams, et al. (1988). "Botulinum toxin A-induced protective ptosis in corneal disease." Ophthalmology 95(4): 473-80.
Putterman, A. M. (1990). "Botulinum toxin injections in the treatment of seventh nerve misdirection." American Journal of Ophthalmology 110(2): 205-6.
Uddin, J. M. and P. D. Davies (2002). "Treatment of upper eyelid retraction associated with thyroid eye disease with subconjunctival botulinum toxin injection." Ophthalmology 109(6): 1183-7.

Transactions 28th Meeting European Strabismological Association, de Faber (ed.)
© 2004 European Strabismological Association, ISBN 90 265 1965 6

The useful of botulinum toxin Type-A in the treatment of chronic sixth ocular nerve palsy

L. Sabetti, MD, L. D'Alessandri, MD, K. Salvatori, Orth, E. Balestrazzi, MD
Eye Clinic of L'Aquila (Italy)
Head: Prof. E. Balestrazzi

Address correspondence and reprint request to:
Lelio Sabetti MD,
Clinica Oculistica,
Dipartimento di Scienze Chirurgiche
Via Vetoio, Blocco 11,
67100 L'Aquila
Tel. +39.0862.319.671 Fax +39.0862.319.672
E-mail: lesabetti@tin.it

ABSTRACT

Objective: to analyze the efficacy of Botulinum toxin Type-A (BTA) injection in the differential diagnosis between paresis vs paralysis.
Methods: 21 patients (12 F; 9 M), mean age 38,1+/-18, with acquired VI nerve palsy (mean 41.7^{Δ} ET near and 45^{Δ} ET distance), have been treated with BTA injection into the ipsilateral medial rectus muscle, 6 months after onset. At 6 months follow up, paresis and paralysis were differentiated and the correct surgical strategy was planned.
Results: At 6 months follow up, 19% of patients recovered the lateral rectus muscle functionality (mean 4^{Δ} ET near, 2^{Δ} ET distance) avoiding the surgical treatment; 23.8% manifested paresis (mean 30.5^{Δ} ET near, 32^{Δ} ET distance) and 57.1% paralysis (mean 40.3^{Δ} ET near, 42.8^{Δ} ET distance). These patients underwent surgery and at 1 year follow up the mean residual angle deviation was respectively: 2.4^{Δ} ET and 1^{Δ} ET.
Conclusions: Botulinum Toxin Type-A injection is an invaluable tool in the differential diagnosis between paresis vs paralysis of the VIth nerve, allowing the correct surgical choice.

Keywords: chronic sixth nerve palsy, botulinum toxin

1. INTRODUCTION

Acquired sixth nerve palsy, is usually a consequence of vascular diseases, diabetes, head trauma or cerebral tumours (Jampolsky, 1976). Diagnosis and management of this neurogenic ocular palsy are often difficult and the poor or unknown clinical history of the patients is not able to help the ophthalmologist.

Generally, before surgical treatment, it is necessary to wait at least for 6-8 months, that is the period after which the paralysis can be considered stable. It is rare a spontaneous recovery of this paralysis while it is frequent the occurrence of a contracture of the joint muscle antagonist, which may disguise the functional recovery of this last. Patients affected manifest esotropia with large angle and adults sees double and are forced to take a wrong position of the head in order to neutralise diplopia, or to use prismatic lenses. If diplopia is not adequately controlled it is required a surgical treatment.

The timing of surgical treatment and the choice of the correct surgical strategy are difficult decisions and the functional result of surgery is often unpredictable.

Boutulinum toxin Type A (BTA) injected in the hyperfunctional muscles causes a flaccid paralysis by preventing the release of acetylcholine at the neuromuscular junction and favours a gradually and physiologic recovery of the hypofunctioned muscles (Scott, 1980).

BTA injection can be used during the waiting period for the spontaneous recovery or for surgery. In fact in case that VI nerve palsy resolves BTA helps in prevent diplopia, while if it is an unresolved palsy, BTA is an invaluable tool in the differential diagnosis between paresis vs palsy, allowing the choice of a correct surgical procedure.

In this study we evaluated the efficacy of BTA injections in 21 patients with chronic sixth nerve palsy.

2. MATERIALS AND METHODS

Between April 1998 and October 2001, 21 patients (12F, 9M; mean age 38.1+/-18 range 10-64 years) with acquired VI nerve palsy underwent ipsilateral medial rectus BTA injections, 6 months after onset.

The mean pre-injection angle deviation was 41.7^{Δ} ET near and 45^{Δ} ET distance.

All patients underwent a complete preoperative ophtalmological and orthoptic clinical examination including: ocular refraction with and without cycloplegia, Goldmann tonometry, biomicroscopy of the anterior segment and funduscopic examinations.

The orthoptic examination evaluated the ocular motility in the nine diagnostic gaze positions, strabismus was measured with the prism and cover test for near and distance fixation. The presence of anomalous head positions; Worth and micro-Worth, 4-dot test, Lang test (I-II), Titmus, TNO, red filter ladder test, Hess-Lancaster screen test and the passive and active duction test were performed. Inclusion criteria were VI nerve palsy more than 6 months after onset, anomalous head position. Exclusion criteria were previous surgical treatments, congenital abnormalities of extraocular muscles and the assumption of drugs interfering with the neuromuscular system in the last 6 months.

In all cases the informed consent was obtained.

Each patient underwent a single injection of BTA (20 UI, BoTX, Dysport®, Ipsen) directly in the ipsilateral medial rectus muscle.

Follow up was performed at 1 and 6 months. At 6 months from enrollment, differential diagnosis between a paresis and paralysis was respectively defined if the affected eye could be actively abducted or not, across the midline.

Patients with paresis underwent a single horizontal rectus muscle procedure; while patients with paralysis underwent a vertical muscle transposition. (Riordan-Eva, 1992).

3. RESULTS

Nineteen per cent of patients manifested a gradually and physiologic recovery of the lateral rectus muscle at 1 month (mean 8^{Δ} ET near, 6^{Δ} ET distance) and at 6 months (mean 4^{Δ} ET near, 2^{Δ} ET distance) follow up. These patients lamented diplopia only within 2 months after BTA injection but it could be neutralised with prismatic lenses. These patients avoided the surgical treatment.
On the contrary, 23.8% of patients manifested paresis at 1 month (mean 25^{Δ} ET near, 27^{Δ} ET distance), and at 6 months (mean angle deviation 30.5^{Δ} ET near and 32^{Δ} ET distance) follow up. These patients underwent horizontal rectus muscles procedure. One year after surgery the mean residual angle deviation was 2.4^{Δ} ET (range 0-4^{Δ} ET).
On the other hand, 57.1% of cases manifested paralysis, at 1 month (mean 37.3^{Δ} ET near, 39.8^{Δ} ET distance) and at 6 months (mean 40.3^{Δ} ET near, 42.8^{Δ} ET distance) follow up. Consequently all of them underwent vertical muscles transposition procedure. At 1 year follow up the mean residual angle deviation was 1^{Δ} ET (range 4^{Δ} ET - 6^{Δ} XT).

4. DISCUSSION

The aim of surgery in paralytic strabismus is to restore the best equilibrium between muscle forces unbalanced by the ocular palsy. Moreover it is necessary to eliminate the eventual presence of diplopia and/or of anomalous head posture.
In the VIth nerve palsy the choice of the surgical strategy depends on the extent of recovery. BTA injection resulted an invaluable tool in this decision.
During the first 3 months after onset of palsy, it is possible to have a spontaneous recovery, but in the following period there is the occurrence of a contracture of the joint muscle antagonist.
Elasticity of deficient muscle is gradually reduced due to a constant elongation with a gradual loss of tonus, hyper extensibility and progressive degeneration of muscles fibres (Kommerel, 1976).
According to the literature, the degeneration become irreversible after one or two years with the reduction in active muscle tension (Rotz). However, as demonstrated in this study, a full recovery (19%), or a partial recovery of the lateral rectus function (23.8%) resulted even in chronic VI nerve palsy (Repka, 1994). BTA injection in acquired sixth nerve palsy, avoids an hyper-contraction of the ipsilateral medial rectus muscle and promote the recovery of the lateral rectus function. This avoids surgical treatment in patients that restore orthotropia by injection alone. Patients that present a persistence of a large angle esotropia with diplopia or anomalous head position, allow a differential diagnosis between a paresis vs paralysis. This is necessary to plane the correct surgical procedure. If the affected eye cannot be abducted beyond the mid-line, the transposition procedure will be required . If the affected eye can abduct, the recession and resection procedure should be sufficient.

5. CONCLUSION

BTA injection can be considered an invaluable tool in the management and diagnosis of VI nerve palsy. On the basis of our results, BTA injection allows a differential diagnosis between paresis vs paralysis, necessary condition to plane the correct surgical treatment and to attain a successful functional outcome.

6. REFERENCES

Jampolsky A.
Management of acquired (adult) muscle palsies.
In: Transaction of the New Orleans Academy of Ophthalmology symposium
On Neuro-ophthalmology. ST.Luis:Mosby,1976

Kommerel G., Oliver D., Theopold M.
Adaptative programming of phasic and tonic components in saccadic eye movements.
Investigation in patients with abdu lens palsy.
Invest Opthalmol Vis Sci 1976;15: 657-660

Repka MX, Lam GC, Morrison NA
The efficacy of botulinum neurotoxin A for the treatment of complete and partially recovered chronic sixth nerve palsy.
J Pediatric Ophthalmol Strabismus.1994 Mar-Apr;31(2):79-83.

Riordan-Eva, Lee J.P.
Management of VI nerve palsy avoiding unnecessary surgery
Eye 1992;6:386-330

Rotz A., Speeg-Schatz C.
Eye Surgery
Swetz & Zeitlinger publication p.339

Scott AB.
Botulinum toxin injection into extra –ocular muscles as alternative to strabismus surgery.
Ophthalmology 1980;87:1044-50

Transactions 28th Meeting European Strabismological Association, de Faber (ed.)

Quantitative E.M.G. of E.O.M in patients with congenital fibrosis of the extraocular muscles (CFEOM1)

C. Schiavi, C. Bellusci and E.C. Campos
Ophthalmology Service, University of Bologna, Bologna, Italy

ABSTRACT: Congenital fibrosis of the extraocular muscles (CFEOM) is a relatively rare eye movement disorder typically inherited in an autosomal dominant fashion. Affected individuals show congenital, bilateral ptosis and restrictive external ophthalmoplegia, with their eyes partially or completely fixed in an infraducted (downward) and strabismic position.

It remains unclear whether this disorder results from a primary myopathic or from a neuropathic process, and whether these two processes can be pathophysiologically related to one another.

We performed the electromyography with quantitative analysis (QEMG) of the extraocular muscles (EOM) in three members of a family affected by CFEOM whose disease gene maps to the locus on chromosome 12 (CFEOM1). QEMG data from the EOM of the affected members provides a further demonstration of a neuropathic process for CFEOM1 involving the superior and inferior division of the oculomotor nerve.

KEYWORDS: Electromyography, congenital fibrosis, extraocular muscle.

1. INTRODUCTION

Congenital fibrosis of the extraocular muscles (CFEOM) is a relatively rare eye movement disorder typically inherited in an autosomal dominant fashion with minimum prevalence estimated as 1 in 230,000. Affected individuals show congenital, bilateral ptosis and restrictive external ophthalmoplegia, with their eyes partially or completely fixed in an infraducted (downward) and strabismic position. Often aberrant residual movements occur on attempts to move the eyes into the restricted field of vision (1). The intra-familial heterogeneity is often possible (2). All family members have markedly reduced vertical movements but the involvement of horizontal muscles varies greatly between family members, as does the involvement of the levator muscle.

Absence of the superior division of the oculomotor nerve with consequent abnormalities of the superior rectus and levator palpebrae superioris muscles has been documented in one autopsy report from CFEOM patient (3). Biopsy specimens of the inferior rectus muscle from individuals with CFEOM are typically reported to contain fibrous tissue, or a mixture of myo-fibers and fibrous tissue.

Restrictive ophthalmoplegia, "stiff" muscles at surgery, and findings of connective tissue in muscle biopsy examination led many to propose that these disorders are the result of a myopathic process with fibrous changes. It remains unclear whether this disorder results from a primary myopathic or from a neuropathic process, and whether these two processes can be pathophysiologically related to one another.

We performed electromyography with quantitative analysis (QEMG) of the extraocular muscles (EOM) in three members of a family affected by CFEOM whose disease gene maps to the locus on chromosome 12 (4). We refer to this genetically defined disorder as "classic CFEOM" to distinguish it from sporadic, autosomal recessive, and clinically variant forms. In this report, we present the preliminary clinical and pathological findings.

2. MATERIAL AND METHODS

The family comprised an affected mother (71 years-old), her affected daughter (50 years-old) and the daughter's affected son (9 years old), (Fig. 1).

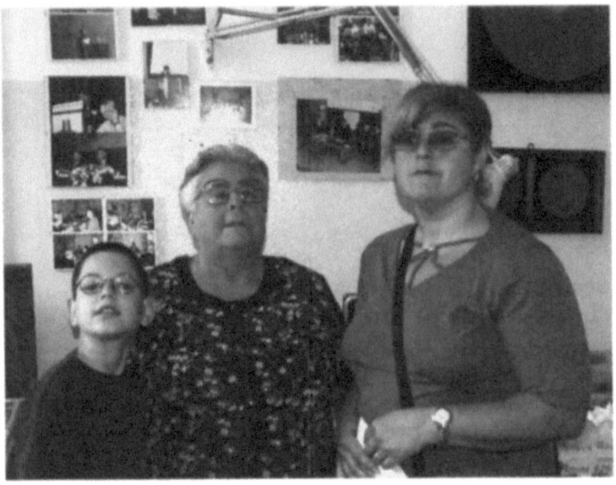

Fig. 1: Family affected by congenital fibrosis of extraocular muscles.

Mother has a second unaffected son. The feature common to all affected members was ptosis with a completely loss of the ocular movements of elevation and depression with other variable manifestations of disorders of ocular motility. Mother exhibited a restrictive esotropia in primary position. On the contrary, daughter and her son showed a restrictive exotropia. All patients showed an anomalous head posture with chin up and aberrant movements on attempt to move the eyes up-ward. A full examination of visual functions and ocular examination was carried out in all the members. None of the family members underwent EOM surgery to correct strabismus or anomalous head posture.

Electromyography with quantitative analysis was performed on EOM of the two adult patients and in the unaffected member. Superior rectus muscle as well medial and lateral rectus muscles were studied. Quantitative electromyography (QEMG) is a general term referring to the technique and conditions used to study the microphysiology of the motor unit (5). It permits the recording of a single muscle fiber action potential. Signal is recorded by using a single concentric needle electrode and the motor unit potential (MUP) is the compound action potential that reflects the electrical activity of the muscle fibers belonging to a single motor unit. During slight voluntary muscle contraction, this compound action potential is characterized by its consistent appearance with regard to shape and amplitude. The relevant parameters may be one or more of the following: amplitude, duration, area, phases and turns. Typically at least 20 MUPs are recorded from each muscle tested (5).

A computerized myograph (Dantec) was used to record the EMG signal and Keypoint program was employed for QEMG analysis. The test was performed by inserting a 30G concentric needle electrode (Oxford Instrument) in a proper position of the EOM, instructing the patient to perform a weak contraction of the muscle and then recording at least 5 seconds of EMG activity. Based on the recorded signal, the examiner selects a MUP to be analysed and adjusts marker positions for the measurements before accepting the results. The selected MUP is stored and the electrode is moved to another insertion depth or in a new EOM position and the procedure is repeated until a sufficient number of MUPs have been analysed.

Subjects were instructed to look in the direction of the minimum EOM contraction (i.e. abduction position for medial rectus EMG) in such a way as to activate only the motor units from the orbital layer of each EOM. The activity of a single motor units was tightly correlated with a given eye position and electromyographic studies showed that orbital layer fibers are recruited before those near the globe. In fact, fibers in the orbital layers have lower recruitment threshold than those in the global layer that are active only in their fields of action (6).

3. RESULTS

The main result of our study is the evidence of electromyographic signs of denervation with the presence of polyphasic potentials found mainly in the superior rectus muscle but also in the medial rectus muscle of all affected members of the family. The QEMG from the lateral rectus muscle was normal.

QEMG data from the superior recti muscles revealed a mean MUP duration (12 msec) significantly longer than normals (4-5 msec) with incidence of polyphasic potential close to 20% (Fig. 2).

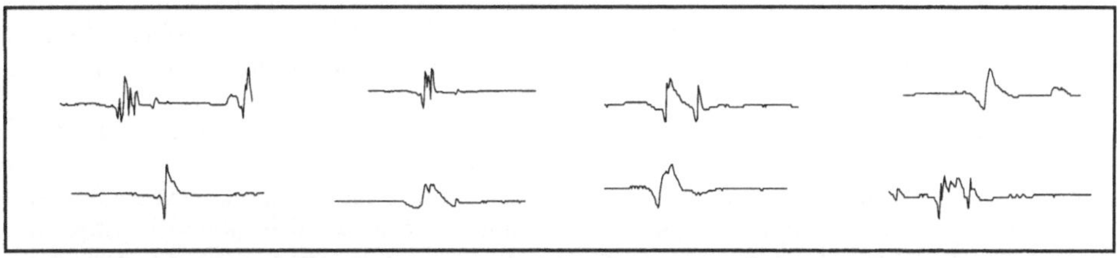

Fig. 2: Typical Motor Unit Potentials from superior rectus muscle of a patient affected by CFEOM1.

The mean MUP duration from the medial recti was 8 msec still longer than normal value (Fig. 3). The incidence of polyphasic potential was 4%, near to that observed in normal EOM.

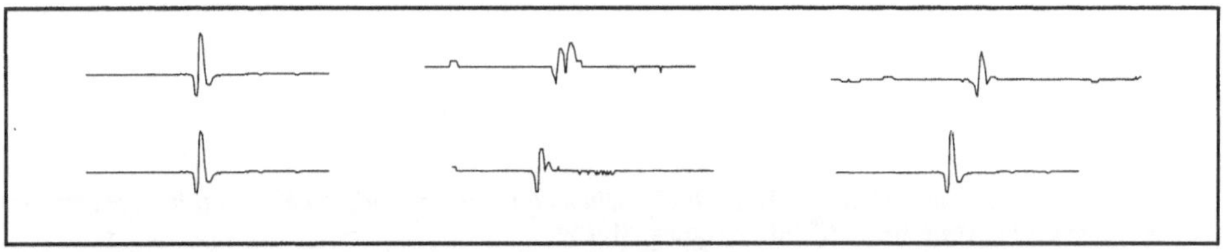

Fig. 3: Typical Motor Unit potentials from medial rectus muscle of a patient affected by CFEOM1.

The electromyographic findings recorded from the lateral recti muscles of two affected members as well as from the EOM of the unaffected member were normal with regard to MUP amplitude, duration and phase (Fig. 4).

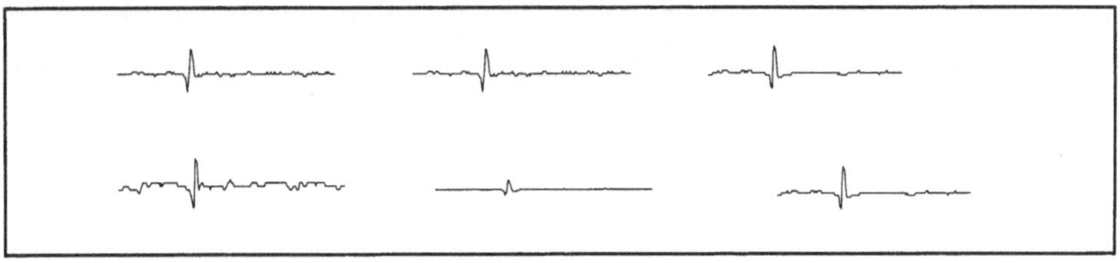

Fig. 4: Typical Motor Unit potentials from lateral rectus muscle of a patient affected by CFEOM1.

4. COMMENT

In the past, EMG has been used extensively to study EOM function. EMG data first convincingly showed that Duane's retraction syndrome was an innervational abnormality, characterized by rectus muscles co-contraction. To our knowledge there is no evidence in the literature about EMG of EOM on patients affected by congenital fibrosis of extraocular muscles (CFEOM). The neuropathologic mechanisms underlying the ocular motility defect in CFEOM are not known. Post-mortem neuropathologic examination of an affected individual from a classic CFEOM1, however, demonstrated an absence of the superior branch of the oculomotor nerve and its corresponding sub-nuclei in the midbrain, and marked abnormalities of the superior rectus and levator palpebrae superioris muscles, normally innervated by this branch (3). The phenotype of our family suggests a similar anatomic defect affecting the superior more than the inferior division of the oculomotor nerve and its corresponding sub-nuclei.

Similar to the findings in families with classic CFEOM1, dysfunction of the superior rectus and levator palpebrae superioris muscles alone does not account for all the ocular motility defects in our family. We cannot determine from the motility examination, if these defects result from abnormal innervation and/or from mechanical restriction secondary to muscle contracture with or without fibrosis (2). In fact, our affected family members have different forms of strabismus: the grandmother had a restrictive esotropia in primary position, on the contrary the mother with her child showed a restrictive exotropia.

QEMG data from the EOM of the affected members provides a further demonstration of a neuropathic process for CFEOM1 involving the superior and inferior division of the oculomotor nerve. The QEMG analysis from the superior rectus muscles showed the largest abnormalities with high incidence of polyphasic potentials. Similar aspects could be found in EMG from peripheral skeletal muscle of patients affected by spinal muscular atrophy (SMA) characterized by degeneration and loss of motor neurons of the anterior horn. Similarly, we can speculate that the pathogenesis of CFEOM could be related to the primitive lesion of mesencephalic oculomotor subnuclei with secondary damage of motor neurons and corresponding extraocular muscles.

Finally, QEMG from the lateral rectus muscle revealed normal electrical activity in both affected members. Therefore, the bilateral absence of abduction with large-angle esotropia seen in one affected member could result from secondary long-standing contractures more than from primary dysfunction of the abducens nerve.

REFERENCES

Von Noorden G.K. and Campos E.C. 2002. *Binocular vision and ocular motility: Theory and management of strabismus.* 6th Ed. St. Louis, Mosby.

Reck A., Manners R., Hatchwell E. 1998. Phenotypic heterogeneity may occur in congenital fibrosis of the extraocular muscles. *Br. J. Ophthalmol.* 82:676-679.

Engle E.C., Goumnerov B.C., McKeown C.A. et al. 1997. Oculomotor nerve and muscles abnormalities in congenital fibrosis of the extraocular muscles. *Ann. Neurol.* 41:314-325.

Engel E.C., Kunkel L.M., Specht L.A. et al. 1994. Mapping a gene for congenital fibrosis of the extraocular muscles to the centromeric region of chromosome 12. *Nat. Genet.* 7:69-73.

Stalberg E., Falck B., Sonoo M., et al. 1995. Multi-MUP EMG analysis – a two year experience in daily clinical work. *Electroenceph. and clin. neurophys.* 97(3):145-154.

Scott A.B., Collins C.C. 1973. Division of labor in human extraocular muscle. *Arch. Ophthalmol.* 90:319-322.

Session 8
Oblique muscles

Transactions 28th Meeting European Strabismological Association, de Faber (ed.)
 ISBN 90 265 1965 6

The surgical Indications and Outcome of Superior Oblique Tendon Spacers

Geh VSY FRCOphth, Dawson E DBO, Lee JP FRCS FRCOphth
Moorfields Eye Hospital, London, UK

ABSTRACT: The indications for the use of superior oblique tendon spacers and the surgical outcomes were reviewed. 11 patients underwent this procedure (12 eyes), 5 for traumatic Brown Syndrome, 4 (5 eyes) for primary Brown Syndrome and 2 for superior oblique overaction. 6 patients (45%) reported improved symptoms following surgery. A good result was achieved for the treatment of superior oblique overaction (100%).There was moderate success for the treatment of primary Brown's Syndrome (50%). Disappointing results were achieved for patients with traumatic Brown's Syndrome (40%); the use of spacers for this condition has not been previously reported.

KEYWORDS: Superior oblique tendon spacer, Brown Syndrome

1. INTRODUCTION

The use of a superior oblique silicon tendon spacer was first described by Wright as a means to produce a more predictable, graded and potentially reversible weakening of the superior oblique muscle. (Wright 1991) He described its use in patients with superior oblique overaction or in primary Brown Syndrome. Conventional methods of superior oblique weakening have included superior oblique tenotomy, tenectomy, recession split tendon lengthening or Z lengthening. However, these techniques have occasionally lead to unpredictable result including consecutive superior oblique palsy. Furthermore, patients with fusion may suffer head tilt, vertical or torsional diplopia or loss of stereopsis following surgery. We describe our experience with the use of silicone superior oblique tendon spacers.

2. SUBJECTS AND METHODS

The case notes of all patients at Moorfields Eye Hospital who have undergone superior oblique tendon spacer surgery by a single surgeon were reviewed. 11 patients underwent this procedure. All patients had unilateral surgery except for 1. Preoperative diagnosis included 5 patients with traumatic Brown Syndrome, 4 patients with primary Brown Syndrome and 2 with superior oblique overaction. Parameters for assessment included length of spacer used, manifest ocular deviation in primary position, subjective symptoms, Hess Charts and fields of binocular vision. Evidence of V or A patterns were also noted.

Manifest ocular deviations were recorded in prism dioptres at near with best corrected vision pre and post operatively. Change in subjective symptoms post operatively were noted as worse, no change, minimal, moderate or good. Pre and post operative visual field were scored as a percentage of normal according to a previously described method. (Fitzsimons 1990) Hess Chart measurements was recorded as improved post operatively if the field in the area of the restrictive muscle was larger or if there was reduction in the A or V pattern.

The surgical technique used was similar to that first described by Wright. (Wright 1991) The superior rectus muscle was identified and hooked via a fornix conjunctival incision. The superior oblique tendon was exposed along the nasal border of the superior rectus. Two 5.0 non absorbable double armed sutures were sutured to the tendon approximately 1.5mm apart. The tendon was cut between the two pre placed sutures and a medical grade silicone 240 retinal band was sewn between the two cut ends. The length of expander used was determined by intraperative forced duction test. This ranged from 3.5mm to 7mm. (Average 4.5mm)

3. RESULTS

Both patients with a preoperative diagnosis of superior oblique overaction (patients 1 and 2) had good improvement in symptoms following surgery including improvement in A pattern on Hess Chart. Patient 2 also had improvement in field of binocular vision patient

Of the 4 patients had a pre operative diagnosis of primary Brown Syndrome, patient 5 and 6 had improved symptoms with less diplopia on upgaze. Both had improvements in field of binocular vision and Hess Chart. Patient 4 noticed no change in symptoms although his Hess chart showed objective improvement. Patient 3 developed consecutive superior oblique weakness and required further inferior oblique disinsertion and inferior rectus recession.

5 patients had a pre operative diagnosis of traumatic Brown Syndrome. Patients 7 and 11 had no change in symptoms. There was no change in the small field of binocular vision and no change in the Hess Chart. Patient 8 developed consecutive superior oblique weakness but refused further surgery. Patient 9 had improved elevation but continued to have diplopia on downgaze. He required contralateral inferior rectus posterior fixation suture. Patient 10 had improved symptoms and Hess Chart.

Table 1. Summary of Results

N	Diagnosis	Band (mm)	Deviation in primary Pre-op	Post-op	Symptoms	Hess	Field (%) Pre	Post
1	RSO+	4	10XT	4X	↑↑↑	better		
2	RSO+	5	12XT11L/R	4XT5L/R	↑↑↑	better	28	66
3	RBrowns	7	2ET 4L/R	8XT 10R/L	↓	worse		
4	RBrowns	?	4XT 6L/R	2ET 2L/R	→	better		
5	Bilat Browns	5L4R	nil	nil	↑	better	35	44
6	RBrowns	?	6ET 2R/L	2ET	↑↑	better	72	83
7	LTr.Browns	?	50XT 5L/R	60XT 4L/R	→	same	10	15
8	RTr.Browns	4	nil	nil	↓	worse	71	28
9	RTr.Browns	3	nil	nil	↑	better	71	49
10	RTr.Browns	5	2ET 12L/R	6X 4L/R	↑	better		
11	RTr.Browns	3.5	10XT5L/R	8XT 4L/R	→	same	6	6

Key: SO=Superior Oblique Overaction, Tr.Browns=Traumatic Browns, ↓= worse, →= no change, ↑=minimal improvement, ↑↑=moderate improvement, ↑↑↑=good improvement.

4. DISCUSSION AND CONCLUSION

Overall 6 patients reported improved symptoms following surgery. (55%). This is in contrast to previously reported success of 94%-100%. (Wright 1991, Stager 1999) We feel that this difference is probably due to the varied case mix of our patients. We achieved good results for superior oblique overaction (100%), moderate success for primary Brown Syndrome (50%) and disappointing results for traumatic Brown Syndrome; (40%) The use of silicone expanders for this condition has not been previously described. This group of patients are difficult to treat. Previous reports of surgery for traumatic Brown Syndrome have achieved only 33% success following 1 operation. (Aylward 1992) The reason for poor success rate in this group of patients may be adhesions or damage around the trochlear region.

5. REFERENCES

Aylward G.W. & Lawson J. 1992. The Surgical Treatment of Traumatic Browns Syndrome.*J Pediatr Ophthalmol Strabismus*; 29:276-283

Fitzsimons R. & White J 1990. Functional Scoring of the Field of Binocular Single Vision. *Ophthalmology*; 91(1): 33-35

Stager D.R. and Parks M.M. 1999. Long-Term Results of Silicone Expander for Moderate and Severe Brown Syndrome (Brown Syndrome "Plus"); *Journal of AAPOS*; 3(6):328-332

Wright K.W. 1991. Superior Oblique Silicone Expander for Brown Syndrome and Superior Oblique Overaction. *J.Pediatr Ophthalmol Strabismus*; 28(2):101-107

Transactions 28th Meeting European Strabismological Association, de Faber (ed.)
© 2004 European Strabismological Association, ISBN 90 265 1965 6

Evaluation of binocular visual function with electrophysiologic and psychophysic tests in Brown syndrome.

Önder Üretmen,Filiz Afrashi,Süheyla Köse,Erkan Ünsal,Kemal Pamukçu
Ege University School of Medicine Ophthalmology Department,35100
Bornova Izmir TURKEY

Objective: To evaluate binocular visual function by determining contrast sensitivity functions, visual evoked responses (VER)and stereopsis levels in patients with Brown syndrome.

Methods: Twelve patients with Brown syndrome were enrolled and compared to 12 normal subjects of similar ages and sex. All cases underwent a full ophthalmologic examination besides a de- tailed strabismological examination. Stereoacuity was measured with Titmus and TNO tests. Cambridge Low Contrast Grading test was used to evaluate contrast sensitivity while VER were recorded with Medelec Neuropto system.

Results: We determined that patients with Brown syndrome had reduced stereopsis levels than normal subjects. It is also determined that both monocular and binocular contrast sensitivity functions were worse in these patients. Comparing VER recorded in the two groups, we established that the latencies were longer and the amplitudes were smaller in patients with Brown syndrome. Binocular enhancement of VER amplitude, though more evident in the control group, was persent in both groups.

Conclusion: In Brown syndrome, partial binocular visual functional abnormalities could be found in addition to the characteristic ocular motility restrictions.

Transactions 28th Meeting European Strabismological Association, de Faber (ed.)
© 2004 European Strabismological Association, ISBN 90 265 1965 6

Results of superior oblique tenotomy for A-pattern strabismus measured with two methods

A.Maino,A.Ansons.
Royal Eye Hospital,Manchester,UK.

Objective:To evaluate the results obtained by superior oblique (SO)posterior tenotomy at the scleral insertion in patients with A-pattern strabismus with moderate to severe SO overaction using the prism cover test and the synoptophore.

Design:Retrospective study.

Methods:We analysed the clinical records of all patients that underwent unilateral or bilateral SO posterior tenotomy performed between 1991 and 2002. Main outcome measures were: extent of A-pattern deviation measured with the prism cover test (PCT)at 6 m and with the synoptophore and grading of the SO overaction (measured on a 9 point system,from –4 to +4). Patients 'ocular deviation was measured in primary position (PP),20 degrees upgaze and downgaze position (synoptophore)and maximal excursion upgaze and downgaze (PCT). All measures were recorded preoperatively and repeated 2 weeks and 3 months after the opera- tion.Statistical analysis was performed using Student 's t-test,repeated measures ANOVA test and simple linear regression.

Results:21 patients with A-pattern exotropia and 8 patients with A-pattern esotropia were in- cluded in the study.2 patients underwent an unilateral procedure. There were 27 who had simultaneous muscle surgery (recession and resection)for horizontal deviation and 3 patients that had superior rectus surgery to correct dissociated vertical deviation (DVD).Mean age was 23 years (range 3 – 44 years)).The results are summarized as follows:

There is a statistically significant change in angle of deviation after surgery.This was demonstrated with PCT (up-downgaze,$p<0.001$;PP-upgaze,$p<0.001$;PP-downgaze,$p=0.012$) and with the synoptophore (up-downgaze,$p<0.001$;PP-downgaze,$p<0.001$)except for the change in angle from primary position to upgaze ($p=0.336$).A significant change in superior oblique function after surgery was found for the left eye ($p=0.012$)but not for the right eye ($p=0.371$).Simple linear regression analysis shows that:1) the change in alignment after sur- gery is correlated to the preoperative deviation ($p=0.002$).2) the measurements obtained with PCT are correlated to the ones obtained with the synoptophore ($p=0.005$).

Conclusions:Although the PCT measurement of the A-pattern is greater than the synoptop- hore measurement,the difference was found not to be statistically significant.The measure- ments obtained with the PCT and the synoptophore correlated well therefore either technique could be used for the assessment of A-pattern strabismus.

Transactions 28th Meeting European Strabismological Association, de Faber (ed.)
© 2004 European Strabismological Association, ISBN 90 265 1965 6

Inferior oblique muscle function : correlation between scleral insertions of inferior, lateral recti and inferior oblique muscles and clinical function of inferior oblique muscle.

D. Denis, E. Hadjadj, J. Conrath, C. Benso
Ophthalmology Department, Hôpital Nord
Marseille, France

ABSTRACT: Primary hyperfunction of the inferior oblique muscle causes elevation of the non-fixing eye in adduction. The goal of this work was to measure the position of the scleral insertion of the inferior oblique muscle compared with those of the lateral and inferior recti muscles and to assess if these measures were correlated to clinical hyperfunction. 122 eyes from 78 strabic children, ranging from 30 to 196 months, 29 boys and 49 girls, 74 esotropia, 48 exotropia , 57 right eyes and 65 left eyes, have been included. This study shows the innervationnal theory to be most likely to explain the hyperfunction of inferior oblique muscle.

Keys Words: Hyperfunction of the inferior oblique muscle, strabismus, innervationnal theory.

1. PURPOSE

Primary hyperfunction of the inferior oblique muscle causes elevation of the non-fixing eye in adduction. The goal of this work was to measure the position of the scleral insertion of the inferior oblique muscle compared with those of the lateral and inferior recti muscles and to assess if these measures were correlated to clinical hyperfunction.

2. PATIENTS AND METHODS

122 eyes from 78 strabic children, ranging from 30 to 196 months, 29 boys and 49 girls, 74 esotropia, 48 exotropia , 57 right eyes and 65 left eyes, have been included.

All measures have been made by the same examiner, with millimetric calliper, during oculomotor surgery, after conjunctival dissection.

Measures were (Figure 1) :

IOALR : distance between the anterior insertion of the inferior oblique muscle and the anterior insertion of the lateral rectus muscle.

IOAIR : distance between the anterior insertion of the inferior oblique muscle and the anterior insertion of the inferior rectus muscle.

IOAL : distance between the anterior insertion of the inferior oblique muscle and limbus.

Clinical function of inferior oblique muscle was graded in this way (Figure 2) :

0 : no hyperfunction
+ : hyperfunction in extreme adduction
++ : hyperfunction in moderate adduction
+++ : hyperfunction between moderate adduction and primary position
++++ : hyperfunction in primary position

3 groups have been defined :

group 1 : include normal function 0 and hyperfunction +
group 2 : hyperfunction ++
group 3 : include hyperfunction +++ and ++++

SPSS 10 statistical software was used for the following statistical tests : Spearman correlation and Kruskal Wallis.

3. RESULTS

122 eyes from 78 strabic children, 29 boys (37, 2 %) and 49 girls (62, 8 %), 74 esotropia (60 %), 48 exotropia (40 %), 57 right eyes and 65 left eyes, ranging from 30 to 196 months have been included.

Hyperfunction of inferior oblique muscle was bilateral in 65 % of cases.

Distribution of eyes in the different groups was :

44, 26 % in group 1
29, 51 % in group 2
26, 23 % in group 3

Means and standard deviation of age, IOAL, IOALR, IOAIR are shown in table I.
Minimal and maximal values of IOAL, IOALR, IOAIR according to function of oblique inferior muscle are shown in table II.
Means and standard deviation of IOAL, IOALR, IOAIR according to function of oblique inferior muscle function are shown in table III.
Spearman correlations between age and the different measures are shown in table IV. There is no correlation between age and the different measures (low correlation coefficient < 0,5).
Distribution of ages according to the 3 groups of hyperfunction are shown in table V (Kruskal-Wallis test). There is no statistically significant difference concerning age in the 3 groups.

Comparison between muscles measurements and clinical inferior oblique muscle function according to the 3 groups of hyperfunction are shown in table VI (Kruskal Wallis test : significant when p<0,05). There is no statistically significant difference between the 3 groups of hyperfunction for IOALR (p:0,389), for IOAIR (p: 0,281) and for IOAL (p: 0,288).

4. DISCUSSION

Hyperfunction of inferior oblique muscle appears between 12 and 18 months and expresses itself by elevation of the non-fixing eye in adduction in 60 to 78 % of congenital esotropia (1, 2, 3, 4). It is bilateral in 90 % of cases although often asymmetrical. It can be isolated or associated

with an alphabetic syndrome. Hyperfunction of the inferior oblique muscle plays an essential role in oculomotor disturbance because of the low tolerance of vertical disturbance.
Our study is in accord with Fink's results (1) who related a distance of 9-10 mm between the anterior insertion of the inferior oblique muscle and the lateral rectus muscle.
Etiopathogenesis of this anomaly has often been discussed and 2 principal theories confront each other :

- Gobin and his theory of the sagittalisation of the inferior oblique muscle. He thinks that the anatomical malposition of the inferior oblique muscle is the primitive anomaly that prevents fusion, this producing secondary innervationnal horizontal deviation (5, 6, 7).
- Other authors [Quéré (8), Pigassou (9, 10), Teissier (11)] think that hyperfunction of the inferior oblique muscle has an innervationnal origin such as latent nystagmus and DVD.

For Quéré (8), the hyperfunction of the inferior oblique muscle is a part of ocular tonic dysregulation. Vertical troubles could have a supra-nuclear origin. For Pigassou (9, 10), the hyperfunction of the inferior oblique muscle could be the exaggeration of physiological function and its importance could be proportional to the degree of adduction. For Teissier (11), there is no correlation between the anatomic insertion of inferior oblique muscle and clinical hyperfunction but his study included only 35 patients.

In this study, we found no correlation between the inferior oblique muscle function and its scleral insertion (and in particular with the distance between inferior oblique and inferior rectus or between inferior oblique and lateral rectus muscles).

There is a statistically significant difference for IOAL but :

- this measure is the most difficult to perform (difficulty to observe at the same time the anterior part of the inferior oblique muscle, which is retro-equatorial, and the limbus, while taking a strictly radial measure).
- furthermore, there is a low variation of the means between the different groups, that has not necessarily a clinical significance but may cause the statistically significant difference because standard deviations are very low (all measures near the mean, quality of measures).

5. CONCLUSION

This study shows the innervationnal theory to be most likely to explain the hyperfunction of inferior oblique muscle.

Table

	Means	Standar deviation	N
Age (months)	71.65	35.42	78
IOAL(mm)	16.1	0.94	122
IOALR (mm)	9.65	0.94	122
IOAIR (mm)	12.94	0.98	122

TABLE I : means and standard deviation of age, IOAL, IOALR, IOAIR

Function	Minimum	Maximum	N
IOAL			
1	14	18.00	54
2	14.5	18.00	36
3	15	18.00	32
total	14	18	122
IOALR			
1	8.00	12.00	54
2	8.00	11.5	36
3	8.00	12.00	32
total	8.00	12.00	122
IOAIR			
1	11.00	16.00	54
2	11.14	14.00	36
3	11.00	14.5	32
total	11.00	16.00	122

TABLE II : minimal and maximal values of IOAL, IOALR, IOAIR according to function of oblique inferior muscle

Function	N	Means	SD
IOAL			
1	54	15.96	0.99
2	36	15.94	0.91
3	32	16.5	0.80
total	122	16.1	0.94
IOALR			
1	54	9.56	0.96
2	36	9.6	0.82
3	32	9.88	1.04
total	122	9.65	0.95
IOAIR			
1	54	13.05	1.07
2	36	12.72	0.88
3	32	13.02	0.91
total	122	12.94	0.98

TABLE III : means and standard deviation of IOAL, IOALR, IOAIR according to function of oblique inferior muscle

		Age	IOAL	IOALR	IOAIR
Age	corr N		0.331 122	0.273 122	0.299 122

TABLE IV : Spearman correlations between age and the different measures

	N	Means	SD
Age 1			
2	54	75.3	38.82
3	36	62.39	33.97
Total	32	72.44	34.43
	122	70.73	36.45

TABLE V : Repartition of ages according to the 3 groups of hyperfunction (Kruskal-Wallis test)

Distances / Function OI	Means's range	Tests used	p
IO AL	1 : 56.86 2 : 56.46 3 : 66.13	Kruskal-Wallis	0,228
IO ALR	1 : 58.67 2 : 59.38 3 : 68.67	Kruskal-Wallis	0,389
IO AIR	1 : 63.56 2 : 54.04 3 : 66.42	Kruskal-Wallis	0,281

Non Significance : p > 0,05

TABLE VI : muscles measurements and clinic inferior oblique muscle function (Kruskal Wallis test)

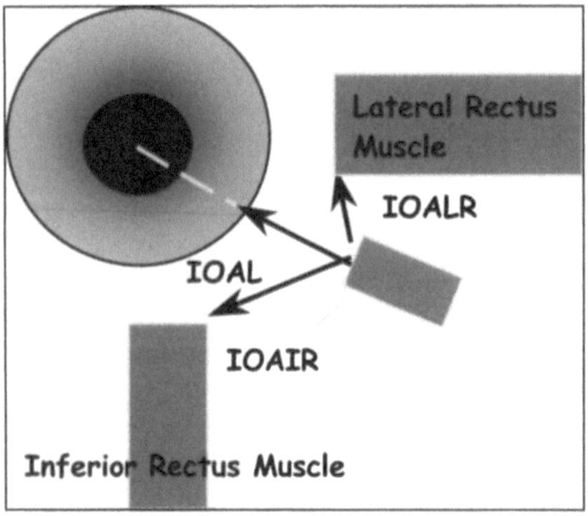

Illustration 1 : the different measures

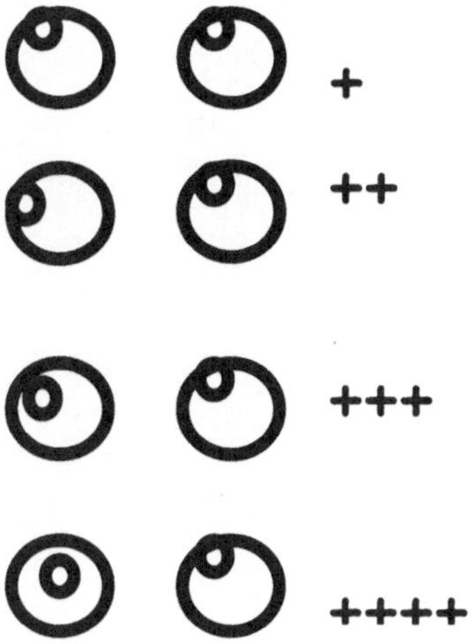

Illustration 2 : grading of clinical function of inferior oblique muscle

Bibliography

1. Fink W.H. The anatomy of the extrinsic muscles of the eye. Strab. Ophthal. Symp. 1950, pp 476.
2. Nelson LB., Wagner RS., Simon JW. Congenital esotropia. Surv Ophthalmol, 1987 ; 31, 363-383.
3. Helveston EM. Techniques and indications for surgery of the superior and inferior obliques muscles. Trans Ophthalmol Soc. UK, 1981, 251-7.
4. Frosini R., LO Monaco G., Campa L. L'élévation en adduction. Rapports avec le strabisme congénital et avec d'autres types de troubles de la motilité oculaire. J. Fr. Ophtalmologie, 1988 ; 11, 37-40.
5. Gobin MH. Anteroposition of inferior oblique muscle in VET. Ophthalmologica, 1964 ; 148, 325.
6. Gobin MH. Sagittalisation des muscles obliques. J. Fr. Orthopt, 1979 ; 11, 153.
7. Gobin MH. Desagittalization of the oblique muscles as a surgical treatment of strabismus. CESSD , Florence, 1982 ; 447.
8. Quéré MA. Les praticiens et les facteurs verticaux. Editions Lissac, 1991, 183 pp.
9. Pigassou-Albouy R. Le muscle oblique inférieur : un muscle pas comme les autres. Bull. Mem. Soc. Fr. Ophtalmol. 1986. p 91-95.
10. Pigassou-Albouy R. Strabisme et motilité extrinsèque. Les Strabismes: tome II: les convergences oculaires, Paris, Milan, Barcelone, Bonn. Editions Masson 1992. p 123-150.
11. Teissier E. Le muscle oblique inférieur. Etude anatomique-clinique et thérapeutique. Thèse pour le diplôme d'état de Docteur en médecine. 1999, 100 pp.

Transactions 28th Meeting European Strabismological Association, de Faber (ed.)
© 2004 European Strabismological Association, ISBN 90 265 1965 6

Clinical results of inferior oblique marginal or z myotomy

S.L. Robbins, W.K. Christian, E.F. Castro & D.B. Granet
UCSD/Abraham Ratner Children's Eye Center, La Jolla, California USA

ABSTRACT

To characterize the role of the marginal or Z myotomy of the inferior oblique muscle, we review a series of patients with small angle hypertropia and inferior oblique overaction having undergone this procedure. Ten patients had inferior oblique Z myotomies performed alone or in conjunction with horizontal strabismus surgery. Our results yielded an average reduction in primary gaze hypertropia of 2.45 - 6.35 PD. The percent reduction of deviation in the three eye positions most effected was consistently 70 - 80%. As evidenced by the standard deviations, many patients had 100% correction of their deviation leaving them orthophoric. There were no overcorrections. Previous overaction of the inferior oblique, measured by duction testing, was improved in all patients. We propose the Z myotomy as another tool in the strabismologist's armamentarium for small angle hypertropia with inferior oblique overaction to predictably decrease the deviation to fusional range or prismatic spectacle fusional range with low risk of overcorrection.

KEYWORDS

Inferior oblique muscle, marginal myotomy, Z myotomy

1. INTRODUCTION

The inferior oblique Z myotomy was originally described by Brown in 1950 and later by Focosi in 1955. The surgical technique we employed was a variation of the 1973 description by de Decker and Kueper. This should not be confused with the 'split tendon lengthening' or sutured myotomy proposed by Crawford in 1976 and later advocated by Ciancia. (Crawford, 1976 & Ciancia, 1977) After prolonged dormancy, the oblique muscle Z myotomy was again examined in two American studies recently. (Mellott, Scott, Ganser and Keech, 2002) (Bardorf and Baker, 2003)

2. METHODS

Ten consecutive patients aged 3 - 83 years old over a 15 month period at the University of California San Diego with small angle hypertropia (3 - 14 prism diopters in primary gaze) and inferior oblique overaction were evaluated. Five patients had inferior oblique Z myotomy as the sole procedure. Five patients underwent inferior oblique Z myotomy along with other horizontal strabismus surgery. No other vertical strabismus procedures were performed concurrently. The range of follow up was 1 week - 8 months; with an average of 4.2 months. A film of our surgical technique was shown. Our Z myotomy technique involved cross clamping the inferior oblique muscle 10 mm apart to include 70% of the muscle belly. The muscle was then cut and cauterized adjacent to the clamps but distal to the blood supply. There were no contiguous muscle fibers after the muscle was cut. The clamps were released allowing the muscle to lengthen. An Afrin-soaked cotton tip applicator was held with gentle pressure on the muscle to help achieve hemostasis.

3. RESULTS

The reduction of hypertropia in the three eye positions most effected expressed in prism diopters and as a percent reduction of the initial deviation is noted in Table 1. Of particular importance is the average reduction of primary gaze hypertropia of 2.45 - 6.35 PD. The percent reduction of initial deviation in all three eye positions was consistently in the 70% range. As evidenced by the standard deviations, many patients had 100% correction of their deviation leaving them orthophoric. There were no overcorrections. Previous overaction of the inferior oblique measured by duction testing improved in all patients.

Table 1. Post Inferior Oblique Z Myotomy - Hypertropia Results in Three Eye Positions

Eye Position	Average Reduction of Hypertropia (Prism Diopters)	Percent Reduction of Initial Deviation
Primary Gaze HT	4.4 ± 1.95 PD	78.4 ± 30.5%
Contralateral Gaze HT	5.5 ± 2.92 PD	70.9 ± 36.5%
Ipsilateral Tilt HT	5.3 ± 3.46 PD	74.7 ± 26.4%

4. CONCLUSIONS

As a lengthening procedure, the Z myotomy appears to reduce the risk of overcorrection due to a percent reduction of motility function rather than by a finite prism diopter correlation. As such, the risk of over-correction is small. Our results clarify the usefulness of the inferior oblique marginal or Z myotomy for mild hypertropias with inferior oblique overaction. We propose the Z myotomy as another tool in the strabismologist's armamentarium for small angle hypertropias with inferior oblique overaction to predictably decrease the deviation to fusional range or prismatic spectacle fusional range with low risk of overcorrection.

REFERENCES

Bardorf, C.M, Baker, J.D. 2003. The efficacy of superior oblique split Z-tendon lengthening for superior oblique overaction. *Journal of AAPOS* 7(2): 96-102.

Brown, H.W, 1950. Surgery on the oblique muscles. In J.H. Allen (ed), *Strabismus Ophthalmology Symposium*. St Louis: C.V. Mosby.

Ciancia, A.O. 1977. Elongacion del tendon del oblicuo superior. XI Panamerican Congress of Ophthalmology, Santiago.

Crawford, J.S. 1976. Surgical treatment of true Brown's syndrome. *American Journal of Ophthalmology* 57:276-280.

de Decker, W. & Kueper, J. 1973. Inferior oblique weakening by marginal myotomy: thermo-electric weakening. *Annals of Ophthalmology* 5: 605-13.

Focosi, M. 1955. La myotomie patielle marginale hans la correition des hyperfonitions legeres tu muscle oblique inferieur. *Bull Soc Belge* 109: 85.

Mellott, M.L, Scott, W.E, Ganser, G.L, Keech, R.V. 2002. Marginal myotomy of the minimally overacting inferior oblique muscle in asymmetric bilateral superior oblique palsies. *Journal of AAPOS* 6(4):216-220.

Transactions 28th Meeting European Strabismological Association, de Faber (ed.)
© 2004 European Strabismological Association, ISBN 90 265 1965 6

Management of adherence syndrome following inferior oblique surgery

B.J. L. Burton, E.L.M. Dawson, J.P. Lee
Department of Strabismus and Paediatrics.
Moorfields Eye Hospital
City Road
London EC1V 2PD.

ABSTRACT: A retrospective review of patients with Adherence Syndrome following strabismus surgery between 1989 and 2001 was performed. All 14 patients were thought to have undergone previous ipsilateral inferior oblique surgery. We usually performed an extensive conjunctival peritomy over nearly 180 degrees recessing the conjunctiva leaving the sclera to repithelialise and in addition recessed the inferior rectus by 2.5-3mm. Only one patient required an additional operation. Of the 11 patients who had undergone surgery at our institution all showed a significant improvement in their symptoms, five were discharged happy, three continue to be followed and three failed to attend further appointments after their initial two week post operation visit. It is not possible to restore normal eye movements in these patients but one can improve their appearance in primary position with single vision. Patients should be given realistic expectations before surgery and the limited aims of surgery must be explained.
KEYWORDS: Adherence syndrome, inferior oblique, conjunctival peritomy

1. INTRODUCTION

The adherence syndrome was described by Marshall Parks who initially felt that surgical disruption of orbital fat led to a restrictive ocular motility pattern (Parks 1978). This typically occurs following inferior oblique surgery or retinal detachment surgery (Wright 1986). More recently he revised his description of the mechanism of the restriction, now suggesting that the fat is not directly involved and that it is in fact the loss of elasticity of the septae in the extraconal space as a result of inflammation which restricts the globes movements (Parks 1986).

At present once adherence syndrome has occurred the prognosis is necessarily guarded, surgery is aimed at moving the diplopia free zone to encompass the primary position and at improving the cosmetic appearance where possible (Parks 1986).

We wish to report the results that can be achieved using more conventional surgical techniques and to highlight the therapeutic use of deliberate conjunctival recession in these patients (Dunlap 1974).

2. SUBJECTS AND METHODS

The diagnostic database of the senior surgeon in the strabismus service at Moorfields (JPL) was reviewed looking at the last twelve years. Fourteen patients were identified who had been diagnosed as having an adherence syndrome following strabismus surgery. The notes were reviewed retrospectively.

The average age was 16 (2 to 61), 11 were female. Unsurprisingly 13/14 patients had previous inferior oblique surgery, which was almost certainly the cause of the restriction in each case, there was no record of which muscles had been operated on in the remaining patient. Six patients had two previous operations and four had three operations prior to referral.

3. RESULTS

The original diagnosis, previous surgery, treatment at Moorfields and outcome of our patients are summarised in tables 1 and 2.

TABLE 1 Summary of preoperative patient characteristics.

Number	Age attended Moorfields	Symptoms	Original diagnosis from referring hospital	Previous Surgery	PCT n
1	12	cosmesis	Left ET with Bilateral IO overaction	L MR recessed, L LR rescted with L IO myectomy	6 BO with 32 R/L
2	10	diplopia	Congenital Left HT	LIO recessed on two occasions, three years later LIO explored and disinserted	10 BO with 12 R/L
3	26	diplopia	Chronic Left SO underaction	LIO myectomy, Five years later RIO myectomy	2BI with 5 L/R
4	5	cosmesis	Left ET	Previous Squint surgery, no details available	35 BO with 26 L/R
5	44	diplopia	Chronic Bilateral SO underaction	LIO disinserted, three years later RIO disinserted	6 BI with 16 L/R
6	4	cosmesis	Congenital Left SO underaction	LIO myectomy	20 BI with 18 R/L
7	2	cosmesis	Right ET and Right HypoT	RMR recessed RLR resected, 3 months later LIO recessed	40 BO with 14 R/L
8	10	diplopia	L ET	Bilateral MR recession, 4 years later bilateral MR Faden sutures, 4 years later LMR recessed with LLR resected, LIO recessed, 2 weeks later LIOmyectomy.	2 BO with 16 R/L
9	6	cosmesis	Congenital Right SO underaction	RMR recessed RLR resected, 1 year later bilateral IO recession, later the same year RIO explored and adhesions cleared	30 R/L
10	61	diplopia on upgaze	Right SO underaction	R IO recession, later same year R IO myectomy, clearance of adhesions and conjunctival recession.	10 BI with 3 L/R

11	4	cosmesis	Left XT	LLR recession LMR resection. One year later L IO recession and resection of LMR.	12 BI with 12 R/L
12	10	parental concern about abnormal head posture	Right ET	Bilat MR recession, 3 years later R MR Faden, L MR resected, R IO recessed	30 BO with 20 L/R
13	8	headache and occasional blurring of vision, no cosmetic problem	Right ET	R MR recession R LR resected, 1 year later L IO myectomy.	6 BO with 27 R/L
14	27	diplopia	Chronic Right SO underaction	R IO recessed (snapped during surgery), 1 year later R IO recessed.	25 BI with 4 L/R

ET= Esotropia, XT=exotropia, SO=superior oblique, IO=inferior oblique, BI= Base in prism, BO= Base out prism, R/L=Right over left, PCTn=Prism cover test near.

TABLE 2 Corrective surgery performed at Moorfields.

Number	First surgery at Moorfields	PCT n	Outcome	Length of follow up after first surgery at Moorfields
1	R IO disinsertion. L IR 3mm recession, L conjunctiva recessed	Not recorded	Improved cosmetically with small persistent Left HypoT and ET. No diplopia, happy with operative result.	2 weeks then DNA
2	L IO adhesions freed, R IO recessed, LIR recessed 2.5 mm, conjunctiva recessed	6 BO with 3 L/R	No diplopia, discharged happy	2 yrs
3	RIO recessed, RIR recessed, conjunctiva recessed	8 BI with 4 L/R	Diplopia on extremes of gaze only, not bothersome, stable for 1 year,	2yrs
4	R IO recessed, R IR recessed 2 mm, conjunctiva recessed	10 BO with 18 L/R	Cosmetically good, discharged happy.	2yrs
5	R IR recessed 3mm on adjustable sutures, conjunctiva recessed	2 BI with 8 L/R	7 months later L IO disinsertion. 2 weeks post op 6 BI with 3 L/R. Minimal head tilt to right, not bothered by diplopia on R elevation and depression, DNA further appointments.	8 month

6	L IO disinserted, L IR 3mm recessed, conjunctiva recessed	8 BI with 8 R/L	Almost no head tilt, good binoc function, Mod exophoria with hyperphoria, discharged happy.	19 months
7	L IR -3mm recession, L MR recession, conjunctiva recessed	20 BO with 8 R/L	Cosmetically good, discharged happy.	4yr
8	L IR 3mm recession on adjustable sutures, L LR recessed on adjustables, conjunctiva recessed	20 BO with 18 R/L	Cosmetically good, discharged happy.	5.5 months
9	L IR -3mm recession, conjunctiva recessed	4 BI with 6 R/L	Cosmetically good at 2 weeks, DNA further appointments.	2 weeks then DNA
10	L IO disinsertion, L SR Faden	10 BI with 3 R/L	Diplopia on R gaze which does not bother him.	3 months
11	R LR -7mm and reinserted down 2/3 muscle width. R MR +5mm and reinserted down 2/3 muscle width	14 BO with 9 R/L	Vision excellent, good cosmesis, stable measurement, residual L ET with hypotropia, no diplopia.	2.5 years
12	None		Cosmetically satisfactory, double vision on upgaze to right. Improved spontaneously since original referral.	No surgery
13	Offered surgery but declined at present			No surgery
14	Offered surgery but declined at present			No surgery

DNA = Did not attend

Our approach was to perform a forced duction test which was positive in all cases. Following this we explored the inferior oblique and inferior rectus. An extensive conjunctival recession was performed followed by dissection of scar tissue and disinsertion of any remaining fibres of inferior oblique with great care taken with haemostasis and trying to avoid further unnecessary surgical trauma. Finally the inferior rectus was recessed 2.5-3mm. Where possible this was done using adjustable sutures, although many of our patients were too young for this technique to be tried. There is a risk of ipsilateral lower lid retraction with this procedure although none of our patients required treatment for this.

In two cases the vertical deviation in primary gaze was not the major problem and in these patients we elected to operate on the other eye. In one case we performed a Faden procedure to reduce diplopia on up gaze, and the other patient had an inverse Knapp procedure combined with a recess resect operation for her exotropia.

Three patients declined surgery, but of the eleven who had an operation at Moorfields five were discharged happy with an improvement in either their diplopia or cosmetic appearance or both. Three did not reattend after their two week post op visit but were all much improved at this early stage. Three patients are still being followed up but all of these showed improvement following surgery and we have no plans for further operations on them at present.

4. DISCUSSION

Adherence syndrome following inferior oblique surgery can be recognised by finding limited upgaze usually in the presence of an ipsilateral hypotropia in primary position which is worse on abduction. There should also be a positive forced duction test although this can be difficult to assess. Some cases may show ipsilateral upper lid retraction.

Prevention is better than cure and the importance of careful surgical dissection, protecting the integrity of the muscle sleeve during vitreo-retinal surgery (Wright 1986), trying to avoid exposing orbital fat and minimising bleeding during strabismus surgery have been highlighted previously (Dunlap 1974).

5. CONCLUSION

Our surgical results show that in expert hands acceptable results can be achieved in most cases of adherence syndrome caused by strabismus surgery.

Patients should be given realistic expectations before surgery, and the limited aims of the surgery should be explained. It is not currently possible to give back normal eye movements once an adherence syndrome has occurred but a reasonable cosmetic result with single vision at least in primary position should be aimed for and is usually achievable.

REFERENCES

Dunlap EA. Surgery of muscle adhesions and effects of multiple operations. Br J Ophthalmol. 1974;58:307-312.

Parks MM. Causes of the adhesive syndrome. In: Symposium on strabismus; Transactions of the New Orleans Academy of Ophthalmology. St Louis: CV Mosby, 1978;269-279.

Parks MM. Discussion of Wright KW. The fat adherence syndrome and strabismus after retina surgery. Ophthalmology 1986;93:411-5.

Wright KW. The fat adherence syndrome and strabismus after retina surgery. Ophthalmology 1986;93:411-5.

Session 9
Paralytic strabismus

Transactions 28th Meeting European Strabismological Association, de Faber (ed.)
 ISBN 90 265 1965 6

Changes in incomitance in acquired unilateral sixth nerve palsy

L. Garnham DBOT & J.P. Lee FRCOphth
Moorfields Eye Hospital, London, England

ABSTRACT Acquired cranial nerve palsy is characterized by typical muscle sequelae. We undertook a retrospective review over eighteen months of acquired unilateral VIN palsy. Twenty-seven patients were identified and 6 patients had a total paralysis of the lateral rectus. The remaining 21 had partial palsy. There were 14 males and 13 females whose ages ranged from 26-87 years. We analysed aetiology, duration and recovery of the palsy, and ocular motility with emphasis on analysis of Hess charts. Five of the six patients with total palsy had no ipsilateral medial rectus overaction and none showed any subsequent recovery. Of the 21 partial palsy patients all except 4 showed complete recovery. Twelve had ipsilateral medial rectus overaction from the onset and the remaining 9 had no medial rectus overaction. Medial Rectus overaction does not always develop in cases of total VIN palsy and further investigation may help clarify this.

KEYWORDS: VIN palsy; ipsilateral medial rectus overaction

1 INTRODUCTION

Acquired cranial nerve palsy is characterized by: -

1) Underaction of the affected muscle
2) Overaction of the contralateral synergist
3) Overaction of the ipsilateral antagonist
4) Inhibitional palsy of the contralateral antagonist

These underactions and overactions occur due to Hering's (1868) and Sherrington's (1894) Laws of innervation and lead to spread of concomitance.

2 METHOD

A retrospective review of patient notes was carried out over an eighteen-month period on patients attending with a recently acquired unilateral VIN palsy. Twenty-seven patients were identified (14 females and 13 females) who had an age range of 26-87 years (mean 51 years). Six of these had a total VIN palsy characterized by an inability to abduct the affected eye beyond the midline. The remaining 21 had a partial VIN palsy.
Aetiology, duration and recovery of the palsy and ocular motility were analysed. Particular study was made of Hess charts, which were plotted in all cases to aid assessment of the development of muscle sequelae. When patients had an area of single vision Fields Of Binocular Single Vision (BSV) were plotted.

3 RESULTS

Five of the six patients with total VIN palsy had no ipsilateral medial rectus overaction and all six patients failed to show any signs of recovery. Of the remaining 21 patients with partial VIN

palsy, 17 showed complete recovery. Ipsilateral medial rectus overaction was seen from the onset in 12 of these patients with partial palsy, including the 4 who have not shown signs of recovery. The remaining 9 had no ipsilateral medial rectus overaction at any time.
Hess chart analysis clearly showed the lack of ipsilateral medial rectus overaction in the 5 cases of total VIN palsy (Fig1). Another case of partial VIN palsy (Fig2) shows fully developed muscle sequelae.

Fig.1

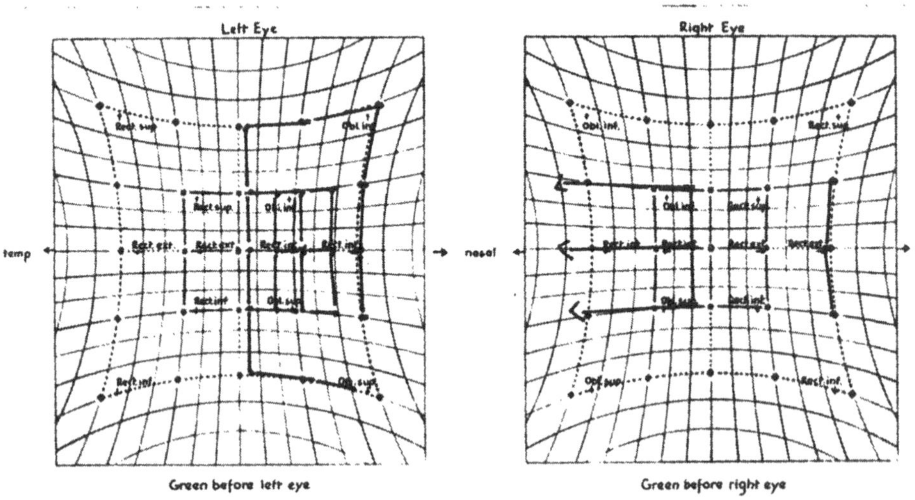

Fig.2

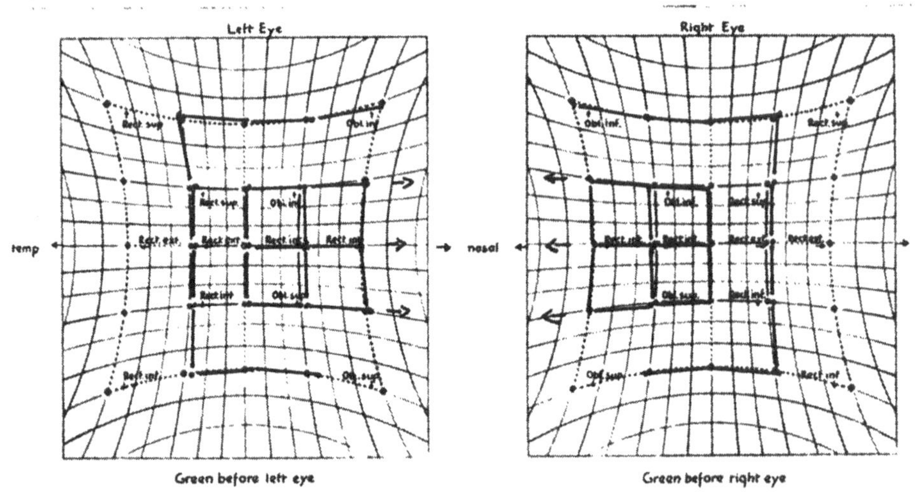

In total VIN palsy with classical muscle sequelae no area of BSV would be expected, however in all 5 cases of ours an area of BSV was found in the direction opposite to that of the affected lateral rectus. Three of these patients adopted an Abnormal Head Posture (AHP) of face turn to make use of this area of single vision.

The aetiology of the VIN palsy in these 5 cases consists of: -
Head trauma, meningioma, Burkitt's lymphoma, carotico-cavernous fistula and one is awaiting the results of an MRI scan. The aetiology of the one case of total VIN palsy with ipsilateral medial rectus overaction was extradural intracavernous aneurysm with a gradual onset over 2 years.

4 DISCUSSION

Why do some cases of total unrecovered VIN palsy show no overaction of the ipsilateral antagonist?
There was no undetected partial IIIN palsy as none of the muscles supplied by either branch of this nerve was underacting. No case had had previous extra ocular muscle surgery nor had any myopathic disease. There was no muscle pathology associated with the aetiology and direct trauma to the muscle to the muscle had not occurred in any case.
It has been suggested by some authors including Guibor (1950) that the patient should be encouraged to fix with the paretic eye to prevent ipsilateral medial rectus overaction in VIN palsy. In our study, however, all 5 patients fixed with their non-paretic eye.

5 CONCLUSIONS

There are some cases of VIN palsy where there is profound paralysis of fibres responsible for ocular rotation, with sparing of fibres responsible for position holding. EMG studies, saccadic velocity, measured forced duction and forced generation testing would help clarify this.

REFERENCES

Guibor, G.B.1950. Some uses of ophthalmic prisms. In J.H. Allen (ed.), *Strabismus Ophthalmic Symposium 1*, St.Louis: The C.V. Mosby Co.

Hering, E. 1868. Die Lehre vom Binocularen Sehen, Leipzig: Wilhem Englemann.

Sherrington, C.S. 1894. Experimental note on two movements of the eyes, J.Physiol. (London)17:27

Transactions 28th Meeting European Strabismological Association, de Faber (ed.)
© 2004 European Strabismological Association, ISBN 90 265 1965 6

Limitation of Opposing Ductions Following Augmented Horizontal Rectus Muscle Transposition

David K. Coats, M.D., Mohamed A.W. Hussein M.D.
Cullen Eye Institute, Baylor College of Medicine, Departments of Ophthalmology and Pediatrics, Texas Children's Hospital, Houston, Texas, United States

ABSTRACT:Purpose: To report the effect on ductions in opposing gaze following total or partial horizontal rectus muscle transposition augmented with posterior fixation sutures to treat vertical gaze misalignment due to cyclovertical muscle palsies. Methods: We reviewed the records of 5 patients who underwent horizontal rectus muscle transposition augmented with posterior fixation sutures for treatment of vertical gaze misalignment secondary to cyclovertical muscle palsy. Results: Four patients achieved excellent alignment in the primary position after 1 operation. One patient required additional surgery for residual deviation with excellent final alignment in the primary position. Ductions in the direction of the palsied muscle improved in all patients. Four patients (80%) developed significant limitation of vertical gaze in the direction opposite that of the palsied muscle.Conclusion: Transposition surgery augmented with posterior fixation is effective in managing vertical misalignment secondary to cyclovertical muscle palsy, improving alignment in the primary position and producing improvement of eye rotation in the direction of the paralyzed muscle. This procedure, however, can produce considerable limitation of ductions in the direction opposite to that of the paralyzed muscle.

KEYWORDS: Augmented transposition, duction limitation

1. INTRODUCTION

Successful use of augmented transposition procedures in the management of vertical misalignment secondary to vertical muscle paralysis has been reported.[1] Reported benefits have included improved primary gaze alignment with modest improvement of eye rotation in the field of action of the paralyzed vertical rectus muscle. The effect of this procedure on ductions in the direction opposite that of the paralyzed vertical muscle has not been reported.

2. METHODS

The records of 5 patients (1-4 previously reported)[1,2] who underwent partial or total horizontal rectus muscle transposition augmented with posterior fixation suture for treatment of vertical gaze misalignment due to cyclovertical muscle palsy were reviewed. The preoperative and postoperative ocular motility status of each patient is tabulated (Table1).

Table 1. Preoperative and postoperative assessment

#	Age (Years)	Diagnosis	Etiology	Preoperative duction	Procedure	Postoperative duction	F/U (months)
1**		Monocular elevation deficiency (OD)	Congenital, idiopathic	-4 Supraduction	FTT to the SR, PFS 15 (OD)	-2 Supraduction 0 Infraduction	23
2	45	Third nerve palsy (OD)	Trauma	-4 Supraduction	PTT to the SR PFS 15 (OD)	-3 Supraduction -3 Infraduction	5
3	4	Monocular elevation deficiency (OD)	Congenital, Idiopathic	-4 Supraduction	FTT to the SR, PFS14 (OD)	-2 Supraduction -3 Infraduction	43
4*	19	Third nerve palsy (OD)	Trauma	-3 Infraduction	PTT to the IR, PFS 15 (OD)	-2 Infraduction -3 Supraduction	9
5	9	Inferior Rectus Palsy (OS)	Blowout fracture	-4 Infraduction	FTT to the IR, PFS 15 (OS)	-2 Infraduction -3 Supraduction	12

SR= Superior rectus IR= Inferior rectus PFS= Posterior fixation suture FTT = Full tendon transposition PTT= Partial tendon transposition * = More than one surgery was needed ** Patient had previous LR recession

3. RESULTS

Mean follow up was 16 months (5 to 24 months). All patients had excellent vertical alignment in the primary position after the transposition surgery with improvement of ductions in the field of action of the palsied muscle. One (patient # 4) required additional surgery for concurrent horizontal and residual vertical strabismus. Four (80%) of the patients developed considerable limitation of ductions in the direction opposite that of the palsied muscle following the transposition surgery with an average duction limitation of –2.5. Patient #1, who did not develop limitation of opposing ductions, had previously undergone lateral rectus muscle recession in both eyes for management of intermittent exotropia.

4. DISCUSSION

The major goals of surgery to treat paralytic strabismus are to improve alignment in the primary position, create a maximum field of single binocular vision and, if possible, to improve rotation of the eye in the direction of the paralyzed muscle. Transposition of part or all of the rectus muscles invariably results in some mechanical restriction to full rotation of the globe in the opposite direction[3] by altering the force vectors of the transposed vertical muscles. Elongating the path of the transposed muscle induces passive elastic force, increasing the tone of the transposed muscles. Contraction of the muscles concerned with movement of the eyes in the opposite direction to that of the paralyzed muscle hence will always face an increased opposing tone. Posterior fixation suture augmentation enhances the tone of transposed muscles by providing additional stretching, contributing to duction limitation on attempted opposite gaze. Limitation of ductions in the opposite direction to that of the transposed muscles following vertical muscle transposition to treat horizontal muscle palsies has not been a problem.[4] The explanation by Clark et al,[5] of horizontal translation of the globe in the direction of horizontal eye movement may help to explain the absence of opposing duction limitation following vertical rectus transposition for horizontal rectus palsy. While translocation following horizontal rectus muscle transposition has not been studied, it may be more limited, and thus could help explain opposing duction limitation following surgery. Whether subtle weakness of the inferior rectus in case two or the superior rectus in case four contributed to postoperative duction limitation is not clear, but possible. It is also unclear why 1 patient did not develop limitation of opposing ductions. Perhaps transposition of the previously recessed lateral muscles produced fewer unwanted restrictive forces than transposition of previously unoperated muscles.

In summary, posterior fixation suture augmented transposition surgery used for treatment of cyclovertical palsy can be associated with considerable limitation of ductions in the direction opposite to that of the paralyzed muscle. Unsuspected paresis of the antagonist rectus muscle may contribute to, but does not entirely explain the problem. Opposing ductions may be especially problematic for superior augmented transposition surgery as downgaze limitation may be more symptomatic.

REFERENCES

Paysse EA, Brady McCreery KM, Ross A, Coats, DK. Use of augmented rectus muscle transposition surgery for complex strabismus. Ophthalmol. 2002;109:1309-1314.

Coats DK, Brady-McCreery KM, Paysse EA. Split rectus muscle modified Foster procedure for paralytic strabismus: a report of 5 cases. Binocul Vis Strabismus Q. 2001;16:281-284.

Metz HS. 20th Annual Frank Costenbader Lecture—Muscle Transposition Surgery. J. Pediatr. Ophthalmol. Strabismus. 1993;30:346-353.

Foster RS. Vertical muscle transposition augmented with lateral fixation. J. AAPOS. 1997;1:20-30.

Clark RA, Demer JL. Rectus extraocular muscle pulley displacement after surgical transposition and posterior fixation for treatment of paralytic strabismus. Am. J. Ophthalmol. 2002;133:119-128.

Transactions 28th Meeting European Strabismological Association, de Faber (ed.)
© 2004 European Strabismological Association, ISBN 90 265 1965 6

Sixth Nerve Palsies as Isolated Mononeuropathies in Patients with Multiple Sclerosis.

J.A. Gonzalez-Martin, V. Trimble, G. Kyle & I.B. Marsh.
Walton-University Hospital Aintree, Liverpool, United Kingdom.

ABSTRACT: 10 patients with clinically definite Multiple Sclerosis that developed isolated sixth nerve palsies are presented. The time course to recovery and different therapeutic options are described.

KEYWORDS: Sixth Nerve Palsy, Multiple Sclerosis, Diplopia.

1 INTRODUCTION

1.1 *Background*

Fairly common ocular manifestations in patients with Multiple Sclerosis are optic neuritis and diplopia due to internuclear ophthalmoplegia. Isolated Mononeuropathies such as sixth nerve palsies are infrequently reported.

1.2 *Frequency of Sixth nerve Palsies in Multiple Sclerosis*

Moster et al (1984) have reported a case series of 49 young adults (age range 15 to 50 years old) with isolated sixth nerve palsies. 6 (12%) of these patients had multiple sclerosis to account for the sixth nerve palsy. Peters et al (2002) published a case series of 45 young adults (age range 20 to 50 years old) with non-traumatic sixth nerve palsy. They found that 11 patients (24%) had multiple sclerosis to account for their palsy. Peters et al argue that their higher prevalence is due to the routine use of magnetic resonance imaging (MRI) that was not used in Moster et al series. It is also of interest to observe Barr et al (2000) series. They report that sixth nerve palsy in young adults (age range 18 to 50 years old) with MS had a particularly low prevalence of only 1.6%. They discuss that a lesion of the sixth nerve nucleus results in an ipsilateral horizontal gaze palsy due to the internuclear neurons which project to the contralateral medial rectus subdivision of the third nerve nuclear complex. Also that as the fascicular fibers pass through the pons they establish relations that would result on sixth nerve palsy associated with other brainstem signs such as ipsilateral facial nerve palsy, conjugate gaze palsy, ataxia and contralateral hemiparesis. These additional signs may be subtle and easy to miss. In our series we estimate that the prevalence of sixth nerve palsy in isolation for the whole population seen with MS in a tertiary referral clinic is 6.5%.

1.3 *Clinically Multiple Sclerosis*

Objective evidence of two episodes of demyelination separated in time by at least one month account for the definition of clinically multiple sclerosis. Traditionally the diagnosis is based in clinical neurological findings being a diagnosis of exclusion for any other neurological complaint that may produce similar symptoms. The findings of the cerebral spinal fluid (elevated proteins, oligoclonal Ig G bands), MRI (demyelination plaques) or abnormal visual evoked potentials are complementary to the clinical examination but not diagnostic as such. Lately the revised criteria for the diagnosis of MS includes MRI amongst others, McDonald et al (2001).

2 METHODS

Patients attending a tertiary referral neurology MS clinic. All patient with any ocular complaint were seen by an orthoptist and ophthalmologist. Only patients with sixth nerve in isolation are included in this study. All patients underwent orthoptist assessment including serial Hess chart to record extraocular movements and fields of binocular single vision.

3 RESULTS

10 patients were entered and followed. 8 females and 2 males. The mean age of the group was 44 years old (range 26 to 71). The mean angle of deviation at presentation was 12Δ base out for near and 17Δ base out for distance. The mean time to recovery or stabilisation of the deviation was 6 months. 4 of the ten patients had spontaneous recovery in a mean time of 6 months. 4 patients underwent botulinum toxin injection to the ipsilateral medial rectus. 2 of these patients showed little or no recovery of the deviation and underwent subsequently surgery consisting on medial rectus recession and latereal rectus resection on the affected eye. 2 patients were managed by permanent prismatic correction alone.

4 CONCLUSIONS

It has been our experience that patients presenting to a neurology clinic with a relapse of MS to include diplopia are in many instances not offered therapeutic help. The concept that the relapsing remitting nature of the MS would produce spontaneous resolution of a sixth nerve palsy that may account for the diplopia is erroneous. We find that spontaneous recovery is not the norm and most patients need some form of intervention. Also that the holistic approach to the care of these patients by means of orthoptist and ophthalmology input in the MS clinics provides significant benefits.

5 REFERENCES

Barr D.2000 Isolated Sixth nerve palsy: an uncommon presenting sign of multiple sclerosis. *J Neurol* 247: 701-4.

McDonald W.I. 2001. Recommended diagnostic criteria for multiple sclerosis: guidelines from the International Panel on the diagnosis of multiple sclerosis. *Ann Neurol* 50: 121-7

Moster, M.L. 1984. Isolated Sixth-Nerve Palsies in Younger Adults. *Arch Ophthalmol* 102: 1328-30.

Peters G. B. III. 2002. Cause and Prognosis of Non-traumatic Sixth Nerve Palsies in Young Adults. *Ophthalmology* 109: 1925-8.

Rose J.W. 1992 Acute VIth cranial nerve dysfunction in multiple sclerosis. Evaluation by magnetic resonance imaging. *J Clin Neuroophthalmol* 12: 17-20.

Transactions 28th Meeting European Strabismological Association, de Faber (ed.)
© 2004 European Strabismological Association, ISBN 90 265 1965 6

The natural history of brainstem ocular motility disorders due to vascular pathology

F.J. Rowe
Division of Orthoptics, University of Liverpool, UK.

C.P. Noonan
Department of Ophthalmology, Warrington Hospital, UK.

ABSTRACT: Introduction/objective To perform a cross sectional study of cases of ocular motility disorders due to brainstem vascular pathology. To review the types of ocular motility disorders documented in these cases and address the natural history of recovery.
Methods Each patient underwent a full Orthoptic and Ophthalmic examination. Complete neurological workup with appropriate CT/MR brain imaging was obtained. Patients with other brainstem pathology such as multiple sclerosis, degenerative or space occupying lesions were excluded.
Results A variety of ocular motility disorders were documented. These included cranial nerve palsies, ophthalmoplegia, nystagmus and abnormalities of saccadic and smooth pursuit movements. Treatment was mostly conservative with occlusion, filters and prisms and provision of support and coping strategies. Nine of the twelve patients were managed conservatively. Two of the nine patients had a return to normal ocular motility status within a 2-month period. Three patients required active intervention (Botulinum toxin (BT) or surgery) in addition to conservative treatment.
Conclusions: 16% (2/12 patients) improved to normal ocular motility status. This occurred within 2 months of initial insult. Eight other patients (67%) had a partial recovery with symptoms relieved either by conservative methods alone or by the addition of BT or surgery.

KEYWORDS: Brainstem, Ocular motility, Vascular pathology

1. INTRODUCTION

Brainstem vascular accidents, result in range of ocular motility disorders dependent on the area within the brainstem affected. These range from nuclear cranial nerve palsies, gaze palsies, nystagmus and eye movement (saccadic, smooth pursuit and vergence) difficulties. The associated general signs and symptoms such as hemiplegia, tremor, central Horner's syndrome and vertigo aid the diagnosis in many cases with confirmation by neuro-imaging of the brainstem area.

Medical advances over the past decade have lead, so it seems, to an increase in the number of patients seen in our clinics with brainstem ocular motility disorders. As a result of this perceived increase, a study was undertaken to review cases with brainstem vascular pathology to document the associated ocular motility problems, treatment given and final outcome.

2. METHODS AND MATERIALS

For the purposes of this study patients with an acute vascular event affecting the brainstem were included. Patients with brainstem symptoms secondary to multiple sclerosis, myasthenia gravis, progressive supranuclear palsy, space occupying lesion and infectious or inflammatory conditions were excluded.

A cross section analysis was undertaken and cases were reviewed over a twelve-month period from March 2002 to March 2003. Twelve cases were identified that adhered to our inclusion criteria. A further 19 cases were excluded. Brainstem pathology was confirmed by neurological examination involving CT but mostly MR imaging. Each patient had a full ophthalmic and orthoptic assessment.

RESULTS

Seven females and five males were reviewed with an average age at presentation of 53 years (range 25 to 78 years). There was little difference in the average age of females (51 years; range 25 to 73 years) and males (56 years; range 42 to 78 years). Vascular lesions were due to infarction in eight cases and haemorrhage in four cases.

The ocular motility disorders included double elevator palsy, internuclear ophthalmoplegia, nuclear or fascicular third nerve palsy, fascicular sixth nerve palsy, gaze palsy and abnormal movement systems of saccades and smooth pursuits. See table 1. Ocular symptoms were reported by each patient either constantly or intermittently and included binocular diplopia, oscillopsia, blurred vision and reading difficulties. There were numerous generalised symptoms including hemiplegia, seventh nerve palsy, hand tremor, and difficulties with balance and speech.

Four of the twelve patients required no treatment. One patient with a unilateral internuclear ophthalmoplegia improved spontaneously over a 6 week period. Three patients were asymptomatic due to suppression in two patients and complete ptosis in one patient. Eight patients received conservative treatment, consisting of prisms, occlusion, or Bangerter filters. Two patients received BT injection, in addition to either occlusion or prisms, one preferring multiple injections and one not benefiting from their single BT injection. One patient had surgery for a double elevator palsy which was successful. The follow-up period at the time of this cross section analysis ranged from 6 weeks to 8 years from presentation (average 2½ years).

Two patients showed no recovery in ocular motility (over a period of 2 and 3 years) although both were asymptomatic, one with the use of prisms. Two patients had full recovery of ocular motility over a period of 6 weeks and 2 months. The remaining patients showed some improvement of ocular motility ranging from minimal (three patients), partial (three patients) and good (two patients) range of eye movement. This recovery was seen over a variable time period of 6 months to 8 years. No patient was symptomatic in the primary position at follow-up due either to the use of prisms or occlusion, presence of suppression or ptosis.

3. DISCUSSION

The ocular motility deficits recorded in these patients were varied. Double elevator palsy is a presumed interruption of supranuclear input from the vertical upgaze areas in the midbrain (Jampel & Fells 1968, Lessel 1975. Patients typically have a hypotropia in the primary position with pseudoptosis and true ptosis. Our two patients had a complete limitation of elevation with hypotropia and pseudoptosis.

A lesion of the medial longitudinal fasciculus (MLF) will result in internuclear ophthalmoplegia (Bronstein et al. 1990) with loss/impairment of adduction of the contralateral eye due to involvement of interneurons from the ipsilateral sixth nerve nucleus to the contralateral medial rectus subnucleus. Vascular events when diffuse cause bilateral internuclear ophthalmoplegia and when more focal cause unilateral internuclear ophthalmoplegia due to the midline separation of the blood supply to the two halves of the brainstem. We reviewed two cases of internuclear ophthalmoplegia, one unilateral and one bilateral with typical characteristics of limited adduction and abducting nystagmus of the contralateral eye. Convergence was retained in both cases. A more extensive lesion of the MLF involving the ipsilateral sixth nerve nucleus will result in a one and a half syndrome with ipsilateral horizontal gaze palsy and ipsilateral loss/impairment of adduction. One of our patients was noted to have a recovering one and a half syndrome in addition to numerous other ocular motility problems.

Four of our patients had a third palsy. Two patients had a nuclear third nerve palsy, one patient had a complete left third nerve palsy and limited movement in the right eye corresponding to contralateral superior rectus involvement and the second patient had a complete right third nerve palsy with a contralateral superior division third nerve palsy. The bilateral defect is due to the anatomy of the nucleus and its fibres. The fibres for superior rectus function pass through the contralateral superior rectus subnucleus without synapse and innervate the contralateral superior rectus (Bienfang 1975). Therefore lesions in this region cause ipsilateral third nerve palsies and contralateral superior rectus weakness. Levator function is under bilateral control at the level of the third nerve nuclei due to the bilateral organisation of the caudal central subnucleus that supplies the levator muscle (Leigh & Zee 1991) and therefore can result in bilateral ptosis. Two patients had a fascicular lesion resulting in a third nerve palsy without pupil involvement but also with a vertical gaze palsy. Fascicular lesions can give additional signs such as hemiplegia, central Horner's syndrome and intention tremor, e.g. Weber's syndrome, Benedikt's syndrome and Claude's syndrome.

Gaze palsies result from involvement of the brainstem nuclei and their projections responsible for generating vertical and horizontal eye movements (Rowe 2003). Vertical gaze palsies commonly result from lesions in the brainstem as bilateral input is required to generate vertical gaze. The nuclei responsible for generating vertical gaze movements are connected via the MLF and posterior commissure and vertical gaze palsies result from lesions to the riMLF and rostral midbrain (Bender 1980, Green 1993, Lagreze 1996). Innervation is unilateral to depressor extraocular muscles but bilateral to elevator muscles. Therefore gaze palsies on elevation are more common. Upward gaze palsies were noted in four of the patients in this study. Horizontal gaze palsies result from lesions involving the sixth nerve nucleus often of a vascular pathology. Seventh nerve involvement can occur with horizontal gaze palsies or sixth nerve palsies because of its close proximity with the sixth nerve (Miller 2002). One patient had a fascicular bilateral sixth nerve palsy with unilateral seventh nerve involvement in association with the ocular motility deficit of abduction.

Disorders of saccades result in abnormalities of initiation, velocity, accuracy and inappropriate saccadic intrusions. Slow saccades may be noted with nerve palsies or drug use. Accuracy disorders may be noted with brainstem or cerebellar disease. Abnormal saccadic eye movements were noted in five patients. Normal smooth-pursuit movements may be replaced by series of small saccades termed "cog-wheeling". This was the case in one patient in this study and smooth pursuit movements were noted as abnormal and jerky in a further three patients.

Skew deviation is an acquired vertical misalignment of the visual axes caused by a disturbance of supranuclear function. (Brandt & Dieterich 1993, Keane 1975). The deviation is more common in unilateral lesions than bilateral lesions and the eye ipsilateral to the lesion is usually the hypotropic eye. Diplopia is often present but no particular extraocular muscle is involved. A comitant skew deviation was noted in one patient in this series. Nystagmus was noted in three patients and included upbeat, downbeat and gaze evoked waveforms. Gaze evoked nystagmus was more prevalent and can be seen during and following recovery of gaze palsies but also with damage to the neural integrators of horizontal and vertical gaze.

A number of our patients did not require ocular treatment due either to symmetrical involvement of eye movements or to resolution of the ocular motility defect. Of those requiring treatment, five patients had conservative options, two had BT A injections with or without prisms or occlusion and one patient had surgery with prisms to correct the small residual deviation.The indications for treatment include binocular diplopia due to strabismus, abnormal head posture for strabismus or to achieve fixation with gaze palsy, and oscillopsia. Prisms can be useful in some cases. However many are unsuccessful due to incomitance and occlusion may be required. BT is useful to ascertain the effect of weakening specific muscles before considering surgery. We had varying success with this in two cases. Surgery was undertaken successfully in one case in our study for double elevator palsy.

As regards the ocular outcome of our patients, ten patients improved of which two had full ocular motility and the remaining eight patients showing minimal, partial or good levels of improvement. Two patients showed no improvement in ocular motility although both patients were asymptomatic in primary gaze, one with the use of prisms. The time period of follow-up in this cross section analysis ranged from 6 weeks to 8 years.

The natural history of our patients could be assessed in nine of the 12 patients who required no treatment or conservative options only. Two patients had full resolution of ocular motility disturbance, one showed minimal improvement, three showed partial recovery and two showed good recovery. Evidence of improvement is encouraging and for those patients with residual binocular diplopia this could be alleviated with prisms or occlusion. In one patient the diplopia was far apart enough to be ignored without requiring prisms and in two patients suppression was demonstrated. Of the three cases that had treatment intervention, all showed improvement of a variable extent. In all patients that showed improvement the general trend was a slower recovery time for those patients with more marked abnormalities of ocular motility such as those patients with combined gaze palsies and cranial nerve palsies.

4. CONCLUSIONS

Of 12 patients with brainstem vascular pathology and ocular motility deficit only two showed no improvement in eye signs. The more extensive the pathology, the more significant the ocular motility disorder and the less likelihood of recovery. There was a variable time period of follow-up and recovery and some patients showed evidence of recovery (even of a minimal extent) after a period of 3-5 years. Most patients were managed appropriately with conservative means of prisms, occlusion or Bangerter filters with only three patients requiring BT or surgery. The natural history is promising and despite many patients demonstrating slow recovery, only two remained static with regard to their ocular motility status. All patients were asymptomatic in the primary position.

REFERENCES

Bender MB. 1980 Brain control of conjugate horizontal and vertical eye movements; a survey of the structural and functional correlates. *Brain*. 103: 23

Bienfang DC. 1975 Crossing axons in the third nerve nucleus. *Investigative Ophthalmology and Visual* Science. 14:927

Brandt T, Dieterich M. 1993 Skew deviation with ocular torsion : a vestibular brainstem sign of topographic diagnostic value. *Annals of Neurology*. 33: 528

Bronstein AM, Rudge P, Gresty MA, DuBoulay G, Morris J. 1990 Abnormalities of horizontal gaze. Clinical, oculographic and MRI findings. II Gaze palsy and INO. *Journal of Neurology Neurosurgery and Psychiatry*. 53: 200

Green JP, Newman NJ, Winterkorn JS. 1993 Paralysis of downgaze in two patients with clinical-radiologic correlation. *Archives of Ophthalmology*. 111: 219

Jampel RS, Fells P. 1968 Monocular elevation paresis caused by a central nervous system lesion. *Archives of Ophthalmology*. 80: 45

Keane JR. 1975 Ocular skew deviation. *Archives of Neurology*. 32: 185

Lagreze W-D, Warner JEA, Zamani AA, Gouras GK, Koralnik IJ, Bienfang DC. 1996 Mesencephalic clefts associated with eye movement disorders. *Archives of Ophthalmology*. 114: 429

Leigh RJ, Zee DS. 1991 *The neurology of eye movements*. Contemporary Neurology Series. P329

Lessel S. 1975 Supranuclear paralysis of monocular elevation. *Neurology*. 25: 1134

Miller NR, Biousse V, Hwang T, Patel S, Newman NJ, Zee DS. 2002 Isolated acquired unilateral horizontal gaze paresis from a putative lesion of the abducens nucleus. *Journal of NeuroOphthalmology*. 22: 204

Pierrot-Deseilligny C, Goasguen J. 1984 Isolated abducens nucleus damage due to histiocytosis X. Electro-oculographic analysis and physiological deductions. *Brain*. 107: 1019

Rowe FJ. 2003 Supranuclear and internuclear control of eye movements. A review. *British Orthoptic Journal*. 60: 2

Table 1 Patient Details

Case	Gender	Age at onset	Vascular pathology	Ocular motility	General signs	Symptoms	Treatment	Follow-up period	Outcome
1	Female	71	Infarct	Double elevator palsy		Diplopia	Prisms	2 years	Static
2	Female	42	Haemorrhage	Unilateral INO		Diplopia		2 months	Full improvement
3	Male	78	Infarct	Double elevator palsy		Diplopia	Prisms Surgery	3 years	Good improvement
4	Male	52	Infarct	Fixation instability, Jerky pursuits Reduced hor & vert saccades Upward gaze palsy		Blurred vision	Prisms Occlusion Filters	3 years	Static
5	Female	41	Haemorrhage	Bilateral INO		Diplopia	Prisms BT A	8 years	Minimal improvement
6	Male	42	Infarct	Complete unilateral III Upward gaze palsy	Difficulty with speech, balance, swallowing	Diplopia	Occlusion BT A	5 years	Minimal improvement
7	Female	73	Infarct	Bilateral nuclear III Spared pupils, No ptosis Reduced vert saccades	Hand tremor	Diplopia		2 years	Partial improvement
8	Male	50	Haemorrhage	Gaze evoked hor & vert nystagmus Upward gaze palsy, Cogwheeling Reduced hor & vert saccades Upbeat/downbeat nystagmus Fixation instability, Sluggish pupils	Difficulty with speech, hemiplegia	Reading difficulties Diplopia		4 years	Minimal improvement
9	Female	38	Infarct	Skew deviation, Jerky pursuits Reduced vert saccades Upbeat nystagmus Gaze evoked hor nystagmus	Dizziness Difficulty with balance Vertigo	Diplopia Blurred vision Oscillopsia	Prisms	18 months	Partial improvement
10	Female	67	Infarct	Complete unilateral III Vertical nystagmus, Jerky pursuits Reduced hor & vert saccades Reduced hor & vert gaze holding Recovering 1½ syndrome Upward gaze palsy	Dizziness Difficulty with speech and balance VII palsy	Diplopia Oscillopsia	Prisms Occlusion	6 months	Good improvement
11	Female	25	Haemorrhage	Bilateral VI	VII palsy	Diplopia	Prisms	6 weeks	Full improvement
12	Male	58	Infarct	Complete nuclear III Contralateral superior division III		Diplopia		1 year	Partial improvement

Transactions 28th Meeting European Strabismological Association, de Faber (ed.)

Long-term follow-up after vertical rectus muscl transposition and botulinum toxin for sith nerve paralysis

Wirth G.M. and Landau K.
Department of Ophthalmology, University Hospital, Zuerich

BACKGROUND: Several procedures for surgical treatment of sixth nerve paralysis have been des- cribed. They include the transfer of the abducting power in the field of action of the lateral rectus and weakening of the medial rectus. We report the long-term outcome in our patients treated with complete transposition of the vertical recti and chemodenervetion of the medial rectus.

METHODS: Charts of nineteen patients, operated on between 9/90 and 4/02, have been reviewed. In addition, all patients were called back for an actual examination. Parameters such as age at on- set of paralysis, duration, etiology, laterality, orthoptic examination before, one, three, twelve months and at last visit after surgery, as well as patient satisfaction were recorded.

RESULTS: Seven patients had tumor compression and 12 patients had trauma causing their sixth nerve paralysis. Two patients died and two were lost to follow up. The mean postoperative follow up was 30 months (range 3 to 107). Generally, the tumor patients had a longer lasting paralysis (mean 72 months)than those with injury (mean 20 months)prior to surgery. Three patients had fully recovered contralateral sixth nerve palsy and in one patient bilateral paralysis persisted. The average preoperative distance deviation was +36 ^ ((range 10 ^ to 60 ^). The induced exoshift at the last visit was 29 ^ ((range 6 to 55). Eight patients were exotropic at the one month follow up, 4 at the 3 month follow up and only one at the last visit. No anterior segment ischemia occurred. Generally, the result of the procedure was well received by the patients.

CONCLUSION: Complete vertical rectus muscle transposition with chemodenervation of the medial rectus is an effective way to treat patients with abducens nerve paralysis and the long-term results of this procedure are stable.

Transactions 28th Meeting European Strabismological Association, de Faber (ed.)
© 2004 European Strabismological Association, ISBN 90 265 1965 6

New methods for quantifying severity of diplopia

Jonathan M. Holmes and Mark J. Kupersmith
Mayo Clinic, Rochester MN, USA and Beth Israel Medical Center, New York NY, USA

INTRODUCTION: In clinical practice, and for clinical trials, it is desirable to have a rapid, inexpensive, simple test to quantify the severity of a patient 's diplopia. The current "gold standard" is the field of single binocular vision, plotted on a Goldmann perimeter. Such equipment is not available in many centers and we therefore developed two new tests that might be used to quantify the severity of diplopia.

METHODS: We developed a brief questionnaire that addresses the frequency and positions of gaze of a patient 's diplopia. The questionnaire yields a symptom score from 0 (no diplopia)to 25 (con- stant diplopia everywhere)and is weighted toward primary position and downgaze. We also devi- sed a new diplopia scoring system based on the office examination, using the head mounted Cervical Range of Motion (CROM)device, which is very portable and easy to use in any examining room. We standardized gaze positions and determined whether the patient had diplopia when fi- xing on distance and near targets. The CROM diplopia exam score ranges from a minimum of 0 to a maximum of 25. These scores can readily be converted to a 0 to 100 scale for direct comparison with other measures. We studied 15 adult patients ages 26 to 65 with acquired diplopia secondary to a variety of conditions, including cranial nerve palsies, thyroid eye disease and supranuclear palsies. We administered our two new tests to each patient and performed a formal field of single binocular vision (diplopia field)on a Goldmann perimeter, which was then scored using established methods from 0 to 100, where zero represents no diplopia, and 100 is diplopia in all fields of gaze. We then compared the scores obtained by each of the 3 techniques, using intra- class correlation coefficients (ICC).

RESULTS: Among our 15 patients, the scores on the "gold standard"diplopia field ranged from 5 to 100. On a parallel scale of 0 to 100, we found a similar range of diplopia symptom scores from 12 to 96, and a similar range of CROM diplopia exam scores from 12 to 96. There was excellent agreement between the diplopia field score and the symptom score (ICC=0. 90)and the diplopia field score and the CROM exam score (ICC=0. 87).

CONCLUSIONS: Our new diplopia symptom score and new CROM diplopia exam score are valid measures of diplopia severity. The tests are easy to administer and require less expensive and less cumbersome equipment than previously available. Future studies will investigate the test- retest reliability of our new tests and their utility in longitudinal clinical evaluation. Our new diplopia symptom score and new CROM diplopia exam score may prove to be valuable outcome measures for future clinical trials in strabismus.

Session 10

Thyroid/Duane's/Varia

Transactions 28th Meeting European Strabismological Association, de Faber (ed.)

Management of Large Vertical Deviations in Thyroid Eye Disease

Cliff Weir[1,2], Alec Ansons[1]

[1]*Manchester Royal Eye Hospital,* [2]*Gartnavel General Hospital, Glasgow, UK*

ABSTRACT: The management of patients with large vertical deviations secondary to thyroid eye disease is problematic. We describe our experience from 7 such patients who underwent ipsilateral inferior rectus recession combined with contralateral superior rectus recession.

KEYWORDS: thyroid eye disease; strabismus

1. INTRODUCTION

Restrictive strabismus is a frequent complication of thyroid eye disease and often requires surgical correction. Certain patterns of ocular motility disturbance are recognised usually involving multiple muscles producing either vertical, horizontal or torsional deviations or combinations of all three. Vertical misalignments are frequently the result of unilateral inferior rectus contracture producing a restriction of elevation of the affected eye. In such patients with small to moderate angles good surgical results can be obtained by performing an ipsilateral inferior rectus recession, preferably with adjustable sutures.[1] However, when larger vertical angles are present, for example greater than 20 prism dioptres (Δ), attempting to fully correct the deviation by performing a single inferior rectus recession can result in underaction of the inferior rectus muscle in down-gaze thereby producing a reversal of the deviation. In addition there is considerable risk of lower eyelid retraction developing post-operatively. In view of this some authors [2], [3] suggest combining an ipsilateral inferior rectus recession with a contralateral superior rectus recession, although they do not comment upon the outcomes of this procedure. Flanders et al. [4] report very good immediate post-operative results in a small group of 6 patients undergoing such surgery. At their last assessment all 6 had an "excellent result", defined as being free of diplopia in both the primary and reading position without the need for prisms. However, the outcomes from this type of surgery in terms of objective measurements of the vertical deviation and the field of binocular single vision (BSV) are not well described in the literature. We therefore report the results of 7 consecutive patients with large vertical deviations secondary to thyroid eye disease who underwent ipsilateral inferior rectus recession combined with a contralateral superior rectus recession.

2. METHODS

The patients were identified from the strabismus database kept by one of the authors (AMA) and all underwent surgery between 1992 and 2002. Four were female and 3 were male, with a mean age of 61 years (range 53-78 years). All patients had been previously assessed by an endocrinologist. Five patients were hyperthyroid initially, 1 euthyroid and 1 hypothyroid, although by the time of their surgery all were euthyroid, having had stable endocrine function for at least 6 months. Two patients had been treated with radioactive iodine, 2 with carbimazole and 1 with thyroxine. Two patients received no treatment. As part of the initial management of their thyroid eye disease 3 patients received radiotherapy and 3 were given oral prednisolone. One patient underwent bilateral orbital decompressions. All 7 patients underwent a full orthoptic and ophthalmic examination, and had stable ocular alignment for at least 6 months prior to surgery. The field of BSV was quantified according to the method of Woodruff et al..[5] No patients had undergone any previous strabismus surgery and none had any other past medical or ophthalmic history that could have also affected their ocular motility.

The surgical technique is as described by Ansons & Davis [2] with the use of adjustable sutures in all cases. Six patients were operated on under general anaesthetic with the adjustment performed approximately 6 hours post-operatively. In 1 patient the procedure was carried out under local anaesthesia, which consisted of topical Benoxinate drops. The adjustment was carried out peri-operatively. The aim of surgery in all cases was to leave each individual under-corrected by between 5Δ and 10Δ in the primary position, with no reversal in downgaze. All patients were followed up for a minimum of 6 months, with 2 patients followed up for 7 years and 11 years respectively

3. RESULTS

Six patients had best corrected visual acuities in each eye of between 6/5 and 6/9. The remaining patient had right and left acuities of 6/24 and 6/12 respectively as the result of previous compressive optic neuropathy. The mean pre-operative vertical angle in the primary position was 30Δ (SD 9Δ; range 18Δ -50Δ) for near, and 32Δ (SD 8Δ; range 25Δ -50Δ) for distance. The mean vertical angle on down-gaze was 25Δ (SD 7Δ; range 16Δ -32Δ). These measurements were not significantly affected by spectacle correction. Two patients also had a significant esotropia, one measuring 70Δ for near and 55Δ for distance, the other measuring 20Δ for near and 30Δ for distance. Again these deviations were not significantly affected by spectacle correction. Four patients had no recordable field of binocular single vision pre-operatively. The remaining 3 patients had a mean BSV score of 44% (SD 4%; range 40-48%).

The mean size of the inferior and superior rectus recessions were 5.6mm (range 3-8mm) and 5 mm (range 3-6mm) respectively. Three patients required adjustment post-operatively. The 2 patients with significant esotropias underwent bilateral medial rectus recessions of 5mm and 3mm respectively, using adjustable sutures. No subsequent adjustment was required.

One week following surgery the mean vertical deviation was significantly reduced to 8Δ (SD10Δ) for near and 9Δ (SD 9Δ) for distance in the primary position, and to 5Δ (SD 8Δ) in downgaze. Approximately 2 months later the mean vertical deviation was 9Δ (SD 9Δ) for near and 9Δ (SD10Δ) for distance in the primary position, and 5Δ (SD 5Δ) in downgaze. At the clinic visit six months following surgery the mean vertical deviation was 6Δ (SD 6Δ) for near and 5Δ (SD 5Δ) for distance in the primary position, and 4Δ (SD 2Δ) in downgaze. One patient showed a reversal of their deviation in downgaze at this visit, with an angle of 5Δ. There was no reversal in the primary position. One patient subsequently underwent a superior oblique posterior tenotomy. For the 2 patients who also underwent bilateral medial rectus recessions were their respective residual esodeviations at this visit were 4Δ and 1Δ for near, and 14Δ and 12Δ for distance. For the 2 patients who were followed up for 7 and 11 years their respective vertical deviations were 17Δ and 9Δ for near, 14Δ and 11Δ for distance in the primary position, and 6Δ and 4Δ in downgaze.

A field of BSV was recordable in 5 patients following surgery. The mean percentage scores were 77% (SD 13%), 75 % (SD 14%) and 81% (SD 12%) at 1 week, 2 months and 6 months post-operatively respectively. The remaining 2 patients achieved single vision in the primary position with the aid of prisms, although these were not required in downgaze. Following surgery 2 patients developed significant lower eyelid retraction of 2mm and 3mm respectively, on the side of the inferior rectus recession. One of these patients is awaiting lid surgery, whilst the other is not troubled by the eyelid retraction.

4. DISCUSSION

This study illustrates that ipsilateral inferior rectus recession combined with contralateral superior rectus recession using adjustable sutures can be effective in the management of large vertical angles in thyroid eye disease. The length of follow up (6 months) for 5 of the 7 patients is relatively short and further assessment will be required to establish the longer term stability of these initial results. It is interesting to note that the size of the vertical deviation in the 2 patients who have been followed up for many years is gradually reducing. This is well described following unilateral inferior rectus recessions, when even reversal of the deviation can occur.[6] One patient in our series developed reversal of the deviation in downgaze, although she remains asymptomatic. This is well reported following inferior rectus recession and is thought to be related to involvement of the ipsilateral superior rectus muscle which was either masked by the more marked restriction of the inferior rectus muscle, or developed as the disease process progressed. The effect of ipsilateral inferior rectus recession combined with contralateral superior rectus recession on objective measurements of the field of BSV has not been documented previously. According to the criteria described by Flanders et al [4] 5 out of 7 patients had an "excellent" result, with no diplopia in the primary or reading position. The remaining 2 patients had a "good" result, with a small prism being required in the primary position to achieve single vision, but not necessary in the reading position. From a functional point of view all 7 patients were pleased with the outcome of their surgery.

Two patients did develop lower eyelid retraction, which is slightly less than the 3 out of 6 described by Flanders et al. [4]who u nderwent a similar surgical procedure. Kushner [8] advocates the technique of advancement of the capsulopalpebral head at the time of inferior rectus recession to reduce the risk of lower eyelid retraction. This option may be considered in future patients.

The surgical management of large angle vertical strabismus in thyroid eye disease is problematic. This article illustrates that combining ipsilateral inferior rectus recession with contralateral superior rectus recession can give encouraging results.

REFERENCES

1 Lueder GT, Scott WE, Kutschke PJ *et al.* Long-term results of adjustable suture surgery for strabismus secondary to thyroid ophthalmopathy. *Ophthalmology* 1992; 99: 993-7.
2 Ansons AM, Davis H. *Diagnosis and Management of Ocular Motility Disorders*, 3rd edn. Oxford: Blackwell Science, 2001.
3 Rosenbaum A, Santiago A. *Clinical Strabismus Management - Principles and Surgical Techniques.* Philadelphia: WB Saunders Co., 1999.
4 Flanders M, Hastings M. Diagnosis and surgical management of strabismus associated with thyroid-related orbitopathy. *J Pediatr Ophthalmol Strabismus* 1997; 34: 333-40.
5 Woodruff G, O'Reilly C, Kraft SP. Functional scoring of the field of binocular single vision in patients with diplopia. *Ophthalmology* 1987; 94: 1554-61.
6 Hudson HL, Feldon SE. Late overcorrection of hypotropia in Graves ophthalmopathy. Predictive factors. *Ophthalmology* 1992; 99: 356-60.
7 Scott WE, Thalacker JA. Diagnosis and treatment of thyroid myopathy. *Ophthalmology* 1981; 88: 493-8.
8 Kushner BJ. A surgical procedure to minimize lower-eyelid retraction with inferior rectus recession. *Arch Ophthalmol* 1992; 110: 1011-4.

Transactions 28th Meeting European Strabismological Association, de Faber (ed.)
© 2004 European Strabismological Association, ISBN 90 265 1965 6

Dosage of Eye Muscle Surgery in Endocrine Orbitopathy

K.-P. Boergen, G. Rudolph, O. Ehrt, P. Kalpadakis
University Eye Hospital, Munich, Germany

ABSTRACT: From 1982 to 1999 eye muscle surgery was performed in 167 patients suffering from endocrine orbitopathy. Recessions were the preferred procedure and topical anaesthesia was used to allow dosage under intact active motility. In 64 patients only one inferior rectus muscle was recessed. This sub-group was analyzed in the respect to functional results, dose-effect correlation and the existence of a learning curve. 95% showed fusion in primary position, 84% had a field of binocular single vision of 10° off primary position and 61% had no double vision within 30°. No dose-effect correlation could be demonstrated. This supports the basic idea that intraoperative dosage improves motility and thus reduces any deviation irrespective of it's preoperative value.

KEYWORDS: topical anaesthesia, eye muscle surgery, endocrine or thyroid orbitopathy

1 INTRODUCTION

Motility problems in chronic thyroid eye disease are caused by fibrosis and /or lipomatosis of the eye muscles, leading to a mechanical restriction of eye movements. Usually the inferior rectus muscles are most involved. Therefore elevation is limited in most cases. Some do suffer from limitation of abduction caused by fibrosis of the medial rectus muscle. After stabilization of the endocrine and orthoptic status for at least 6 months surgical rehabilitation should be planned in all patients suffering from double vision or a marked chin elevation. Since eye movements are mechanically restricted the primary aim of any surgery is normalization of motility and not correction of squint angles. Therefore recessions of the most involved muscle is the preferred procedure. Common rules for the dosage can not be applied as the elastic properties of the eye muscles are severely altered. This problem can be overcome in three different ways:

- preoperative determination of the amount of recession
- intraoperative dosage using active or passive motility
- postoperatively with adjustable sutures.

Since 1982 we routinely use intraoperative dosage under topical anaesthesia and have reported on this procedure several times (1-3, 7). The purpose of this paper is to evaluate all cases operated between 1982 and 1999 with respect to functional results and dose-effect correlation. Since all patients have been operated by the same surgeon the personal learning curve can be analyzed.

2 PATIENTS AND METHODS

From 1982 to 1999 167 patients with endocrine orbitopathy were operated under topical anaesthesia. Details of the surgical procedure can be found in previous publications (1-3, 7). After checking passive and active motility the muscle was hooked, put on sutures and carefully detached from the sclera. Then the patient was asked to look into the direction opposite to the action of the muscle e.g. upwards in case of an elevation deficit after detachment of the inferior rectus muscle. The muscle was reattached to the sclera in this position.
The functional results were evaluated in all 167 patients. In a sub-group of 64 patients only one inferior rectus muscle was recessed. These cases were examined with respect to dose-effect correlation and learning curve. In a sub-group of ten patients the effect of a one muscle procedure on motility was documented using the measurement of monocular excursion as described by Kestenbaum.

3 RESULTS

3.1 *Motility changes*

In 10 patients improvement of elevation and the change of depression after recession of one inferior rectus muscle was determined 1 or 2 days after operation and after three months (Fig. 1a and b). Immediately postoperative, elevation was improved but depression reduced. After 3 months there was a further improvement of elevation and a reduction of the limitation of depression.

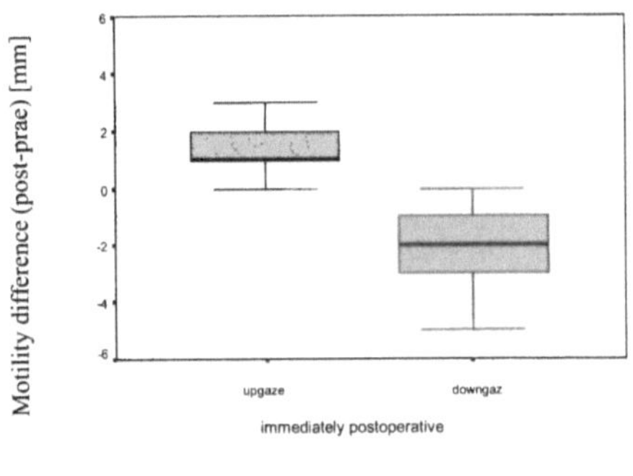

Fig. 1a. (see text)

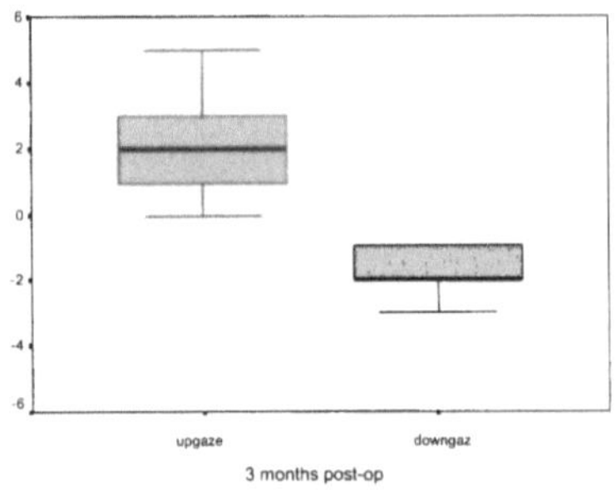

Fig. 1b. (see text)

3.2 *Functional results*

The field of binocular single vision (BSV) was analyzed in all 167 cases how underwent one or several operations. 95% of the patients showed fusion in primary position. 84% had BSV within the central 10° and 61% within 30°.

3.3 *Dose-effect correlation*

The effect of a single inferior rectus recession in 64 patients on the vertical deviation in primary position, up- and down-gaze is shown in Fig. 2a, the relation between dosage and effect in Fig. 2b.

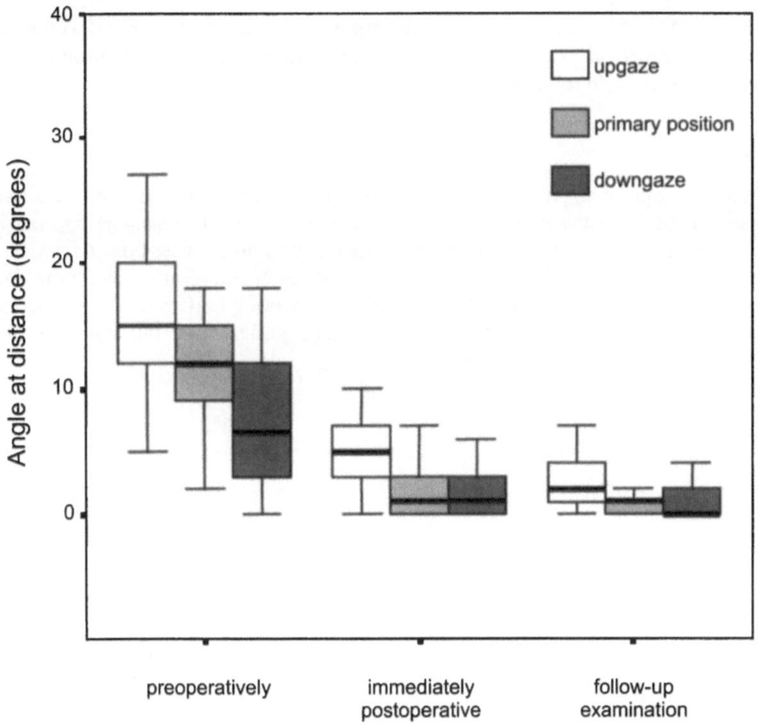

Fig. 2a: (see text)

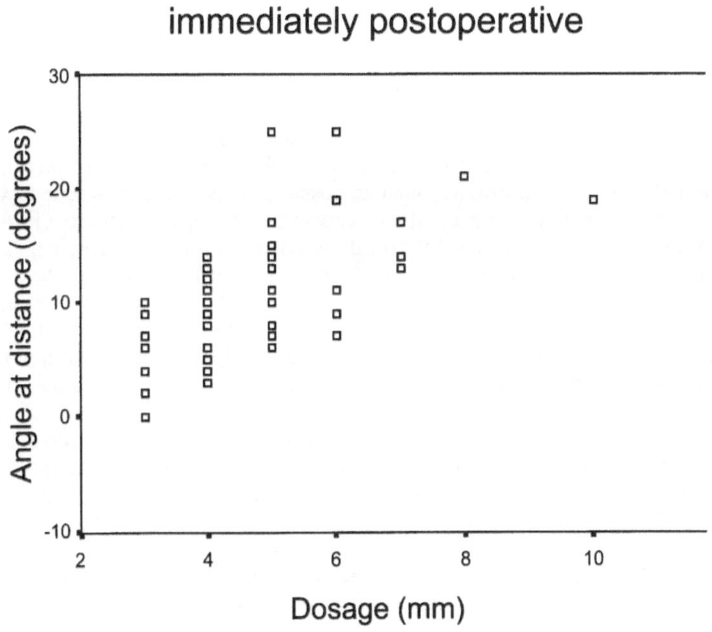

Fig. 2b: (see text)

Although there is a graded effect on the angle in different positions of gaze (Fig. 2a) the effect of any amount of recession varies a lot (Fig. 2b) so that no dosage recommendation can be derived from the preoperative angle of deviation.

3.4 *Learning curve*

The sub-group of patients operated on one inferior rectus muscle only was divided into two groups: patients operated before (group A) and after 1992 (group B). The dosage applied is documented in fig. 3. There is a tendency for a reduction of the amount of recession. After 1992 recessions of more than 6 mm were no longer used and recessions of only 3mm done more frequently. But the difference between the two groups is statistically not significant. The reduction of the preoperative angle at distance (Fig. 4) shows less scattering after 1992 but again the difference between group A and B is not significant.

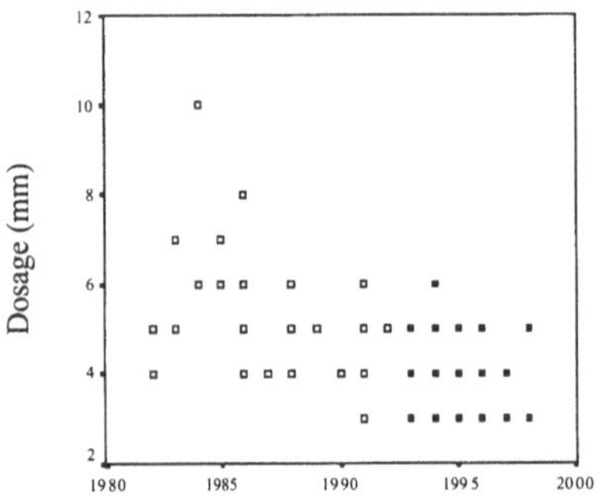

Fig. 3 (see text)

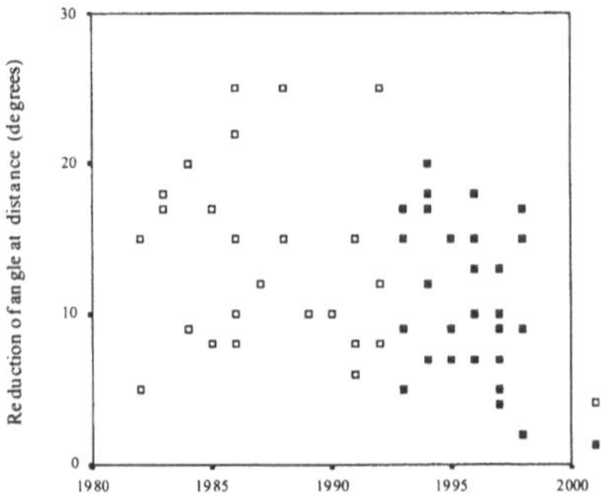

Fig. 4 (see text)

4. DISCUSSION

Eye movements in chronic stages of endocrine orbitopathy are often mechanically restricted due to fibrosis and/or lipomatosis of the eye muscles. Therefore the primary aim for functional rehabilitation is the normalization of motility as much as possible. This was also stressed by a recent study (10). The authors compared two groups of endocrine orbitopathy patients: in one group surgery aimed at an improvement of motility, in the second at an angle correction. The first group showed significantly better functional results. Our study underlines these results.

Topical anaesthesia allows an optimal determination of the amount of recession in the operation room. As active motility is intact the patient is able to look into the direction of motility restriction. This gives a direct indication of how much a muscle should be recessed. Since not only the eye muscles but other orbital tissues as well are involved in the fibrotic process a complete normalization of motility is often not possible even with very large recessions.

The latter have furthermore a high risk of primary over-correction but also of a secondary over-effect caused by shrinkage of the antagonist. This risk can be minimized by doing the dosage under intact active motility. Although there might be an over-effect in primary position and limitation in down gaze immediately postoperative this usually improves over the time and causes no permanent problem.

There is a large variability of the angle reduction achieved by the same amount of recession. Therefore clear dosage recommendations can not be derived from preoperative deviations. There seems to be a small personal learning curve over the years. We found a tendency for smaller recession with time. After 1992 the recession of 6 mm was never exceeded.

The manipulation on the eye muscle under topical anaesthesia is very well tolerated by the patient. The oculo-cardiac reflex is absent so that no bradycardia or even heart arrest disturbs the patient and the surgeon.

In summary, eye muscle surgery under topical anaesthesia is a safe and very successful procedure for the adequate dosage of recessions and the improvement of motility in patients with endocrine orbitopathy.

5. REFERENCES

Boergen, K.P. 1981. Operation in Oberflächenanästhesie bei endokriner Orbitopathie. Klin. Monatsbl. Augenheilkd. 178: 453-456.

Boergen, K.P. 1993. Squint operation under topical anesthesia in endocrine orbitopathy. Strabismus 1: 167-172.

Boergen, K.P. 1993. Schieloperation in Tropfanästhesie bei endokriner Orbitopathie Z. Prakt. Augenheilkd. 14: 301-305.

Coats, D.K., Paysse. E.A., Plager, D.A., Wallace, D.K. 1999. Early surgery for thyroid ophthalmopathy. Ophthalmology 106: 324-329.

Esser, J. 1994. Endokrine Orbitopathie. Ophthalmologe 91: 3-19.

Hahnenkamp, K., Honemann, C.W., Fischer, L.G., Duriex, M.E., Mühlendyck, H., Braun, U. 2000. Effect of different anesthetic regimes on the oculocardiac reflex during strabismus surgery. Pediatr. Anesth. 10: 601-608.

Kalpadakis, P., Rudolph, G., Boergen, K.P. 2002. Dosierung muskelchirurgischer Eingriffe in Tropfanästhesie bei Patienten mit endokriner Orbitopathie. Ophthalmologe 99: 941-945.

Kose, S., Uretmen, O., Emre,S., Pamukcu, K. 2002. Recession of the inferior rectus muscle under topical anesthesia in thyroid ophthalmopathy. J. Pediatr. Ophthalmol. Strabismus 39: 331-335.

Krzizok, T., Efinger, K. Kaufmann, H. 1993. Dosierbarkeit von Augenmuskeloperationen bei endokriner Orbitopathie. Z. Prakt. Augenheilkd. 14: 273-279.

Nguyen, V.T., Park, D.J., Levin. L., Feldon, S.E. 2002. Correction of restricted extraocular muscle motility in surgical management of strabismus in Graves' ophthalmopathy. Ophthalmology 109: 384-388.

Transactions 28th Meeting European Strabismological Association, de Faber (ed.)
 ISBN 90 265 1965 6

Bilateral duane's syndrome Type I in siblings: Case report

C. Schiavi, M. Fresina, F. Quagliano & E.C. Campos.
Ophtalmology Service, University of Bologna, Bologna, Italy

ABSTRACT: Duane's retraction syndrome type I is a congenital eye movement disorder. The syndrome is unilateral in 82%. Most cases are sporadic, but familial cases have been estimated at 10% by most authors. We report a case of two siblings both with bilateral Duane's syndrome type I. To our knowledge, several examples of bilateral familial Duane's syndrome exist in literature. Hereditary patterns of Duane syndrome and familial occurrence with dominant inheritance patterns have been described. Abnormalities on chromosomes 4, 8 and 22 have been associated with Duane's retraction syndrome. Certainly, Duane's syndrome occurs in autosomal dominant mode; this case is therefore, a new germinal mutation. The other possibility is that it is an autosomal recessive mode and we think there are only few cases suggesting this mode of inheritance. We report our experience about these new cases.

KEYWORDS: Duane, syndrome, familial, bilateral, autosomal, recessive.

1. INTRODUCTION

Stilling-Türk-Duane retraction syndrome is a restrictive syndrome classified by Huber in three types according to electromyographic studies(9). Yet, both horizontal recti muscles are involved with variable degree in each type. Probably, Huber's classification includes clinical variations of the same entity.

Duane's syndrome type I is characterised by globe retraction and narrowing of the palpebral fissure on attempted adduction, limitation of abduction and occasionally also of adduction. Commonly associated are elevation or depression in adduction. It represents about 5% of all cases of strabismus(4).

Aetiology of the syndrome is not completely understood, probably depending on the combination of structural anomalies and paradoxical anomalous lateral rectus innervation of the affected eye due to misdirection of axons destined for the medial rectus(8,12,16). Duane's syndrome is generally unilateral (82%). In this instance a more common occurrence in the left eye (59%) and in females (58%) has been recorded. Duane's syndrome can also be bilateral (18%)(13). Most cases are sporadic, but up to 10% are familial, usually with autosomal dominant inheritance(6,10,18,20). Chromosomal loci for genes contributing to Duane's syndrome have been suggested at 4q, 8q, 22q (Gutowski 2000; Chew et al., 1995; Cullen et al., 1993)(1,3,7).

Several autosomal dominant syndromes with dysmorphic features are associated with Duane's syndrome. The high incidence of associated anomalies in affected patients may suggest that a common genetic defect is responsible. Molecular genetic studies are necessary in order to confirm this hypothesis. The association with other congenital abnormalities suggests that a teratogenic stimulus during the first four to ten week of embryogenesis may be of etiologic significance (Pfaffenbach et al., 1972)(14) in sporadic case of Duane retraction syndrome.

Several examples are recorded in the literature where cases of bilateral Duane's syndrome occurred in a family involving some members with an autosomal dominant mode (Türk 1896; Wolff 1901; Lodberg 1935; Waardenburg et al., 1961; Sevel et al., 1974)(11,15,17,19,20).

A non-dominant bilateral familial case of Duane's syndrome has not been described as yet.

2. CASE REPORT

We report on a family with origins in Vicenza, Italy. Affected members of the family comprise two siblings: a girl aged 11 years (patient 1) and her brother aged 6 years (patient 2); both parents were examined and found to be free of ocular signs and symptoms.

Patient 1 was examined when she was a 4 year old girl. Her eye motility examination confirmed the presence of bilateral Duane's syndrome with absence of abduction in both eyes, restriction of adduction in either eye, bilateral narrowing of the palpebral fissure and retraction of the globe in adduction. An upshoot of the right eye in levoversion and a downshoot of the left eye in dextroversion was present. An esotropia of the right eye of 25 dioptres in primary position and a V pattern caused an anomalous head posture with chin down (Fig. 1). Anterior and posterior segments of the eye were normal. During the first visit visual acuity was 5/6 in the right eye and 6/6 in the left one. The girl had normal binocular vision in the anomalous head posture with stereopsis at the TNO test. Surgery was performed two months after the first visit.

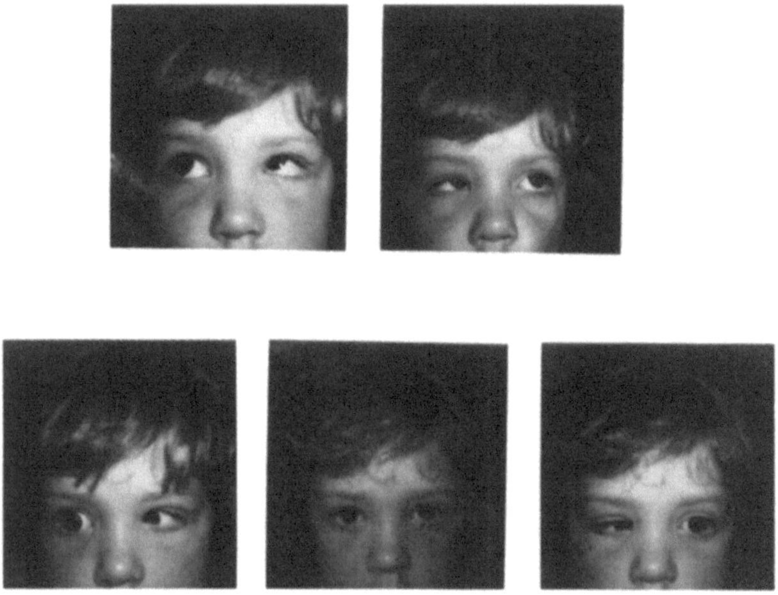

Fig. 1: patient one. Ocular motility before first surgery.

1st Surgery: Recession of both inferior oblique muscles of 9 millimetres associated with 4 mm recession of the medial rectus of the right eye and 3 mm recession of the medial rectus of the left eye. Head posture normalised after surgery. Visual acuity was 6/6 in both eyes. 1 hour of occlusion of the left eye was prescribed. The girl had been examined yearly for 6 years and when she was 10 years old a second surgery was performed in order to reduce the effect of eye retraction in adduction.

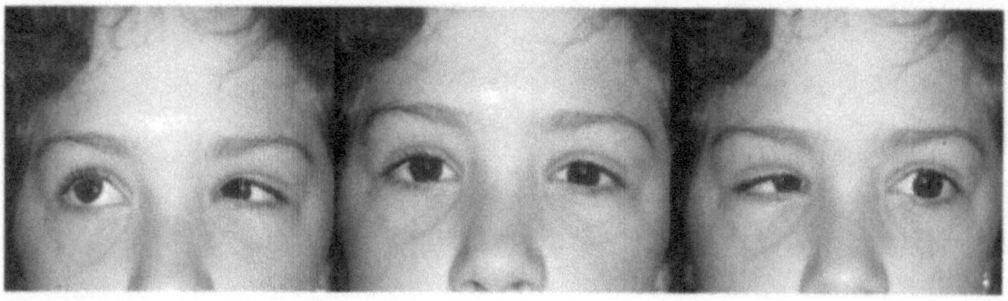

Fig. 2: patient one. Ocular motility before second surgery.

2nd *Surgery:* Right eye: further recession of the medial rectus of 5 mm and 4.5 mm recession of the lateral rectus; left eye: further recession of the medial rectus of 5 mm and 5 mm recession of the lateral rectus.

Postoperatively, there is orthophoria in primary position, no anomalous head posture (Fig. 3), significant reduction of the eye retraction in adduction and of upshoot and downshoot (Fig. 4). Her visual acuity is 6/6 and normal binocular vision and stereopsis are retained.

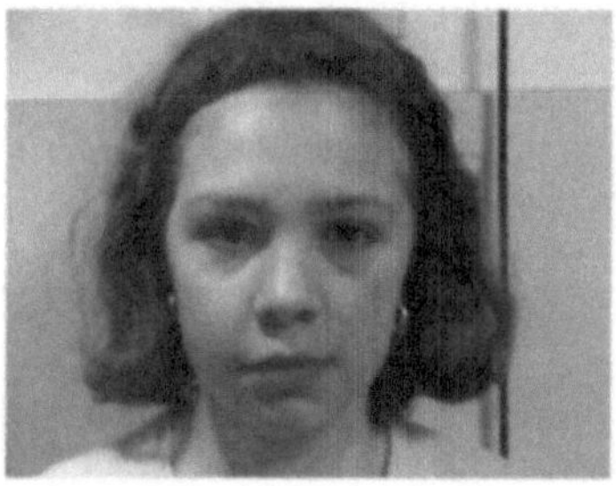

Fig. 3: patient one. Normal head posture after surgery.

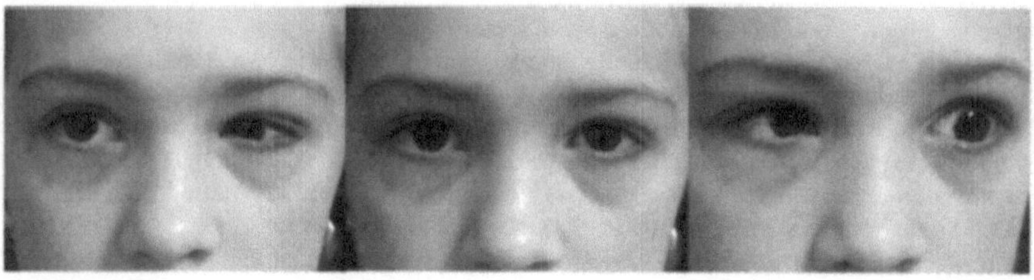

Fig. 4: patient one. Ocular motility after second surgery.

Patient 2 was first examined when he was 20-months old. His eye-motility examination revealed the presence of bilateral Duane's syndrome with absence of abduction in both eyes, restriction of adduction in either eye, bilateral narrowing of the palpebral fissure and retraction of the globe in adduction (Fig. 5). Orthophoria with stereopsis were present in primary position and the head posture was normal (Fig. 6). No pathological features were present in both eyes. When he was 5 years old visual acuity which was 6/6 bilaterally. Now he is 6 year old and at the moment no surgical approach is recommended.

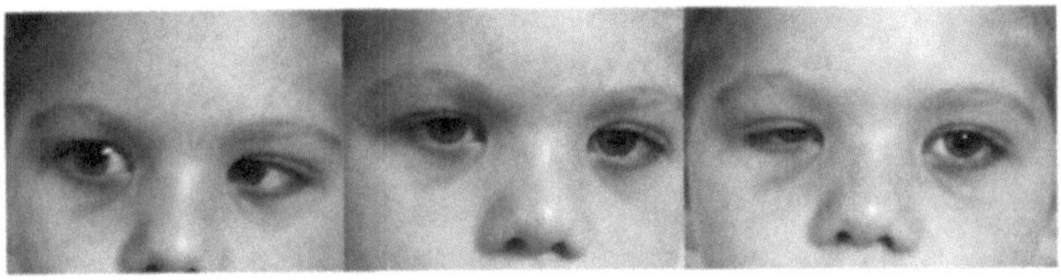

Fig. 5: patient two. Ocular motility.

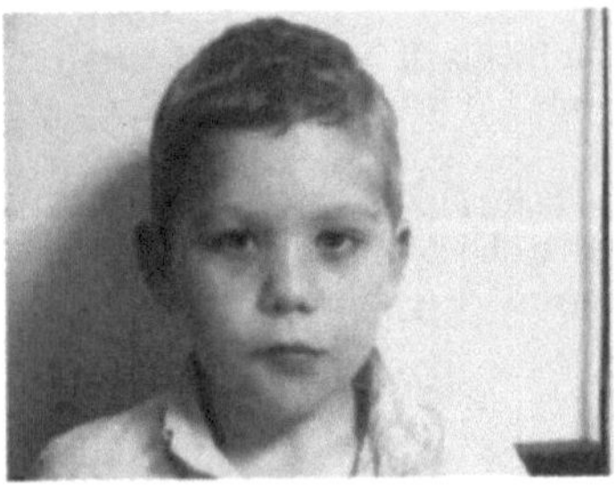

Fig. 6: patient two. Normal head posture.

3. DISCUSSION

To our knowledge, Sevel (1974) provided the first review on bilateral familial Duane's syndrome cases. Sevel's personal contribution is the description of a mother, her son and his two children with Duane's syndrome, that suggests an autosomal dominant inheritance.

Hereditary patterns of Duane's syndrome and familial occurrence with dominant inheritance patterns have eventually been described by several authors[1,2,5,6,10,18]. Abnormalities on chromosomes 4, 8 and 22 have been associated with Duane retraction syndrome [1,3,7].

Two cases of probable autosomal recessive monolateral Duane's syndrome, in two siblings, have been reported by Discepola et al (1987)[5].

No cases of bilateral autosomal recessive Duane's syndrome exist in literature. Our family is unusual in that the condition occurred in siblings, both with bilateral Duane, and not in their parents. Therefore, even if Duane's syndrome certainly occurs in an autosomal dominant mode, our cases could be the result of a new germinal mutation. The other possibility is that they represent the expression of an autosomal recessive mode. However, there are not enough cases for suggesting this mode of inheritance.

Although further investigation is necessary, with molecular genetic studies, the present report can be an addition to our knowledge on heredity of Duane's syndrome.

REFERENCES

Chew, C.K. Foster, P. Hurst, J.A. Salmon, J.F. 1995. Duane's retraction syndrome associated with chromosome 47q27-31 segment deletion. *Am J Ophthalmol* 119(6): 807-809.

Chung, M. Stout, J.T. Borcchert, M.S. 2000. Clinical diversity of hereditary Duane syndrome. *Ophthalmology* 107: 500-503.

Cullen, P. Rodgers, C.S. Callen, D.F. Connolly, V.M. Eyre, H. Fells, P. Gordon, H. Winter, R.M. Thakker, R.V. 1993. Association of familial Duane anomaly and urogenital abnormalities with a bisatellited marker derived from Chromosome 22. *Am J Med Genet* 1;47(6): 925-930.

De Respini, P.A. Caputo, A.R. Wagner, R.S. Guo, S. 1993. Duane's retraction syndrome. *Surv Ophthalmol* 38: 257-288.

Discepola, M.J. Polomeno, R.C. Zeesman, S. Kaplan, P. Williams, F. 1987. Autosomal recessive Duane's retraction syndrome. *Can J Ophthalmol* 22(7): 384-386.

Fodor, F. Marthaa, I. Fodor, A. 1978. In Deller, M.m. Weiss, J.B. (eds). *Retraktion-Syndrome in drei generationem. Acta Strabologica*: 85-89. Lausanne: C.E.R.E.S.

Gutowski, N.J. 2000. Duane's syndrome. *Eur J Neurol* 7(2): 145-149.

Hotchkiss, M.G. Miller, N.R., Clark, A.W. Green, W.M. 1980.Bilateral Duane's retraction syndrome. A clinical-pathologic case report. *Arch Ophthalmol* 98: 870-874.

Huber, A. 1974. Electrophysiology of the retraction syndrome. *Br J Ophthalmol* 58: 293-295.

Klein, D. Franceschetti, A. 1964. Humangenetik. In Becker PE (ed): *Missblidungen und Krankheiten des Auges*: 50. Stuttgart: L Georg Thieme Verlag KG.

Lodberg, C.V. 1935. Zwei Falle con Angeborenem Abduktionsdefekt mit Bulbusretraktion. Verhoef ophthal Ges, 23 Hospitalstidende. *Zbl ges Ophthalmol* 33: 354-358.

Miller, N.R. Kien, S.M. Green, W.M. Clark, A.W. 1982. Unilateral Duane's retraction syndrome type I. *Arch Ophthalmol* 100: 1468-1472.

Noorden GK von, Campos EC. 2002. C.V. Mosby (ed) *Binocular Vision and Ocular Motility. Theory and Management of Strabismus. 6th Edition*. St. Louis.

Pfaffenbach, D.D. Cross, H.E. 1972. Duane's retraction syndrome and associated congenital malformations. *Am J Ophthalmol* 73:442-446.

Sevel, D. Kassar, B.S. 1974. Bilateral Duane Syndrome. Occurence in three successive generations. Arch Ophthalmol 91(6): 492-494.

Tillack, T.W. Winer, J.A. 1962. Anomaly of the abducens nerve. *Yale J Biol Med* 34: 620-629.

Türk, S. 1896. Uber Retrakionsbewegungen der Augen. *Dtsch Med Wochenschr* 22:199-204.

Türk, S. 1899. Bemerkungen zu einem Falle von Retraktion des Auges. *Cbl Pract Augenheilk* 23: 14-17.

Waardenburg, P.J. Franceschetti, A. Klein, D. 1961. Blackwell Scientific Publications Ltd. *Genetics and Ophthalmology*: 423-424. Oxford: England.

Wolff, J. 1901.The occurence of retraction movements of the eyeball together with congenital defects in the external ocular muscles. *Arch Ophthalmol* 34:297-309.

Transactions 28th Meeting European Strabismological Association, de Faber (ed.)

An unusual cause of diplopia as the presenting sign of breast carcinoma

M. Spiritus[1], A. Boschi[1], M-Ch. Many[2], A. Finck[1], A. Escarmelle[1], Ch. Lefebvre[3], Th. Duprez[4], P. Van den Bergh[5], P. Kamgang Semeu[3], J. Klastersky[6], M. Wirix, Ch. Daumerie[7].

Dept. of [1]Ophthalmology, [2]Histology, [3]Medicine, [4]Neuro-Radiology, [5]Neurology, [7]Endocrinology Université Catholique de Louvain, Brussels, Belgium; [6] Dept. of Medicine and Oncology, Institut Jules Bordet, Brussels, Belgium.

ABSTRACT: Enlargement of one or more EOMs with limitation of ocular motility is most frequently observed in thyroid associated orbitopathy and idiopathic inflammatory orbital pseudotumor; it may also be encountered in association with systemic disorders (vasculitis, granulomatous inflammation etc...). In a 47-year-old woman, presenting with a 4-months history of double vision, diplopia was the unique revealing sign of primary breast carcinoma. EOMs involvement with paraneoplastic process or metastases due to breast carcinoma is extremely rare. Differential diagnosis between those two potential sub-entities is discussed together with other causes for EOMs thickening.

KEY WORDS: Diplopia, orbital myositis, breast cancer, extraocular musles metastasis, paraneoplastic phenomenon.

OBJECTIVE: To highlight paraneoplastic or metastatic involvement of the EOMs in a breast carcinoma as a rare cause of diplopia

CASE REPORT: A 47-year-old woman was referred for evaluation of a 4-months history of vertical diplopia mainly in downgaze and horizontal diplopia on left lateral gaze, with retrobulbar strain on attempted eye movements and heaviness of her left upper eyelid. She was able to see one object by lowering her chin of 15° to look upward. The patient had no previous ocular complains and denied any significant medical history of trauma.

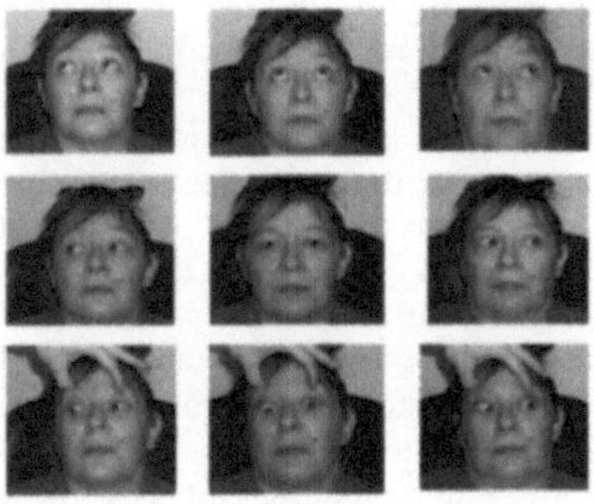

Fig 1

Corrected visual acuity, pupils, visual fields, lid function, slit-lamp examination of the anterior segments, funduscopic examination and intraocular pressure were unremarkable. Examination of ocular motility revealed a left hypertropia of 5^{D}in primary position that increased up to 20-25 $^{\Delta}$ in downgaze and right hypertropia of 6^{Δ} in upgaze. Examination of ductions and versions revealed 1-/ 3- left up- and downgaze deficits, and 1- limitation of left abduction (fig 1). Forced ductions were not performed. Exophthalmometry (Hertel) showed 19 mm OD and 20 mm OS with a 102-mm base. There was no significant decreased retropulsion. Orbital computed tomography (CT) scan (not illustrated) and pre-contrast coronal T1-weighted (T1-W) magnetic resonance (MR) imaging (Fig. 3a) disclosed fusiform enlargement of the left levator and superior rectus muscles, left medial rectus muscle and right lateral rectus muscle, which displayed moderate hypersignal intensity on the T2-weighted images (T2-W) (Fig. 3b). Coronal and axial transverse T1-W images after IV perfusion of paramagnetic contrast agent showed intense and homogeneous enhancement of the involved muscles, but without abnormal foci within them. Tendons at muscle insertions of the enlarged muscles were normal as well as the orbital fat (fig.2, fig.3a-b).

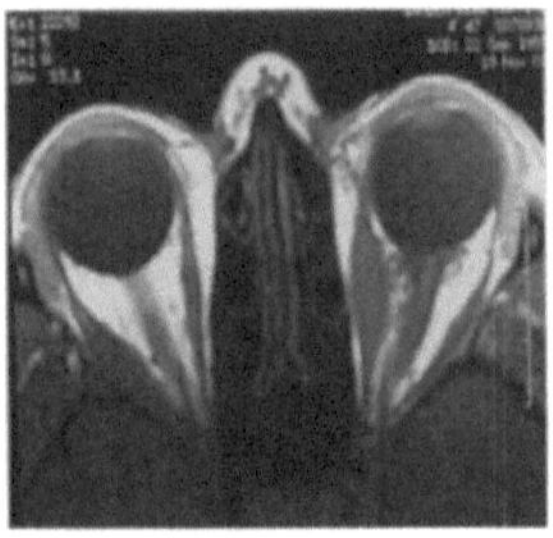

Fig.2- MRI in the axial plane at the initial stage

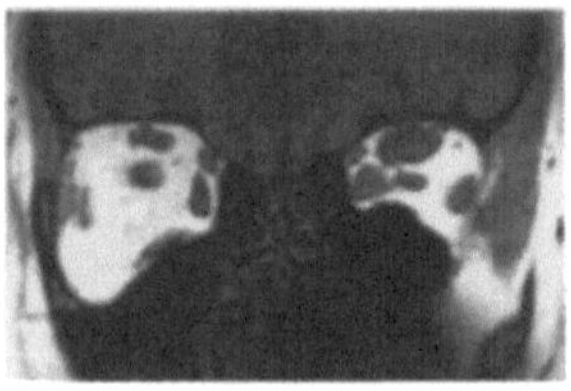

Fig 3a

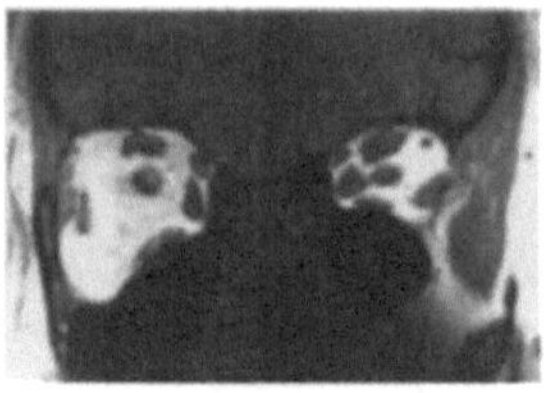

Fig 4a

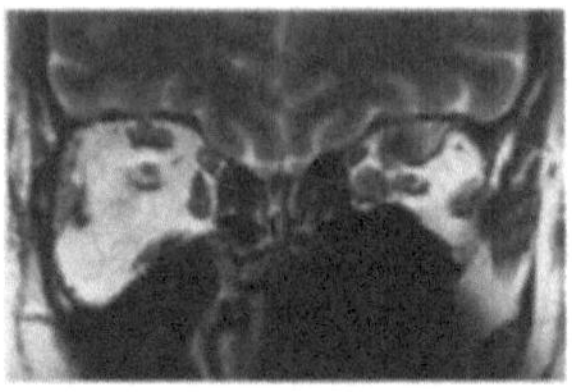

Fig 3b

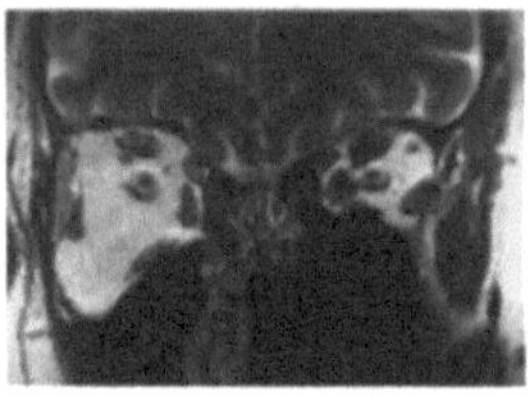

Fig 4b

Fig 3 and 4- MR images in the coronal plane
Fig. 3 a-b: initial stage;
Fig. 4 a-b after the 5th chemotherapeutic cycle

Legend fig 2-4:
Fig. 2: enlargement of the right lateral rectus and the left medial rectus muscles.
Fig. 3a : T1-W spin-echo image showing enlargement of the LSR and LMR muscles.
Fig. 3b: T2-W fast-spin-echo image showing relative hypersignal intensity within involved muscles.
Fig. 4a. T1-W spin-echo image involved muscles have decreased in size when compared to pre-treatment status.
Fig. 4b. T2-W fast-spin-echo image involved muscles have decreased signal intensity when compared to pre-treatment status.
Fig 3a and 3b: similar slice location as in fig. 4a and 4b respectively, to allow comparison.
Image distorsion of the inferior border of the left orbit is due to prosthetic dental material.

Clinical and laboratory workup showed normal results from thyroid testing; no antibodies against thyrotropin receptor (TSHR) were detected in the serum. Further physical examination revealed the presence of a cervical mass and induration of the right supero-external breast soft tissue. Fine-needle aspiration biopsy of the breast soft tissue demonstrated lobular breast carcinoma. An extensive workup detected neck, thoracic, and abdominal metastatic foci but no brain metastasis. Additional laboratory assessment, including muscular enzyme levels in the serum, were within the normal range, except for serum levels tumor markers: CA15,3:70U/ml, (N: F <25); CEA: 4,9ng/ml, (N: </=3). A biopsy of the left medial rectus muscle *via* a conjonctival incision was performed before treatment. The specimen designed for immunohistochemistry did not demonstrate any cells expressing the TSH receptor, at the opposite of what is observed in all cases of thyroid associated orbitopathy (TAO) (fig.5-6). Histological studies of respectively two other specimens of the same muscle, however very tiny, showed normal muscle fibres with a diameter between 8-25 μm, no inflammatory cells, fibroblasts were rare with a moderate fibrotic reaction between the muscular cells (fig 7-8). The patient was treated by multi-agent chemotherapy: FEC -5-fluorouracile, epirubicine and cyclophosphamide- with satisfactory result. After five months of treatment –after the 5th chemotherapeutic cycle-, the patient reported subjective improvement of her diplopia. Our findings supported her impression. Her general condition was satisfactory, with involution

of the cervical mass and almost complete remission of her cancer. Upon examination, she was

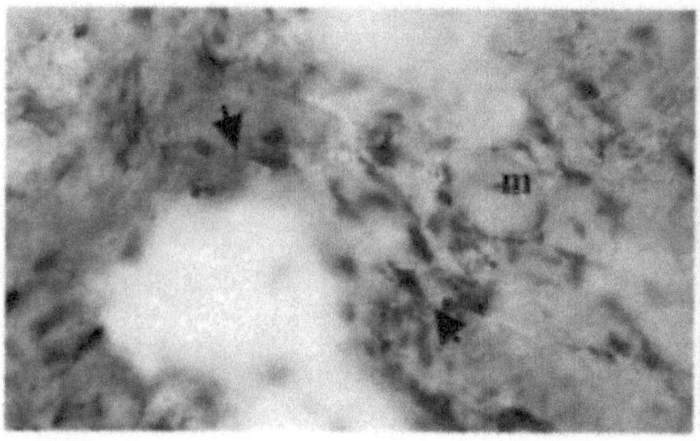

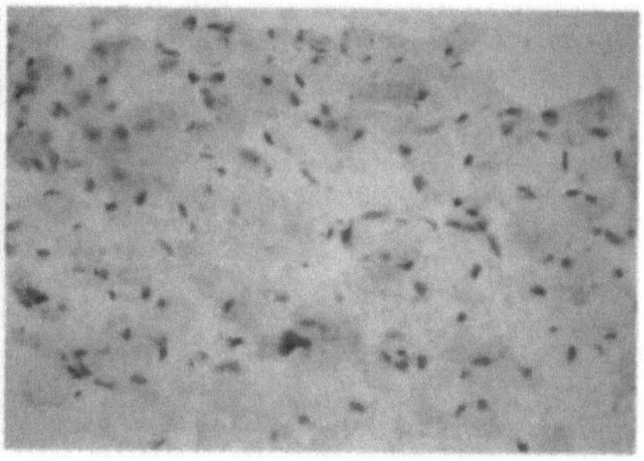

Fig 5 Fig. 6

Figures 5-6: Immunodetetion of TSH receptor on sections of EOMs-

Fig. 5. Patient with TAO: elongated fibroblast-like cells are positively stained (arrows); they are located in the collagen bundles between the muscular cells (m) (x400). Fig 6. Patient with paraneoplastic syndrome: there are no cells expressing the TSH receptor (x230).

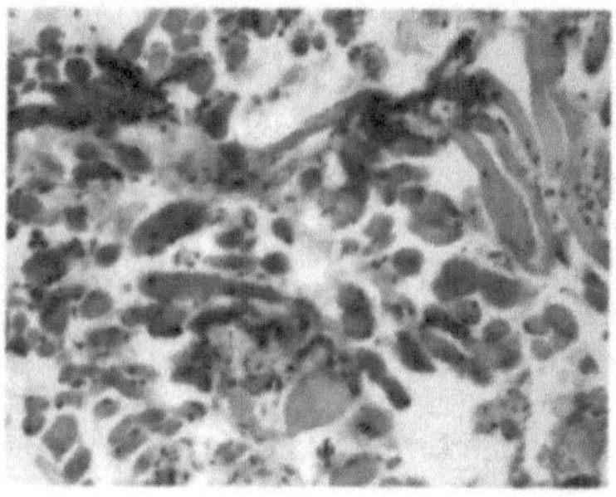

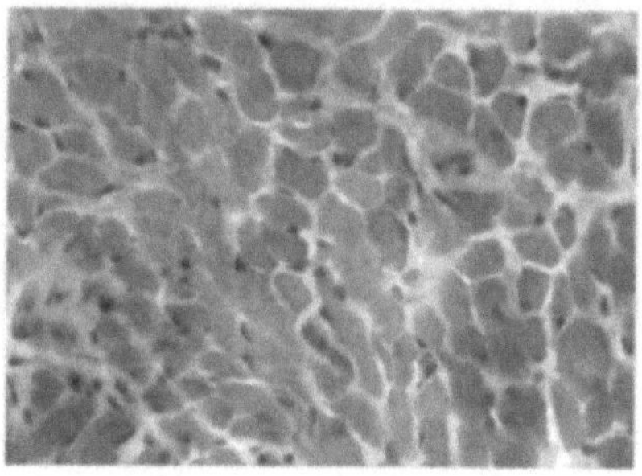

Fig 7 Fig 8

Figures 7-8: Histological studies of the LMR muscle sections in our patient

Fig 7 shows no inflammatory reaction; fibroblasts are rare with a moderate fibrotic reaction between the muscular cells. Formalin-fixed, paraffin-embedded sections
(x200). Fig 8 shows normal fibres muscles with diameter between 8-25μm. No inflammatory cells are present. Hematoxylin-eosin-stained section.

orthophoric at far and near, with stereopsis of 60 seconds of arc on the TNO test in primary position. A left hypertropia of 8 $^{\Delta}$ remained in downgaze and of 14 $^{\Delta}$ in left downgaze; the deficit of elevation and depression of her left eye had improved (fig 9). In the same way, after the 5th chemotherapeutic cycle, the involved muscles had decreased in size on the T1-W images, and in signal intensity on the T2-W images, when compared with the initial images (fig.4a-b).

DISCUSSION: In our patient, we made the diagnosis that diplopia due to EOMs involvement, appeared as the primary presentation of disseminated metastatic breast carcinoma confirmed by biopsy of breast soft tissue. Orbital CT and MRI showed significant and fusiform enlargement of several EOMs exhibiting homogeneous enhancement after paramagnetic contrast agent perfusion. No focal expansive lesion was identified within diseased muscles; the bone structure of the orbits was unremarkable, and the optic nerves appeared intrinsically normal. Besides impaired ocular motility, eye examination remained normal in both eyes.

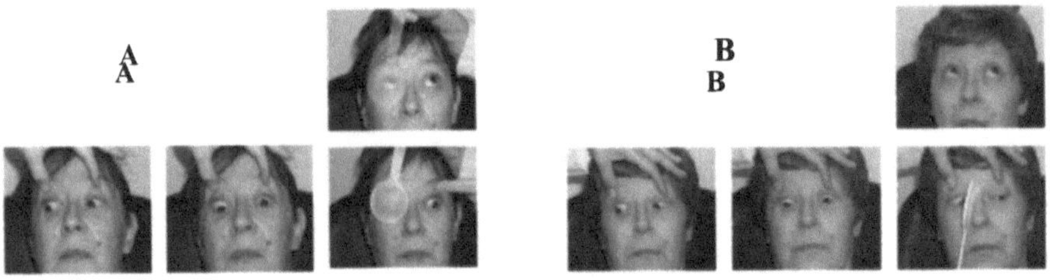

Fig 9.. A. before treatment; B. after the 5th chemotherapeutic cycle. Five months follow-up since diagnosis was made.

Enlargement of EOMs with limitation of ocular motility and periorbital discomfort is most frequently seen feature of TAO and idiopathic inflammatory orbital pseudotumor; it may also be encountered in association with systemic disorders (vasculitis, granulomatous inflammation etc…). In our patient, there was no dysfunction of the thyroid. Currently, cellular autoimmune reaction against TSHR is the most popular pathogenic mechanism of Graves' disease; THSR have also been identified in orbital tissues (Heufelder, 1995; Förster *et al.* 1998). In a former paper, we reported that TSHR immunoreactivity (TSHRI) was found in all EOMs samples from TAO patients and that TSHRI in EOMS seemed to be specific to TAO (Spiritus *et al.* 2000). More, TSHRI might even be found in EOMs of patients with TAO without antibodies against TSHR detected in the serum (Boschi *et al.* 2003). No cellular autoimmune reaction against TSHR was found neither in the serum or the EOM of this patient. In another connection, there was no clinical or laboratory evidence for idiopathic inflammatory orbital syndrome (orbital pseudotumor) or orbital systemic inflammatory condition in our patient. Imaging studies in our patient demonstrated that the orbital fat and the tendon of the enlarged muscles were not involved, contrary to what is usually seen in patients with orbital inflammation.

In cancer patients, diplopia results most frequently from orbital and/or brainstem metastasis, less frequently from metastasis in EOMs, although breast carcinoma appears to have a greater propensity than other malignancies for EOMs metastasis (in Capone, 1990); more rarely orbital myositis has been reported as a possible paraneoplastic phenomenon (Harris *et al.* 1994, Spraul *et al.* 1996, Finol *et al* 2001).

In our patient, orbital CT-scan and MR imaging showed intense and homogeneous enhancement of the belly of several EOMs, without abnormal foci within them, suggesting myositis rather than metastatic involvement of the EOMs. Biopsy of two specimens of the enlarged LMR muscle did not contain cells with a malignant appearance confirming EOM metastasis; on the other end, the muscles fibers appear normal without inflammatory reaction. We must admit that histological studies were not contributive or did not corroborate the results of CT scan- and MR images. Not to say that, as the muscles samples were very small, our findings must be taken cautiously and they do not exclude the possible association between the ocular motility dysfunction and breast carcinoma in our patient. Other authors have drawn the attention that a metastatic orbital breast carcinoma may masquerade as an orbital inflammatory syndrome with non diagnostic cythopathology obtained from fine-needle aspiration biopsy specimens of the orbital tissue. More, bilateral orbital involvement does not lessen the possibility of metastatic breast carcinoma; lobular breast carcinoma, as in our patient, shows a greater tendency toward multicentric involvement (Toller *et al.* 1998).

Paraneoplastic syndromes are defined as disorders evolving at a distance from the primary or metastatic cancers. These entities apparently result from circulating antibodies and/or humoral substances released from the cancer (Minna *et al.* 1982). Involvement of a single or multiples EOMs consisting in a paraneoplastic phenomenon may be the first clinical manifestation in cancers (Harris *et al.* 1994, Spraul *et al.* 1996, Finol *et al* 2001). So far, circulating antibodies against EOMs serving to recognize the paraneoplastic nature of the clinical signs, which frequently develop before the cancer is diagnosed, have not yet been identified.

Out of a literature review, breast cancers ranks third most frequent neoplasm associated with dermatomyositis (polymyositis) (Mebazaa *et al* 2003), which are well-known paraneoplastic phenomena in cancer patients (Manchul *et al.* 1985, Lakhanpal *et al* 1986). To our knowledge, paraneoplastic involvement of the EOMs associated with breast cancer has not yet been reported in the available literature. The clinical manifestations as well as the imaging studies and, the favorable response to chemotherapy in our patient are supporting a cancer causality of the EOMs involvement. Even if the histological studies are not contributive, we believe that the orbital manifestations encountered in our patient might be suggestive of a paraneoplastic phenomenon.

CONCLUSION: The possibility of paraneoplastic or metastatic involvement of EOMs should be kept in mind in patients presenting with diplopia due to ocular mobility limitation, together with peri-orbital discomfort and EOMs enlargement, in spite the rarety of the condition.

REFERENCES:

Boschi A., Daumerie Ch., Spiritus M. *et al.* 2003: Quantification of cells expressing the thyrotropin receptor in extraocular muscles in thyroid associated ophthalmopathy. Correlation with the serum level of autoantibodies and with the evolution of the disease. VII International Symposium on Graves' ophthalmopathy. February 6-8, 2003. Pisa, Italy. Stamperia e Legatoria Pisana.

Capone, Jr. A., Slamovits TL. 1990. Discrete metastasis of solid tumors to extraocular muscles. *Arch Ophthalmol.* 108: 237-243,

Finol H.J., Marquez A., Navas E. *et al* 2001. Extraocular muscle ultrastructural pathology in the paraneoplastic phenomenon associated with retinoblastoma. *J Exp Clin Cancer Res.* 20 (2): 281-285.

Förster G., Otto E., Hansen C. *et al.* 1998.Analysis of orbital T cells in thyroid-associated ophthalmopathy *Clin Exp Immunol,* 112: 427-434.

Harris G.J., Murphy M.L, Schmidt E.W. *et al.* 1994. Orbital myositis as a paraneoplastic syndrome. *Arch Ophthalmol.* 112: 380-386.

Heufelder AE. 1995. Involvement of the orbital fibroblast and TSH receptor in the pathogenesis of Graves'ophthalmopathy. *Thyroid,* 5: 331-340.

Lakhanpal S., Bunch T.W., Ilstrup D.M. *et al* 1986. Polymyositis – dermatomyositis and malignant lesion: does an association exist? *Mayo Clin Proc,* 61: 654-653.

Manchul L.A., Jin A., Prtichard K.I. 1985. The frequency of malignant neoplasms in patients with polymyositis – dermatomyositis. A controlled study. *Arch Intern Med,* 145:1835-1839.

Mebazaa A.,Boussen H., Nouira R. *et al* 2003. Dermatomyositis and malignancy in Tunisia: a multicenter national retrospective study of 20 cases. *J Am. Acad. Dermatol* 48: 530-534.

Minna J.D., Bann P.A.Jr, 1982. Paraneoplastic syndromes. In: Cancer. Principles and Practice of Oncology, ed. DeVita, V.T.Jr. Hellman, S., Rosenberg S.A.. Philadephia J.B. Lippincott, p1476-1517.

Spiritus M., Boschi A., Daumerie Ch. *et al.* 2000. Thyrotropin receptor immunoreactivity in extraocular muscles of patients with thyroid associated ophthalmopathy compared to no thyroid inflammatory orbital diseases and "normals". Trans. 25th Meeting European Strabismological Association (ESA) Jerusalem, Israel, September 1999, ed. by M. Spiritus. Swets & Zeitlinger, Lisse, The Netherlands, p. 220-225.

Spraul C.W., Lang G.E., Lang G.K. 1996. Orbitale Myopathie bei metastasiertem malignem Paragangliom: eine Paraneoplasie? *Klin. Monatsbl. Augenheilkd*: 209:153-157.

Toller K.K., Gigantelli J.W., Spalding M.J. 1998. Bilateral Orbital metastases from breast carcinoma. *Ophthalmology* 105: 1897-1901.

Author's address: M. Spiritus, Cliniques St-Luc, UCL, 10, Hippocrate Avenue, B-1200 Brussels

Transactions 28th Meeting European Strabismological Association, de Faber (ed.)
© 2004 European Strabismological Association, ISBN 90 265 1965 6

Acquired distance esotropia associated with myopia

H. A. Webb & J. P. Lee
Moorfields Eye Hospital, London, England

ABSTRACT: Von Graefe (1864) and Bielschowsky (1922) described acquired progressive esotropia, with larger angle for distance than near, associated with moderate myopia. This is unlike the esotropia seen in patients with high myopia. *Methods:* We reviewed notes, finding 26 cases, age range at first presentation 37-74 years, mean of 55.5. Myopia was from –0.75 to –10.00DS, mean of –5.50 each eye. Eighteen wore glasses, 8 mainly contact lenses. All complained of horizontal diplopia. Seventeen (65%) were treated with prisms, gradually increasing in power. *Results:* Six patients (23%) continued with prisms. Seven patients (27%) had BTXA to one medial rectus muscle, successfully in 2 cases. Seventeen (65%) underwent surgery (mainly medial rectus recession, lateral rectus resection) with relief of diplopia and discarding prisms. Five patients suffered a recurrence usually at 11 years. *Conclusion:* This unusual sub-type of strabismus is a benign entity, responding well to prism correction, or surgery.
KEYWORDS: Acquired, Esotropia, Myopia

1 INTRODUCTION

Von Graefe (1864)[1]and Bielschowsky (1922)[2] described a syndrome of acquired progressive esotropia, with larger angle for distance than near, associated with moderate myopia. We present a series of 26 patients with this condition, which is unlike the esotropia seen in patients with high myopia.

Von Graefe concluded that the causation was reading without glasses, leading to overaction of the medial rectus muscles. He recommended 1) spectacle correction, 2) base out prisms, 3) surgery (graded medial rectus tenotomy).

Bielschowsky noted the characteristic late onset, with diplopia initially for far distance fixation and good binocularity for near. He ascribed it to close-work combined with a 'neuropathic personality'. He recommended no surgery on the medial recti, but lateral rectus resections.

We managed the majority of our patients with adjustable unilateral medial rectus recession and lateral rectus resection.

2 METHODS

We reviewed the notes of 26 patients with this condition, 14 female and 12 male. The age range at first presentation was 37-74 yrs, with a mean of 55.5yrs.

The levels of myopia were from –0.75DS to –10.00DS, with a mean of –5.50DS each eye. (Shown in fig.1).

Eighteen patients mostly wore glasses while eight were mainly were contact lens corrected.

All patients presented with complaints of horizontal diplopia and the duration of these symptoms ranged from 6 months to 31 years with a mean of 9 years. All had esotropia or symptomatic esophoria at 6metres. The near deviation ranged from 2 to 45 prism dioptres, mean 15, and distance deviation from 8 to 45 prism dioptres, mean 22 (Shown in fig.2). Ocular movement

testing showed slight/small bilateral limitations of abduction in 18 cases and unilateral limitation of abduction in 3 cases. Four cases had an associated vertical deviation and motility was described as full in 5 cases.
Seventeen (65%) had been treated with prisms with a gradual increase in power.

3 RESULTS

Six patients (23%) continued with prisms, although surgery has been offered in 3 cases. Seven patients (27%) had botulinum toxin to 1 medial rectus muscle. In 2 cases this proved successful maintenance therapy. The remaining 5 either hated the induced over-correction or found the effect did not last long, so have gone on to have surgery. Seventeen patients (65%) have undergone surgery, mainly having ipsilateral medial rectus recession and lateral rectus resection using adjustable sutures, two had this combined with an inferior oblique recession, for an associated vertical element. One patient had bilateral medial rectus recessions with a lowering of the insertions to collapse an associated V eso pattern. One patient had an ipsilateral medial rectus recession carried out at another hospital prior to presentation to the authors. The surgery provided relief of diplopia and discarding of prisms.

4 FOLLOW-UP

These patients have been followed up for between 1 and 16 years with a mean of 6.5 years. Three patients required further surgery for a recurrence 10-12 years after the first procedure. Two of these had their previous surgery at other hospitals, this includes the patient who had a single medial rectus recession. Another is using prisms for a recurrence after 11 years. One patient has suffered an early recurrence 6 months after surgery, the reason for which is not entirely clear and neurologists are investigating other possible causes. As this seems to be a progressive/recurrent condition patients need to be advised that their symptoms may return. Our cohort, of mean follow up 6.5years, suggests that this might be around the 11 year mark.

5 CONCLUSION

This unusual sub-type of strabismus is a benign entity, in which the pathology is unclear. It responds well to prism correction, or surgery in cases who wish to wear contact lenses or whose prisms become inconveniently strong.

REFERENCES

1. Graefe, A. von: Über die von myopia äbhangige Form convergirenden Schielens und deren Heilung, Graefes Arch. Ophthalmol. 10:156-175, 1864
2. Bielschowsky, A.: Das Einwärtsschielen der Myopen, Ber. Dtsch. Ophthalmol., Ges. 43:245-8, 1922

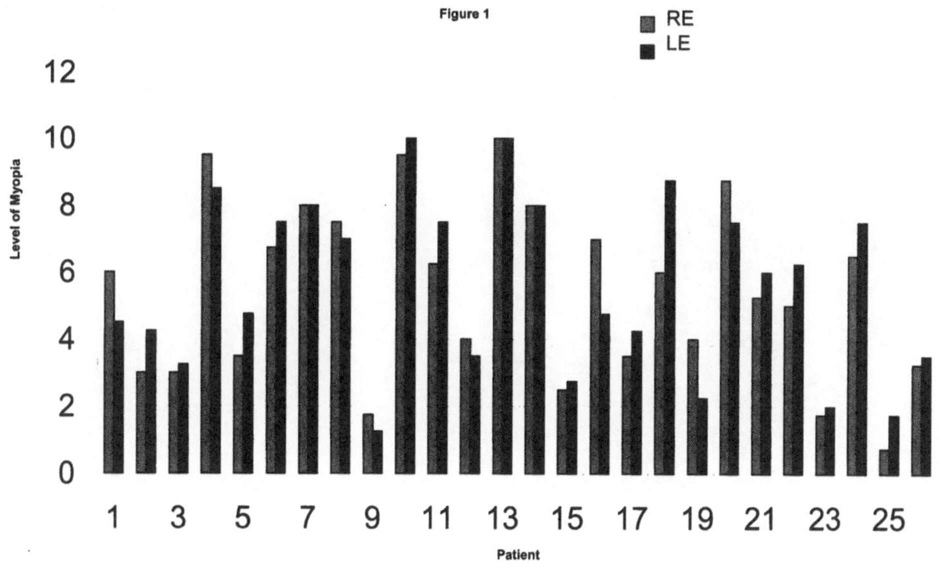
Figure 1
RE
LE
Level of Myopia
12
10
8
6
4
2
0
1 3 5 7 9 11 13 15 17 19 21 23 25
Patient

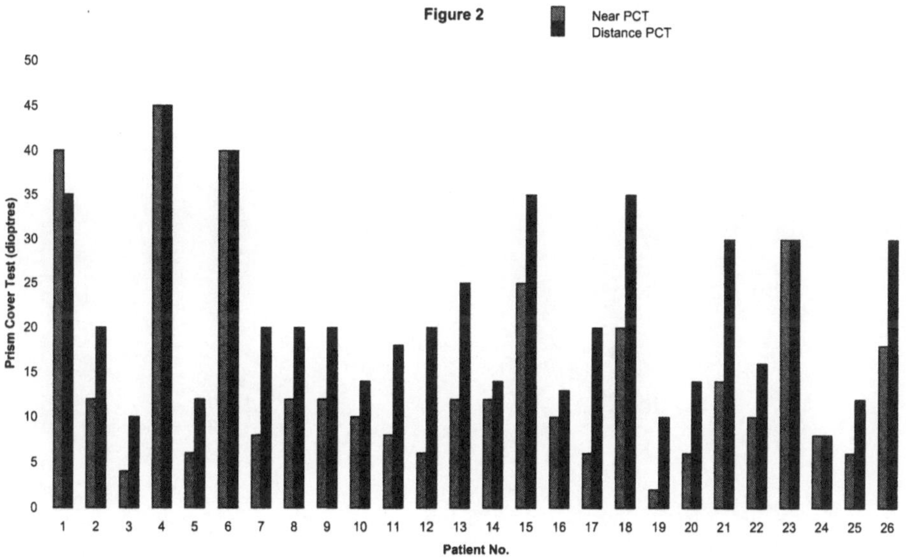
Figure 2
Near PCT
Distance PCT
Prism Cover Test (dioptres)
50
45
40
35
30
25
20
15
10
5
0
1 2 3 4 5 6 7 8 9 10 11 12 13 14 15 16 17 18 19 20 21 22 23 24 25 26
Patient No.

Session 11
Varia

Transactions 28th Meeting European Strabismological Association, de Faber (ed.)
© 2004 European Strabismological Association, ISBN 90 265 1965 6

The eso trend following heroin detoxification

A.Y. Firth
Academic Unit of Ophthalmology and Orthoptics, University of Sheffield, Sheffield, UK.

S. Pulling, M.P. Carr & A.Y. Beaini
Detox 5, Harrogate Clinic, Ripon Road, Harrogate, UK.

ABSTRACT: The angle of deviation was measured using the prism cover test at near (33cm) and distance (6m) before the start and at the end of a 5 day detoxification programme. In a subgroup of patients (n=38) measurements were also recorded on lateral gaze at distance. Eighty-three participants were seen pre detoxification (aged 27.1±4.6 years) and 69 post detoxification. A significant change in the distance angle of deviation in the eso direction was found ($p<0.001$), but the change in near angle was not significant. Right gaze measurements showed a median change of +2Δ (range -12Δ to +10Δ), not significant ($p=0.098$) and left gaze measurements showed a median change of +2Δ (range -8Δ to +10Δ), significant ($p=0.01$). A trend towards development of distance esotropia following detoxification from heroin and / or methadone appears to be present. However, the mechanism for this trend is probably not due to 6th nerve involvement as the increase in incomitance is considered too small to be clinically significant and it is suggested that the increase could be due to decompensation of pre-existing incomitance.

KEYWORDS: Heroin, diamorphine, methadone, detoxification, esodeviation.

The full study from which this short report has been taken will be published elsewhere.

Transactions 28th Meeting European Strabismological Association, de Faber (ed.)
© 2004 European Strabismological Association, ISBN 90 265 1965 6

Principles in Training for Subspecialty Ophthalmic Care in Developing Countries

T Otis Paul MD*, R Scott Foster MD, Bradley Black MD

**Chief, Division of Pediatric Ophthalmology, Oakland Children's Hospital, 5275 Claremont Avenue, Oakland, California 94618, USA*

ABSTRACT: This paper describes general ophthalmic as well as specialized strabismic care programs for developing countries as developed by the authors, and the training principles involved. Over the past three decades Drs. Paul, Black, and Foster have evolved program formats, guidelines, and requirements to provide sorely needed ophthalmic care in developing countries. Initially largely organized toward service, these programs eventually shifted toward teaching in the field of pediatric ophthalmology and strabismus. They consist of consultations, lectures, and demonstration surgeries and require three major principles in place: appropriate technology, empowerment, and sustainability. The best way to facilitate programs that generate better health care in developing countries largely depends on which phase of recovery the country currently experiences, how the training principles apply, and how best to assist the countries.

1. INTRODUCTION

1.1 Over the past few decades the authors have visited a number of developing countries in Europe, Africa, Asia and the Americas, providing both general ophthalmology care and specialized consultation, teaching and service. The programs initially were largely oriented toward cataract surgery and glaucoma care in more rural areas, then towards teaching in the field of pediatric ophthalmology and strabismus in large city hospitals. There seems to be a never-ending amount of service needed in these countries, although, over time, the ability of colleagues to provide service to their own people has increased. However, as the cataract backlog is reduced, there develops an interest in learning specialized ophthalmic concepts and surgery techniques.

Volunteers visiting a developing country should not make assumptions based on previous visits because perceptions and conditions in the country vary. It is essential to have good communications with colleagues in the country visited.

There have been three major principles observed in medical mission trips:

1. That there is appropriate technology based on the existing infrastructure and that the needs are determined at both local and national level.

2. That there is 'empowerment' of the physicians and paramedical personnel in the country. This should include informal teaching in the clinic, working together with colleagues in the operating room, as well as formal lectures and courses at centers of medical education.

3. The project should have sustainability. Equipment should be donated to local organizations, such as Lions Clubs, Rotary Clubs, or Orbis International with support organizations placed in those Clubs so that return trips can be organized more effectively. There is a need, also, for colleagues in these countries to come for further training in more developed countries. This provides the greatest amount of 'multiplier effect', as then a person can return to his or her own country and devote his or her career to service in ophthalmology - particularly pediatric ophthalmology and strabismus, the specialty interest of the authors.

2. APPROPRIATE TECHNOLOGY

2.1 A general guideline is to support the improvement in technology in a developing country is step by step, rather than to bring in the latest technology, which may remain unused. For example, phakoemulsifiers at small hospitals in the poorly served periphery (e.g., rural areas) may be used, with much support, for success by the visiting specialist, after which it may be placed under a dust cover for years. In countries where the water supply is not clean, sediment in the water supply typically contaminates the lens of lasers, reducing effectiveness and ultimately the use of the laser. It is best to work with colleagues in these countries to select what is appropriate. Surgical instruments are most commonly needed.

Empowerment of Physicians and Paramedical Personnel

Most people in the developing world, including physicians, are so used to diminishing resources and an unresponsive government that they may have given up trying to establish new programs. It is, therefore, important to empower the physicians and other personnel to improve this situation. Service programs can bring in visiting specialists with expensive equipment and highly trained technicians to do a large number of operations or procedures in a short period of time. These programs leave a clear and inappropriate message that visiting doctors can carry out various procedures and the local doctors cannot. Should this type of visit continue as the developing country progresses, the service organizations can easily run into more and more problems, formally and informally.

The inability of getting goods through customs, for instance, tends to occur where local organizations have not been asked to participate and cooperate with mission service trips. Some countries, such as Mexico, restrict the type of volunteer organizations allowed by requiring letters of support from local Mexican physicians or local medical societies - before any organization is allowed to work within that country. It is important to ask questions constantly of those participating in medical service visits – is it appropriate and will it provide empowerment?

Program Format and Caveats

A typical program format that we have evolved over the years is to provide first consultation, second lectures, and third demonstration surgery. Lectures are done both formally as well as informally. Demonstration surgery is done together with colleagues of the country, working with them on patients within their own practice. The policy of coming in with inexperienced visiting surgeons is entirely inappropriate, suggesting that they have come simply to practice their surgical techniques.

Another common mistake is to allow very important people from the local villages and cities to come in and receive care from the visiting 'experts'. These typically are those who could afford to pay for private care locally. Providing care to these people provides a direct loss of revenue to the local physicians. This should be avoided whenever possible, and patient referred to the local ophthalmologist to be seen in consultation, and allow that person to bill for services. An important rule in making any decisions in developing countries is to include not only the local ophthalmologists in these decisions, but actually adopt their preferences whenever possible.

Project Sustainability

One of the other important concepts to share is that of the 'spirit of volunteerism'. In many developing countries, the ability to help people beyond the local family or village unit is poorly accepted. This can be addressed by suggesting the formation of volunteer organizations by the local ophthalmologists, which has been done in Zimbabwe in the form of residents doing cataract camps in local villages and in Nicaragua by the formation of an organization called Fundacion Ayudemos Aver, where local ophthalmologists provide volunteer services for screening and surgery on the last Friday of every month. Their transportation and supplies are organized through either the local Lions or Rotary Clubs. Also, organizations like Fundacion Ayudemos Aver, working with local Lions and Rotary Clubs and Orbis International, are a great source of support in the organization and planning of future visits as well as fundraising for equipment and supplies purchase. Basic surgical instruments are most often needed. Commonly local service clubs will provide funds (~£2000) for purchase of a set of instruments. These can be donated and procured with the help of a local chapter in the host country.

CPR and Developing Countries

Sadly, many developing countries can be recovering from war and, in the early stages of recovery, have three phases (called 'CPR') through which the country progresses in restoring health care for the people.

The first phase is that of crisis and chaos ('C'). At times like this any help will be useful and does not have to be coordinated with local doctors as much as in the later stages. However, help at this time can be dangerous to volunteers as the country may still be effectively a war zone. Eye care may largely be related to trauma.

The second phase of recovery would be characterized by peace with poverty ('P'). Government resources have largely been devoted to providing the most efficient aid for indigenous diseases and epidemics. Unfortunately, many governments provide very small amounts of their countries resources to the health care of their people. In this stage of recovery, public health measures are most needed with basic health training and distribution of health resources. Health funding from outside sources is still most appropriate.

The third phase is that of recovery and resourcefulness ('R'). Medical schools are typically started or revived at this stage, and then ophthalmology training is re-established. The training model may include educating ophthalmology technicians along with ophthalmic surgeons. Specialty care is then taught at teaching hospitals, usually in large cities. Until this phase is reached, children's needs are usually ignored. Well-documented childhood starvation at times of drought or political crisis illustrates this. As concerns pediatric ophthalmology, these conditions are manifest as lack of childhood screening programs in cataract camps, as lack of general anesthesia services, lack of equipment in hospitals, and in the lack of pediatric ophthalmology and strabismus management skills by general ophthalmologists.

Once in the recovery phase, ophthalmologists have begun to address the backlog of war injuries, industrial trauma and cataracts, and are more able to help in pediatric care. This phase is the most appropriate for teaching pediatric ophthalmology and strabismus surgery.

3. ACKNOWLEDGEMENTS

The authors wish to thank Smith-Kettlewell Eye Research Institute, California Pacific Medical Center, University of California San Francisco, and the Pacific Vision Foundation for their support of fellows in their training, and are delighted to report that all of them have returned to their countries for service to their own citizens. We are grateful to Orbis International, for their support, which has led the way with educational based programs in developing countries. Many thanks to the Mission Support program of Alcon Laboratories for their repeated donations of sutures and medications.Lastly a special note of gratitude is given to the members of the San Francisco Rotary Club for their generous funding of the purchase of many sets of surgical instruments.

REFERENCES

A Proposal to Rotary International to join the Foundation of the American Academy of Ophthalmology in creating a partnership to fight global blindness. March 2000.

Sommer A. Organizing to prevent third world blindness. *Am J Ophthalmol* 1989; 107(5): 544-546.

Schwab L, Whitfield R. Appropriate ophthalmic surgical technology in developing nations. *Ophthalmic Surgery* 1982; 13(12): 991-993.

Woods J, Kiely J. Short-term international medical service. *Mayo Clinic Proc* 2000; 75: 311-313.

Hodes R, Kloos H. Health and medical care in Ethiopia. *New Eng J Med* 1988; 319(14): 918-923.

First Presented at the Jampolsky Fellows meeting, April 2000, sponsored by Smith-Kettlewell Eye Research Institute, San Francisco,2318 Fillmore Street, California 94115, USA

Transactions 28th Meeting European Strabismological Association, de Faber (ed.)
© 2004 European Strabismological Association, ISBN 90 265 1965 6

Management of Motility Disorders in Patients with Spinocerebellar Ataxia Type 3

Th.B.Kerkhof, CO, E.R.P.Brunt, MD and J.W.R.Pott, MD
Department of Ophthalmology and Neurology,University Hospital Groningen
The Netherlands

ABSTRACT
Spinocerebellar ataxia (SCA) is an inherited neurodegenerative disease , which can be accompanied by ocular motility disorders . Especially SCA type 3 is known for divergence insufficiency. We retrospectively examined our records for patients with SCA type 3 and evaluated the prevalence and management of motility disorders.

1. INTRODUCTION

Spino Cerebellar Ataxia (SCA) is also known as Machado-Joseph disease . It is a representative of the heterogeneous group of Autosomal Dominant Cerebellar Ataxia (ADCA). In ADCA the mutation is an expanded cyosine-adenine-guanine(CAG) nucleotide repeat. SCA type 3 is the most frequent mutation (30-35 %). The onset is after childhood.
Symptoms observed include cerebellar,pyramydal and extrapyramydal signs and ophthalmoplegia. There is a variable spectrum of clinical characteristics, including gait and limb ataxia, dysarthria and oculomotor disturbances.
More specific, the ocular findings described in literature are:
-nystagmus
-normal horizontal saccades
-vertical gaze disorders
-decreased smooth pursuit
-decreased optokinetic nystagmus
-decreased vestibulo-ocular reflex with fixation
-optic nerve atrophia
-divergence insufficiency
Divergence insufficiency is described as an esotropia and diplopia only at distance and single binocular vision at near. Little can to be found on the management of divergence insufficiency.

2. MATERIAL AND METHODS

Retrospectively, we looked at the frequency of divergence insufficiency in patients with SCA, the age of onset, the management and results, and the supposed progression of the disease.
At our neurology departement 80 patients are known with SCA, of which 29 patients had SCA type 3. The patients with SCA type 3 were seen at our department.

19 patients with SCA type 3 had complaints of binocular vision caused by divergence insufficiency (66%). They all had esotropia and diplopia at distance.

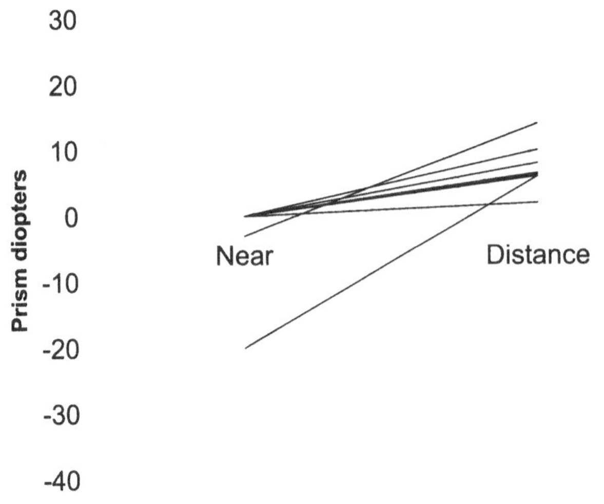

Their mean age was 50 years. The age of onset of symptoms of diplopia was 43 years.

3. RESULTS

Two patients preferred no treatment at all (mean angle at near 5 PD base out, and at distance 14 PD base in)
Twelve patients were stable with prisms , during a mean follow-up of 3.2 years (0-17yrs).
Their mean deviation at distance was 14.5 PD base out, they needed a mean correction of 7 PD base out. Only two patients needed stronger prisms, despite the progressive nature of SCA.
The remaining five patients were in progressive need of prisms during a mean follow-up of 3.2 years (1-10yrs), and eventually needed surgery. The mean deviation at distance was 16 PD base out at the time of their surgery. Three patients had a bilateral medial recession (BMR).One patient had a unilateral medial recession and one patient had a bilateral resection of the lateral rectus muscle, subsequently after a BMR. Post-operatively, all patients needed a slight prism correction, but were free of diplopia.

CONCLUSION

There is a high incidence of divergence insufficiency in patients with SCA type 3. The mean age of onset was 43 years. Despite the progressive nature of the disease, most patients do well with a prism-correction. The few patients with a more progressive nature of their disease may eventually need surgery, our preferred procedure is a BMR. Orthoptic management with prisms, or surgical intervention can establish acceptable binocular single vision in this group of patients.

4. BIBLIOGRAPHY

During S.J., Jen J.C., Demer J.L.: Ocular motility in genetically defined autosomal dominant cerebellar ataxia. American Journal of Ophthalmology.2002; 133,5: 718-721.

Warrenburg van de B.P.C. et coll.: Spinocerebellar ataxias in the Netherlands. American Academy of Neurology.2002:.....

Paulson H.L. et coll.: Intranuclear Inclusions of Expanded Polyglutamine Protein in
Spinocerebellar Ataxia Type 3. Neuron.1997; 19: 333-344.

Riva A., Bradac G.B. :Primary cerebellar and spino-cerebellar ataxia an MRI study on 63 cases. Jurnal of Neuroradiology.1995; 22: 71-76.
Buttner N. et coll. : Oculomotor Phenotypes in Autosomal Dominant Ataxias.Arch Neurology. 1998 ; 55 : 1353-1357.
Klockgether T. et coll. : Repeat lenght and disease progression in spinocerebellar ataxia type 3. Lancet. 1996; 348:830.
Thomas A.H.: Divergence insufficiency. Journal of AAPOS. 2000; 4:395-361.
Haberhausen G., Damian S.M. et coll. : Spinocerebellar ataxia typ3 (SCA3) is genetically identical to Machado-Joseph disease (MJD). Journal of Neurological Sciences.1995; 132: 71-75.

Transactions 28th Meeting European Strabismological Association, de Faber (ed.)

The development and treatment of V-pattern and upshoot in adduction in cyclic esotropia

J. W. R. Pott a , T. B. Kerkhof a , D. Godts b and J. T. H. N. de Faber c
University Hospital Groningen, Netherlands a , University Hospital Antwerpen, Belgium b , the Eye Hospital Rotterdam, Netherlands c .

OBJECTIVE: Cyclic esotropia is a regularly recurring esotropia, usually present in an alternate day pattern. The V-pattern has been described as one of the characteristics of cyclic esotropia1. The aim of the present study is to describe the development and treatment of V-pattern and upshoot in adduction in patients with cyclic esotropia.

METHODS: Three patients with cyclic esotropia are described in retrospect. All patients underwent bilateral medial recession, while one patient additionally had a weakening procedure of both inferior oblique muscles.

RESULTS: All patients developed a V-pattern and upshoot in adduction. After strabismus surgery, normal eye alignment with some signs of binocularity was reached in all three patients. Moreover, the V-pattern and upshoot in adduction completely resolved.

CONCLUSION: V-pattern and upshoot in adduction was seen in all patients with cyclic esotropia in the stage that fusion was disrupted. Loss of fusion has been suggested earlier as a cause of V-pattern and upshoot in adduction2, 3. The present study shows that in cyclic esotropia restoration of fusion by a bilateral medial recession, without weakening of the inferior oblique muscles, also resolves the V-pattern and upshoot in adduction.

REFERENCES

Helveston EM. Cyclic strabismus. Am Orthoptic J 1973;23 :48-51. 2.
Guyton, DL, Weingarten, PE. Sensory torsion as the cause of primary oblique muscle overacti on/underaction and A and V-pattern strabismus. Binocul Vis Eye Muscle Surg Q 1994;9: 209-236. 3.
Brodsky. MC, Donahue SP. Primary oblique muscle overaction. The Brain throws a wild pitch. Arch Ophthalmol: 2001;1307-1314.

Posters

Transactions 28th Meeting European Strabismological Association, de Faber (ed.)
© 2004 European Strabismological Association, ISBN 90 265 1965 6

Thyroid ophtalmopathy manifesting as superior oblique paralysis

V.OĞUZ, M.YOLAR, H. PAZARLI, S. ÖZKAN
DEPARTMENT OF OPHTHALMOLOGY OF THE FACULTY OF MEDICINE OF CERRAHPASA ,UNIVERSITY OF ISTANBUL

ABSTRACT
The thyroid ophtalmopathy may sometimes present as an imbalance of oculomotor muscles. The aim of this study is to investigate the cases that manifest as a paralysis of the superior oblique and to bring an approach to pathogenesis. This study included 7 cases with thyroid ophtalmopathy imitating paralysis of the superior oblique and giving the anamnesis relevant with the signs or symptoms of Graves disease. All the patients showed binocular vertical diplopia at primary position and a paralysis of the superior oblique. Among all our patients showing a binocular vertical diplopia and with an anamnesis which was not compatible with the paralysis of the 4th nerve, we observed a hypertropia of 4 to 26 PD and an upshoot in adduction in the same eye. An excyclotorsion less than 10° was observed in 3 of 7cases. This clinical picture can be interpreted as a transformation of the previously asymptomatic paralysis of superior oblique into symptomatic state as a result of a decrease of fusion due to Graves disease.

Keywords: Graves disease, ophthalmopathy of Graves, Paralysis of the superior oblique muscle, Myopathy.

1. INTRODUCTION

In the thyroid ophthalmomyopathy, involvement of the extraocular muscles (40%) is among the most frequent 3 conditions, one of which is palpebroretractile syndrome (25,8-90%) and the other being exophtalmus (30-60%) [1-4]. The involvement of the extraocular muscles due to thyroid orbitomyopathy is often accompanied with diplopia,as well [1,5,6]. It has been already known that in this patology the inferior rectus muscle has been involved most frequently, and followed by medial rectus and external superior muscles, the involvement of oblique muscles being more rare [4,7,8]. The thyroid ophtalmomyopathy may imitate various oculomotor imbalances and this pathology has to be considered
within the differential diagnosis in all cases showing an ophthalmoplegia [9]. As in the thyroid ophtalmomyopathy the involvement of the inferior rectus is the most frequent, often appearing with a vertical diplopia [4,5].
Furthermore one of the most common causes of vertical diplopia is the paralysis of the superior oblique [4,9]. During the course of thyroid ophtalmopathy, the myopathy may be added to the other signs of the thyroid disease [10], and the ophtalmopathy may also present in the form of an oculomotor imbalance [9]. The aim of our study was to evaluate the cases who had been presented with a paralysis of the superior oblique and to bring an approach to their pathogenesis.

2. MATERIALS AND METHODS

Seven patients composed of 4 females and 3 males who had been followed in the Department of Ophthalmology of the Cerrahpasa Faculty of Medicine of the University of İstanbul were followed up. The ages of the cases ranged between 27 and 72 years, the mean age being

50,28±18.09 years. All of these 7 cases who had been presented with a paralysis of the superior oblique muscle showed a binocular vertical diplopia at primary position. The history of the disease reminded systemic signs or symptoms which may be attributed to Graves disease in all these cases, for a further examination the coexistance of the following conditions were investigated as the previous reports[11,12]:

Diffuse hypertrophy of the thyroid gland and increase in the I^{131} fixation in the scintigraphy,

Hyperthyroidy proven by an increase in T3 and T4 levels and a weak response of TSH by TRH test,

Presence of TRAC (TSH receptor antibody) .

A complete examination of the ocular motility, prism and cover test, Hess screen test , Parks' three-step test and diplopia test with to red glass and the double test with the rods of Maddox for the evaluation of torsion were perfomed. Also, MRI of the orbita, exophtalmometry with Hertel exophthalmometer and the examination of the eyelids were done. In addition to fundus examination, visual field examination with Goldmann perimeter and color vision evaluation were all carried out for neuroophthalmologic evaluation. Neurological examinations and tensilon test were also performed whenever it was considered to be necessary. Routine blood chemistry tests and arterial blood pressure measurementwere done.

3. RESULTS

In all patients who showed a binocular vertical diplopia and whose history does not reveal any sign of the 4th nerve paralysis, we observed a hypertropia from 4 to 26 PD in each eye and an upshoot in adduction, along with the positivity of Bielchowsky test. MRI examinations exhibited bilateral involvement of the inferior recti which was milder in the eye showing an upshoot in adduction in 7 cases. Involvements of various degrees were observed in other oculomotor muscles but there existed no restriction at any position of gaze. An excyclotorsion of less than 10° was observed in 3 of 7 cases. No pathology that may cause 4th nerve paralysis was found in the neuroophthalmologic examinations.

4. DISCUSSION

It is known that the oblique muscles are rarely involved in thyroid ophtalmomyopathy , and the studies investigating the involvement of these muscles are also rare [8,9,13-15]. Additionally, there are only a few studies about the cases who present with a paralysis of the superior oblique simulating the superior oblique involvement as an initial sign of the thyroid ophthalmopathy[9]. In this study the cases arising as a paralysis of the superior oblique muscle and at the same time showing an involvement of the inferior oblique were evaluated. The relationship between the paralysis of the superior oblique and the thyroid ophtalmopathy can be explained in 5 different ways [9]. The most plausible explanation is that probably the paralysis of the superior oblique precedes Graves disease rather than being a result of this disorder. It becomes symptomatic by the diminution of fusion due to the Graves disease [13]. In our 7 patients whose history did not include any cause of the paralysis of the 4th nerve, the most acceptable assumption is the preceding asymptomatic paralysis of the superior oblique that becomes symptomatic after decompensation by diminution in fusion related to the disease.

The second possibility is the early myopathy of the inferior rectus of the eye responsible for the apparent paralysis of the superior oblique [9]. This condition may be interpreted as a subclinic infiltration presenting in the inferior oblique, and spreads through the neighbouring tissues and by the Lockwood ligament to the inferior oblique while inducing a hyperfonction in the latter. It is quite reasonable for such a condition of inferior rectus involvement in two eyes that is less severe in the eye which shows an upshoot in adduction, but this assumption does not explain the absence of inferior oblique hyperfunction of the eye in which the inferior rectus has been severely involved.

The third possibility is the isolated compression of the trochlear nerve at the apex of the orbit especially in cases who show an optical neuropathy. As none of our 7 cases presented a sign due to an optical neuropathy, such an explanation could not be stated for these cases. Besides, the best of our knowledge no case of oculomotor imbalance of neurogenic origin in the thyroid ophtalmomyopathy has been described.

The fourth possible explanation is the coexistence of the paralysis of the 4th nerve with myasthenia. However the absence of a vaxing and vaning deficit and the negative results obtained by the tensilon test which had been considered to be necessary in some of our cases did not indicate such a coexistence in our patients.

The fifth possibility to consider would be an idiopathic vasculopathy of the 4th nerve preceding the ophtalmomyopathy but we did not encounter any clinical signs which reinforced such an assumption [9].

The involvement of the inferior rectus may cause a controlateral hyperdeviation which has a peak in upper gaze position. The occurence of such a controlateral hyperdeviation of the eye showing an upshoot in adduction may be due to a more severe involvement of the inferior rectus in other eye.

Trobe had reported 30 cases of excyclotorsion out of 33 cases (90,9%) with the paralysis of the 4th nerve along with 8 out of 15 (53,4%) with thyroid ophtalmopathy. The relatively low number of the cases with excyclotorsion in our series, being 3 out of 7 (42,9%), is an evidence against the diagnosis of the 4th nerve paralysis while it supports the diagnosis of thyroid ophtalmopathy [16].

In conclusion, this clinical picture may be interpreted as the progression of a previously asymptomatic paralysis of the superior oblique into a symptomatic state and this progression is the result of the diminution of fusion due to the Graves disease. It is also probable that the inflammatory infiltration involving the inferior oblique of the eye with a previously asymptomatic paralysis is the triggering factor of the decompensation of this paralysis.

REFERENCES

Wiersinga Wm, Smith T, Van Der Gaag R, Mourits M, Korneef L: Clinical presentation of Graves' ophthalmopathy. Ophthalmic Res, 1989; 21: 73-82

Vangheluwe O, Ducasse A, Vaudrey C, Maes B, Delisle MJ: Prévalence de l'ophtalmopathy dans la maladie de Basedow.Suivi des malades a un an apres la dècouverte de leur hypothyroidie. J Fr Ophtalmol. 1994; 17: 331-338

Bartley GB, Fatourechi V, Kadrmas Ef, Jacobsen SJ, Ilstrup DM, Garrity Ja, Gorman Ca: The incidence of Graves' ophthalmopathy in Olmsted Country, Minnesota. Am J Ophthalmol. 1995; 120: 511-517

Ducasse A, Schlienger JL: Pathology du système endocrinien. In: Flament J, Storck D (eds), Oeil et pathologie générale. Paris, Masson 1997, pp. 339-374

Sergot RC, Glaser JS: Graves ophthalmopathy. A clinical and immunologic review. Surv Ophthalmol 1981; 26: 1-21

Evans D, Kennerdell JS: Extraocular muscle surgery for dysthyroid myopathy. Am J Ophthalmol, 1989; 95: 767-771

Eggers Hm : Vertical Other strabismus. In: Diamond GR., Eggers HM, eds. Strabismus and Pediatric Ophthalmology. London, Mosby, 1991:12.1-12.9

Char DH. Thyroid eye disease. New York, The USA: Churchill Livingstone Inc; 1990

Moster Ml, Bosley Tm, Slavin Ml, Rubin SE: Thyroid ophthalmopathy presenting with superior oblique paresis. J Clinical Neuroophthalmol. 1992; 12:94-97

Von Noorden G: Binocular vision and ocular motility.St Louis, Mosby, 2002

Oğuz V, Çakirer D, Yolar M, Pazarlı H.: L'èvaluation de la myopathie de Basedow a l'IRM. Ophtalmologie 1998; 12:112-116

Oğuz V,Yolar M, Yetik H, Çakirer D, Uysal O, Pazarlı H.: L'interet de l'IRM dans le traitement de la myopathie de l'orbitopathie dystyroidienne. J Fr Ophtalmol. 2001; 24:842-846.
Knapp P: Special types of muscle anomalies associated with Graves' disease. Ophthalmology, 1979; 86: 2081-2084
Hughes Ds, Beck L, Hill R, Plenty J: Dysthyroid eye disease presenting have Brown' s syndrome. Acta Ophthalmol. 1993; 71:262-265
Nishida Y, Tian S, Isberg B, Tallstedt L, Lennerstrand G: Orbital MRI measurements of tissues in dysthyroid ophthalmopathy. Graefes Arch Covering Joint Exp Ophthalmol. 2001; 239: 824-831
Trobe Jd : Vertical Cyclodeviation and acquired strabismus. Arch Ophthalmol 1984 ; 102 : 717-720

Address of the Author:
Velittin Oguz M.D.,
Department of Ophthalmology,Cerrahpaşa Faculty of Medicine,
University of Istanbul 34303, K.M.Pasa Istanbul, Turkey

Transactions 28th Meeting European Strabismological Association, de Faber (ed.)
© 2004 European Strabismological Association, ISBN 90 265 1965 6

Factors influencing success of botulinum toxin treatment in exotropia: preliminary results

Vinciguerra A., Liberali T., Pensiero S., Cordaro C., Perissutti P
Department of Ophthalmology Istituto "Burlo Garofolo" Trieste
**Department of Ophthalmology Istituto "La Nostra Famiglia" Udine*

ABSTRACT: Objective. To analyse the factors influencing the favourable outcome of botulinum toxin treatment of exotropia. Methods. Nineteen exotropic patients aged between 13-274 months were treated with simultaneous bilateral injections of 20 U of botulinum A toxin (Dysport, Ipsen Ltd, Maidenhaed, England). 12 patients underwent 1 bilateral injection and 7 underwent multiple bilateral injections injected under electromyographic monitoring with audible and visible trace. Patients were followed up for 24 to 60 months after the last injection. The following parameters were analysed: aetiology of exotropia (primary or consecutive), size of exotropia, convergence weakness, potential binocular vision, age of first injection, transient overcorrection (eso shift). Results. The results of our study are summarized in Table1. Motor success was obtained in 12 (67%) and 13 (72%) patients for distance and near vision respectively (Table 2). Convergence weakness. We have compared a basic exotropia group with a convergence weakness group. In the basic exotropia group mean preinjection deviation decreased of 21 and 16 Prismatic Diopters to 6 and 4 PD for distance and near deviation respectively with a percentage of correction of 69 % both for distance and near vision. In the convergence weakness group deviation decreased of 17 and 21 PD to 11 and 12 PD for distance and near vision respectively with a percentage of correction of 43% (Table 3). Potential binocular vision. The mean percentage of correction was 48% and 51% for distance and near vision respectively for patients without preoperative binocular vision. For patients who had preoperative binocular vision the mean percentage correction was 64% and 52% for distance and near vision respectively. Transient overcorrection (eso shift). The mean percentage of correction was 75% and 68% for distance and near respectively for patients with transient overcorrection (Table 4), increasing to 86% and 76% for basic exotropia group. The mean percentage of correction was 58% and 56% for convergence weakness group. Conclusion. Our preliminary results suggest that convergence weakness, transient post injection overcorrection (eso shift) and preoperative fusion are useful predictors of the favourable outcome of botulinum toxin treatment of exotropia.
KEYWORDS: exotropia, botulinum toxin, strabismus.

INTRODUCTION

Botulinum toxin treatment for strabismus is a valuable alternative to traditional surgery. Although esotropia is considered more responsive to botulinum toxin treatment than exotropia (1), controversies still exist about the results with regard to the type of exotropia. The purpose of this this study was to analyse the factors influencing the favourable outcome of botulinum toxin treatment of exotropia

METHODS.

Nineteen exotropic patients aged between 13-274 months were treated with simultaneous bilateral injections of 20 U of botulinum A toxin (Dysport, Ipsen Ltd, Maidenhaed, England). 12 patients underwent 1 bilateral injection and 7 underwent multiple bilateral injections injected under electromyographic monitoring with audible and visible trace. Patients were followed up for 24 to 60 months after the last injection. The following parameters were analysed: aetiology of exotropia (primary or consecutive), size of exotropia, convergence weakness, potential binocular vision, age of first injection, transient overcorrection (eso shift).

RESULTS.

The results of our study are summarized in Table1. Motor success was obtained in 12 (67%) and 13 (72%) patients for distance and near vision respectively (Table 2).
Convergence weakness. We have compared a basic exotropia group with a convergence weakness group. In the basic exotropia group mean preinjection deviation decreased of 21 and 16 Prismatic Diopters to 6 and 4 PD for distance and near deviation respectively with a percentage of correction of 69 % both for distance and near vision. In the convergence weakness group deviation decreased of 17 and 21 PD to 11 and 12 PD for distance and near vision respectively with a percentage of correction of 43% (Table 3).
Potential binocular vision. The mean percentage of correction was 48% and 51% for distance and near vision respectively for patients without preoperative binocular vision. For patients who had preoperative binocular vision the mean percentage correction was 64% and 52% for distance and near vision respectively.
Transient overcorrection (eso shift). The mean percentage of correction was 75% and 68% for distance and near respectively for patients with transient overcorrection, increasing to 86% and 76% for basic exotropia group. The mean percentage of correction was 58% and 56% for convergence weakness group.

CONCLUSION.

Our preliminary results suggest that convergence weakness, transient post injection overcorrection (eso shift) and preoperative fusion are useful predictors of the favourable outcome of botulinum toxin treatment of exotropia

REFERENCES

Abbasoglu OE, Sener EC, Sanac AS. Factors influencing success and dose-effect relation of botulinum toxin treatment. Eye 1996; 10: 385-391.

Spencer RF, Tucker MG, Choi RY, McNeer KW. Botulinum toxin management of childhood intermittent exotropia. Ophthalmology. 1997 Nov;104(11):1762-7.

Hallet M. One man's poison - Clinical applications of botulinum toxin. N Engl J Med 1999; 341: 118-1201.

Osako M, Keltner JM. Botulinum A toxin (Oculinum) in ophthalmology. Surv Ophthalmol 1991; 26: 28-46.

Mc Neer K.W, Tucker MG, Spencer RF. Botulinum toxin managment of Essential Infantile Esotropia in Children. Arch Ophthalmol 1997; 115: 1411-1418. 4. Wagner RS Frohman LP. Long term results: botulinum for sixth nerve palsy. J Pediatr Ophthalmol Strabismus 1989; 26: 106-108

Lee JP, Harris S, Cohen J, Cooper K, MacEwen C, Jones S. Results of a prospective randomized trial of botulinum toxin therapy in acute unilateral sixth nerve palsy. J Pediatr Ophthalmol Strabismus 1994; 31: 283-286

Scott AB, Magoon EH, Mc Neer K.W, Stager DR. Botulinum treatment of childhood strabismus. Ophthalmology 1990; 97:1434-1438.

Transactions 28th Meeting European Strabismological Association, de Faber (ed.)
© 2004 European Strabismological Association, ISBN 90 265 1965 6

Ocular oscillation and visually dependent postural control in congenital nystagmus

G. Savino, A. Salerni, D. Colucci, M. Manzulli, F. de Rossi, A. Dickmann
Department of Ophthalmology, Catholic University of Sacred Heart, Rome, Italy

ABSTRACT: Postural control is impaired in patients affected by congenital nystagmus and this impairment could be related to a reduction of visual cues. Our objective is to verify whether the changes in postural control are due to ocular oscillations or to reduced visual acuity. The patients were 19: 9 affected by congenital nystagmus, and 10 healthy subject. In healty subjects we reduced visual acuity to the level of patients affected by congenital nystagmus by applying Bangerter's filters. Both groups were submitted to complete stabilometric evaluation. A statistical analysis was performed. Control group: The sensory analysis showed a reduced visual score with Bangerter's filters compared with the primary position. Congenital nystagmus group: we observed that a statistically significant improvement of the overall postural control was present in the blocking position vs. the primary position. Comparison between the two groups: no significant differences between blocking position of patients and the 3 different positions in controls. The impaired postural control in patients affected by CN is mainly due to ocular oscillations, with reduced visual acuity creating a secondary effect.

KEYWORDS: congenital nystagmus, dinamic posturography, blocking position

1. First paragraph

The visual, somatosensory and vestibular systems together contribute to the maintenance of postural equilibrium. Afferent inputs interact and the information is analysed centrally by cerebellum, cerebral cortex and basal ganglia. The final result of this analysis is the generation of motor outputs aimed at maintaining postural control.
Postural control is impaired in patients affected by congenital nystagmus (2) and this impairment could be related to a reduction of visual cues (3). Congenital nystagmus patients represent a reliable experimental model to study the influences of reduced visual cues on postural control. The problem which arises is whether the observed postural control impairment is related to the ocular oscillations themselves or to reduced visual acuity, since both conditions may be responsible for a reduced vision-dependent postural stabilization (4)
Aim of this study is to verify whether the changes in postural control in our group of patients are due to ocular oscillations or to reduced visual acuity, since both conditions may be responsible for a reduced vision dependent postural stabilization.

1.1 MATERIALS AND METHODS

The patients of this study were nine patients (mean age: 23.3 y.) affected by congenital nystagmus with anomalous head position, and ten healthy subjects (mean age:25.6 y.) as controls. The control group had good visual acuity, orthophoria and normal ocular motility.
All patients presented with bi-directional jerk nystagmus characterized by a slow, accelerating phase. We therefore excluded all that patients with symptoms or signs suggesting any neurologic, otologic or orthopedic diseases. We observed the blocking position in laterodeviated gaze in 8 patients of the 9, while in the nineth it was present in sursumduction gaze.
The mean binocular visual acuity obtained in the blocking positon was 6/12 (minimum visual acuity: 6/21, maximum visual acuity: 6/75).
Ocular oscillations were also be inhibited or reduced (and the hanomalous head position corrected) by prisms. The mean power of the prisms applied to correct the abnormal position of the head was 20 Dp (range 10-30 Dp).
All patiens were submitted to record the nystagmographic curve, using a magnetic search coil (EPM S3000 Scalar).
In healty subjects we reduced visual acuity to the level of patients affected by congenital nystagmus by applying Bangerter's filters to a mean value of 6/12.
Both groups of patients underwent a complete postural evaluation with dynamic posturography (Euitest, Neurocom Int. Inc., Clackamas, Oregon, USA) performed when the subject standing on a dual forceplate within a visual surrounding. The sensory organization test (SOT) consists of six different conditions in which eyes, platform surface and visual field were submitted to changes.
The composite equilibrium score (ES), which indicates the range of angle of sway with respect to the earth vertical, was computed for each condition.
Sensory analysis, which calculates the relationship among the equilibrium scores in the six conditions, identifies the sensory dysfunction and individual preference for different inputs: somatosensory (test condition 2/1), visual (4/1), vestibular (5/1), and vision preference (3+6/2+5).The patients was asked to gaze at a screen (10x10 cm) which was placed within the platform in a predetermined position and to fixate, during evaluation, a structured stimulus.
All patients were evaluated as follows:
Head in primary position
Head in primary position and gaze rotated to the position of blocked nystagmus
Head in primary position with prisms that block or reduce ocular oscillations
Also the control group was submitted to complete stabilometric evaluation in the following conditions:
Head in primary position and without filters
Head in primary position and gaze rotated in lateroversion
Head in primary position during application of Bangerter's filters.
The data obtained for both groups were compared and were analysed using the SPSS statistical pack-age and employing non-parametric tests for unpaired samples (Mann-Whitney U test) to compare data between groups, and for paired samples (Wilcoxon) to compare data within each group.

1.2 RESULTS

Control group:
In normal subjects the gaze position did not modify the postural control (composit).
The sensory analysis showed a reduced visual score with Bangerter's filters compared with the primary position.
Congenital nystagmus group:

In nystagmic patients we observed that a statistically significant improvement of the overall postural control (composite) was present in the blocking position vs. the primary position (also the visual cues showed a significant difference).

Comparison between the two groups:

Comparison of the position of maximum nystagmus in nystagmic patients with the three positions of the control subjects has revealed, for the composite parameter and the visual parameter, a significant difference between the position of maximum nystagmus and two positions of vision of normal subjects: primary gaze position (composite,p: 0.047; visual cues p:0,020) and laterodeviated gaze (composite,p: 0.044; visual cues p:0.023). On the other hand, there was no difference, for the composite parameter, between the position of maximum nystagmus and the position of control subjects when filters were used (p: 0.313), the visual parameter instead tended toward significance (p:0.066).

Moreover, no significant differences were observed, neither at univariate nor at multivariate analysis, between the position of blocked nystagmus (patients with congenital nystagmus) and the different positions of gaze of controls.

1.2.1 CONCLUSIONS

Our data show a reduced visually dependent postural stabilization when ocular oscillations are present, while no significant deficits related to postural control were observed in congenital nystagmus patients when ocular oscillations are inhibited by blocked nystagmus position or wearing prisms.

Particularly significant is the difference observed when comparing the group of patients placed in a position of maximum nystagmus to the control group of patients when the Bangerter filters were applied to the latter. The postural behaviour of the two groups did not differ for any of the variables considered except for the visual afferences. In fact, in these positions of gaze, the latter are reduced in both groups of patients, but more markedly in the group of patients suffering from congenital nystagmus. Such an observation may be attributed to the conditions of reduced vision, which is presumably lower in patient with maximus nystagmus, infact the binocular visus of the control group with filter applied was similar to the mean binocular visus of the nystagmic patients in block gaze position. Nevertheless we could not exclude that also plays an important role the nystagmic ocular motion. The ocular motion, infact, causes oscillopsia and consequent attempts to compensate it.

This result is in accordance with the observations made by the authors cited above and leads to the suggestion that ocular motor activity reduces visual sensitivity. A possible explanation is that, during involuntary eye movements, a temporary down-regulation of the visual cortex occurs (9).

Our data support the role of ocular oscillations in visual dependent postural impairment recovered under any condition when ocular oscillations were abolished, despite differences in visual acuity.

It can be concluded that the impaired postural control in patients affected by CN is mainly due to ocular oscillations, with reduced visual acuity creating a secondary effect.

Tab. 1. Means and standard deviations of the parameters obtained for each visual condition in the control subjects. (The sensory analysis showed a reduced visual score with Bangerter's filters compared with the others position).

		Composite	Somatos	Visual	Vest.	Pref.
Primary	mean	78,8	0,99	0,88	0,72	0,97
	S.D	2,44	0,02	0,05	0,05	0,04
Lateral	mean	80,2	0,98	0,87	0,76	0,96
	S.D	5,24	0,03	0,04	0,07	0,05
Filters	mean	76,7	0,99	0,85	0,72	0,94
	S.D	7,13	0,01	0,05	0,11	0,04

Tab. 2Means and standard deviations of the parameters obtained for each visual condition in the nystagmic patients. (a statistically significant improvement of the overall postural control (composite) was present in the blocking position vs. the primary position, also the visual cues showed a significant difference).

		Composite	Somatosens.	Visual	Vest.	Pref.
Primary	Mean	74.1	1,01	0,77	0,65	0,96
	S.D	4.56	0,02	0,06	0,08	0,07
Block	Mean	77.2	1,01	0,82	0,74	0,99
	S.D	4.71	0,05	0,09	0,09	0,06
Controlat.	Mean	72.5	1	0,76	0,67	0,92
	S.D	8.78	0,03	0,14	0,13	0,10

Tab. 3 Statistical analysis results: comparison between maximum nystagmus position vs. primary position of the control group. (Comparison of the position of maximum nystagmus in those patients with congenital nystagmus with the primary position of the control subjects has revealed, for the composite parameter and the visual parameter, a significant difference).

Anova test	Univar. Test	Significance
Composite		0.047
Multivariate		0.214
	Somatosensorial	0.712
	Visual	0.020
	Vestibular	0.299
	Preferential	0.156

Tab. 4 Statistical analysis results: comparison between maximum nystagmus position vs. laterodeviated position of the control group. (Comparison of the position of maximum nystagmus in nystagmic patients with congenital nystagmus with the laterodeviated gaze of the controls has revealed, for the composite parameter and the visual parameter, a significant difference).

Anova test	Univar. Test	Significance
Composite		0.044
Multivariate		0.086
	Somatosensorial.	0.293
	Visual	0.023
	Vestibular	0.081
	Preferential	0.250

Tab. 5 Statistical analysis results: comparison between maximum nystagmus position vs. primary position of the control group with visual acuity reduced by means of Bangerter's filters. (there was no difference, for the composite parameter, the visual parameter instead tended toward significance).

Anova test	Univar. test	Significance
Composit		0.313
Multivariate		0.174
	somatosensorial	0.624
	visual	0.066
	vestibular	0.354
	preferential	0.467

2 REFERENCES

Mergner, T. and Rosemeier, T., Interaction of vestibular, somatosensory and visual signals for posture control and motion perception under terrestrial and microgravity conditions., Brain Res. Rev., 28 (1998) 118-135.

T. H. Brandt, The relationship between retinal image slip, oscillopsia and postural imbalance in :Functional Basis of Ocular Motility Disorders, G. Lennerstrand, D. S. Zee and E.L. Keller, eds, Pergamon Press, Oxford, New York, 1982, 379-385.

S. Di Girolamo, W. Di Nardo, A. Cosenza, F. Ottaviani, A. Dickmann and),G. Savino,The role of vision on postural strategy evalueted in patiens affected by congenital nystagmus as an experimental model, J Vest. Res. 9 (1999) 445-451.

W. Paulus, A. Straube and T.H.Brandt,Visual stabilization of posture:physiological stimulus characteristics and clinical aspects, Brain 107 (1984) 1143-1163.

T.H. Brandt, Vertigo:ist multisensory syndromes,Springer-Verlag, London 1991.

M. Dieterich and T.H. Brandt, Impaired motion perception in congenital nystagmus and acquired ocular motor palsy, Clin. Vision Sci. 1 (1987) 337-345.

W. Buchele, T.H.Brandt and D. Degner, Ataxia and oscillopsia in downbeat-nystagmus vertigo syndrome,Adv Oto-Rhino-Laringo 30 (1983) 291-297

A. Straube, W. Paulus, J Quintern and T:H: Brandt, Visual ataxia induced by eye movements: posturographic measurements in normals and patients with ocular motor disorders, Clin. Vision Sci. 4 (1989), 107-113.

R. Wenzel, P. Bartenstein, M. Dieterich, A. Danek, A. Weindl, S. Minoshima, S. Ziegler, M. Schwaiger and T.H. Brandt, Deactivation of human visual cortex during involuntary ocular oscillations. APET activation study, Brain 119 (1996), 101-110.

Transactions 28th Meeting European Strabismological Association, de Faber (ed.)
© 2004 European Strabismological Association, ISBN 90 265 1965 6

Prediction of visual outcome after treatment in children with amblyopia in dependence of initial monocular and binocular functions

I.M.Boychuk
Filatov Institute of Eye Diseases, Odessa, Ukraine

ABSTRACT: The initial monocular and binocular functions were observed to determine which of them have influence on visual outcome after treatment in children with amblyopia.

Children with refractive (90), anisometropic (112) and unilateral strabismic amblyopia (98) aged 5-8 y.o. were observed. Monocular(38) and binocular(6) functions before treatment and improvement of vision (Δv) after treatment were evaluated with the program Statistics for Windows 98. Improvement of visual acuity (Δv) after treatment depended on different initial factors: in refractive amblyopia on critical flicker fusion by phosphen(CFFph) of both eyes and threshold of stereoacuity (SA); in anisomrtropic on CFFph of sound eye and threshold of (SA) and in strabismic on degree of eccentricity of fixation in amblyopic eye, on CFFph and mesopic vision of the sound eye, Starlight test (Hirai et al. 1998) and positive (SA) by test Lang II.

Above mentioned indices allowed to establish quantity rates of expected results(Δv).
KEYWORDS: initial monocular and binocular functions, amblyopia, treatment

1 Amblyopia is a developemental disorder of the infantile visual system and is often associated with strabismus and ametropia. About 3-4% of children in Western Europe and 2-6% in the other countries of the world are affected with it. Prevention and treatment of amblyopia are of great importance for improving visual acuity and stability of the position of the eyes. Animal experiments have clearly identified two main amblyopiogenic factors, that is visual deprivation and abnormal binocular interaction between unequal visual input. Demer and coworkers confirmed this facts in patients, applying PET (von Noorden & Campos, 2002). Some factors of visual outcome after treatment are known to the clinicians, that is: initial vision of amblyopic eye (the higher the better), its monocular fixation (less eccentric the better) and age of the treatment starting (the earlier the better). To determine the main factors of monocular and binocular vision which were correlating with visual improvement and decreasing of deviation after applied treatment in children with amblyopia this work was conducted.

2 MATERIALS AND METHODS

98 children with monolateral strabismic, 112 with anisometropic and 90 with refractive amblyopia aged 4-8 years old were observed. All children had transparent mediae and fundus without disorders. Observed children (300) with different kind of amblyopia were treated in clinical department of laboratory of functional methods of investigation and binocular disturbances of vision in the Filatov Institute of Eye diseases. Patients underwent pleoptic and orthoptic treatment averaged 2-3 courses during the year. Analysis of obtained data of monocular and binocular functions before and after treatment statistically was performed using "Statistics" version 5,0 for Windows 98. Structure of investigated visual functions of both eyes are presented in Table 1

Table 1. Observed monocular and binocular factors.

Monocular functions of both eyes	Binocular functions
Visual acuity	Worth Dot test
Refraction (dptr)	Sinoptophore (junction, fusion)
Threshold by maculotest	Test Lang II (arc sec)
Threshold of electrical sensitivity by phosphen (mA)	Starlight test in three positions of gaze
	Angle of deviation (prism.dptr)
Critical flicker fusion by phosphen (Hz)	
Light sensitivity of cones (log units)	
Light sensitivity of rods (log units)	
Colour thresholds (red, green, blue)	
Mesopic vision	
Monocular fixation	

3 RESULTS

In the group of children with refractive amblyopia significant correlations were established between visual acuity improvement (Δv) and initial visual acuity (VA) of amblyopic eye Rs = 0,87 and critical flicker fusion by phosphen Rs = 0,68 of the better eye. In the group with anisometropia significant correlations were found between (Δv) and critical flicker fusion by phosphen of the better eye in cases with central fixation Rs= – 0,79 and in cases with macular fixation Rs = 0,9. Children with strabismic amblyopia had following significant correlations between (Δv) and initial vision of amblyopic eye: Rs = 0,84; initial threshols on red colour of both eyes Rs = - 0,65; critical flicker fusion by phosphen of the sound eye Rs = 0,7 andmonocular fixation (MF), Rs = 0,93. Decreasing of deviation (Δd) correlated with mesopic vision of fixating eye(MV) Rs = 0,86, with Starlight test in three positions of gase Rs = - 0,74, p = 0,06; Lang II Rs = - 0,87, p = 0,02. Comparison of factors in groups with different improvement of vision in dependence of fixation in children with anisometropic amblyopia is presented in Tables 2,3.

Table 2. Newman Keuls Test (Breakdown & one way ANOVA) for visual improvement in dependence of initial data in children with central and parafoveal fixation and anisometropic amblyopia.

Tests	F	Δvis = / <0,1 n=27	Δvis =/ >0,2 n=57	P1,2
Threshold by phosphen of better eye	15,5	67,2±2,0	48,0±1,5	0,004
Critical flicker fusion by phosphen of better eye	14,2	48,6±3,2	61,2±2,8	0,005
Light sensitivity of better eye	16,03	1,96±0,2	2,38± 0,1	0,004
Threshold by Lang Test II	8,27	0	400±50,0	0,000
Starlight test	11,23	1,5 ±0,5	2,6 ±0,4	0,004

It is obvious from the presented data that better results (Δvis = / >0,2) are obtained in those cases where indices of above mentioned in the Table 2 functions of the sound eye are better , stereovision is positive and interaction between the eyes in the binocular field is better, exist in more than two positions of gaze (P1,2 <0,05).

Table 3. Newman Keuls Test (Breakdown & one way ANOVA) for visual improvement in dependence of initial data in children with macular fixation and anisometropic amblyopia.

Tests	F	Δvis = / <0,1 n=21	Δvis =/ >0,2 n=7	P1,2

Refraction of better eye	8,27	1,06± 0,5	0,28 ± 0,12	0,02
Threshold by Lang Test II	10,6	0	420 ± 178,8	0,000
Starlight test	16,0	1,8 ±0,9	2,6 ±0,5	0,03

The presented data allow to claim, that in this group of children best results (Δvis = / >0,2) were received in cases with weak almost emmetropic refraction of better eye, positive stereoacuity by Lang Test II, interaction between the eyes in the binocular field in more than two positions of gaze (P1,2 <0,05).

Degree of improvement of vision and decreasing of angle of deviation in the group with strabismic amblyopia are presented in the Table 4 and 5.

Table 4. Newman Keuls Test (Breakdown & one way ANOVA) for visual improvement in dependence of initial data in children with strabismic amblyopia

Tests	F	Δvis = 0,15 n =56	Δvis =0,38 n=42	P1,2
Monocular fixation* of amblyopic eye	10,2	2,5 ±0,5	1,0 ±0,02	0,01
Critical flicker fusion by phosphen of sound eye	10,2	40,0 ±2,1	45,0 ±0,5	0,02
Threshold by Lang Test II	11,2	0	520 ± 80,0	0,0001
Starlight test	10,0	1,0± 0,5	2,5 ±0,5	0,02

*Central fixation = 1, parafoveal =2, macular =3

As it following from the presented data, better results after treatment were observed in those children who had central fixation, higher values of critical flicker fusion by phosphen, positive stereoacuity by Lang Test II and interaction in binocular field in 2-3 positions of gaze before treatment (P<0,05).

Table 5. Degree of deviation decreasing in dependence of initial data in the group with strabismic amblyopia

Tests	F	Δdev = 4,0 n =86	Δdev =7,8 n=12	P1,2
Threshold by Lang Test II	10,4	0	520 ± 80,0	0,01
Starlight test	16,0	1,0± 0,5	2,5 ±0,5	0,02

Presented results allow to conclude that decreasing of deviation (7,8 prism.dptr.) were achieved in cases with positive Lang Test II and binocular interaction of eyes in 2-3 positions of gaze (P<0,05).

4 CONCLUSIONS

Monocular factors of central vision such as critical flicker fusion by phosphen of sound eye and central monocular fixation of amblyopic eye, positive threshold by Test Lang II and binocular interaction of eyes in 2-3 positions of gaze by Starlight test suggest visual improvement (Δvis = / >0,2) in all kinds of amblyopia and decreasing of deviation (Δdev) not less than 7,8 pr.dptr. in children with strabismic amblyopia.

It is interesting to mark that functions of the better eye plays significant role in prognosis of treatment results.

REFERENCES

Hirai T., Ito Y., Tsuzuki K.&. Sato M. Binocular field of strabismus measured by starlight test. In: Advances in Strabismology .Proceedings of the VIIIth Meeting of the International Strabismological Association in Maastricht, the Netherlands,1998: 61-64

2.Noorden G. & Campos E. Binocular Vision and Ocular motility. Theory and Management of Strabismus. Mosby, 2002: 286 .

Transactions 28th Meeting European Strabismological Association, de Faber (ed.)

Idiopathic Progressive Strabismus Fixus in the absence of significant myopia

MK Raynor, A Maino, AM Ansons
Manchester Royal Eye Hospital, U.K.

CASE HISTORY

31-year-old Asian female presented to our unit in 2000 complaining of;

- cosmetically unacceptable squint
- discomfort from abnormal head posture (AHP)
- diplopia

She had no squint in childhood. Her symptoms began 6 years prior to presentation and gradually deteriorated over this period. This progression is documented photographically.

EXAMINATION

Refraction and acuity

- Right -2.00/+0.50 x 45 6/6
- Left -1.75/+1.00 x 155 6/6

Forced Duction Test (FDT) performed in clinic

- Right +4 to abduction
- Left Full abduction

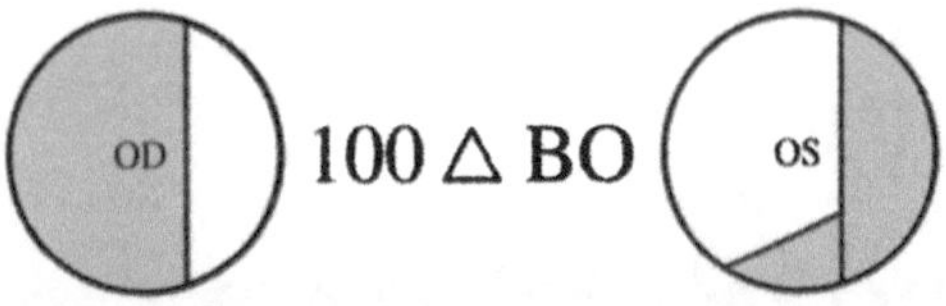

Fig 1 Ocular movements on presentation

Objective torsion measurement

- Right = 8□excyclo
- Left = 12□excyclo

INVESTIGATIONS

- Thyroid function tests: Normal
- Immunology screen: Negative
- Acetylcholine receptor Ab: Negative
- MR scan: No intraorbital or intracranial lesion

TREATMENT

Botulinum toxin (Dysport)
□ □ 4 units to right medial rectus
□ □ 4 units to left medial rectus

Produced an improvement in ocular alignment, reduced AHP and diplopia no worse. BSV – left suppression with Bagolini

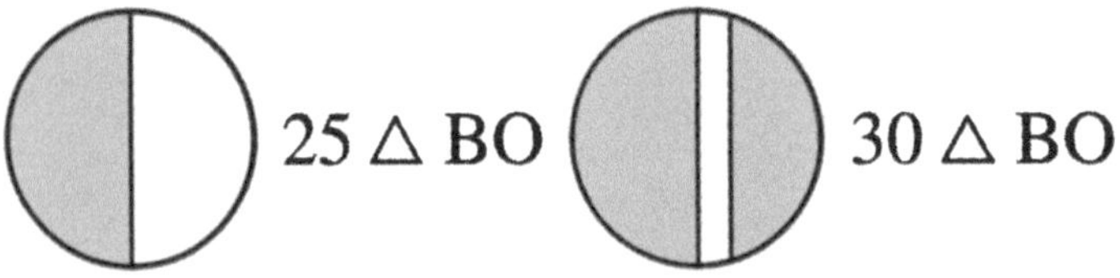

Fig 2 at 1 week post BT

SURGERY

FDT at time of surgery
□ □ Right +3 to abduction
□ □ Left +1 to abduction
Procedure
□ □ Right medial rectus recession of 11mm on adjustable
□ □ Right lateral rectus resection of 4mm on adjustable
□ □ Left medial rectus recession of 9mm on adjustable

POST-OP 1 WEEK

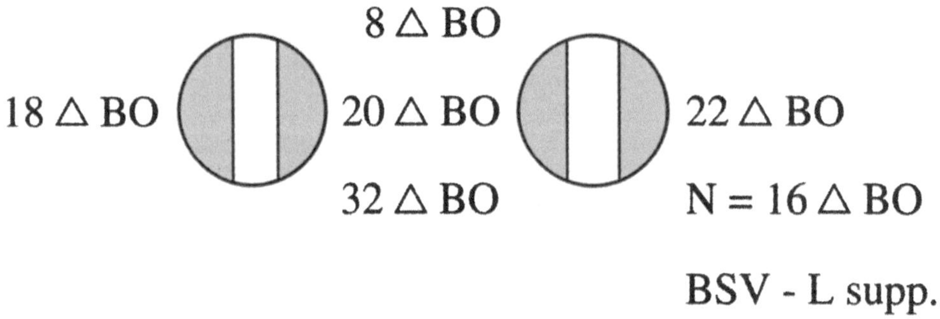

Fig 3 Ocular movements improved at 1 week post op

18 MONTHS POST-OP

There had been some regression with recurrence of the esotropia and AHP.

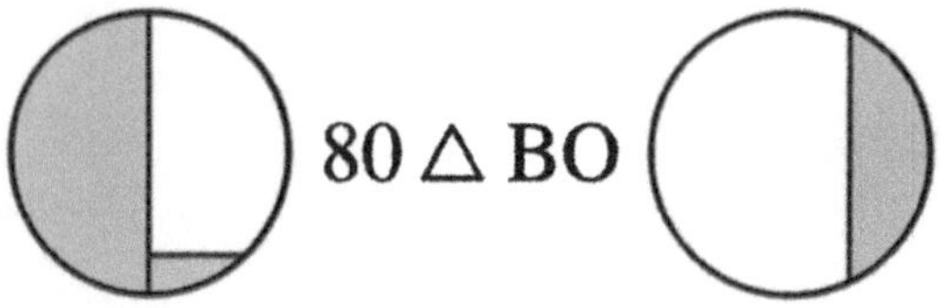

Fig 4 showing eye movements at 18 months

The plan is to repeat BT injections to the medial recti as necessary.

DISCUSSION

Strabismus fixus is a rare progressive condition that may either be congenital or acquired[1]. It typically results in extreme adduction of both eyes causing disabling diplopia. The marked deviation of the globe can cause strangulation of the blood supply with a risk of ocular ischaemia, optic atrophy and central retinal artery occlusion. The acquired form is rare in the absence of high myopia or a history of trauma[2]. There is one case report of strabismus fixus secondary to amyloidosis[3].

The case we describe exhibits none of these factors and appears to be idiopathic.

Our patient has benefited from surgery although there has been regression; her strabismus will be managed by repeated BT injections.

REFERENCES

von Noorden GK. Binocular vision & ocular motility: theory & management of strabismus. St Louis, Mo: Mosby. 6th edition. 471-473

Martinez L. A case of fixed strabismus. Am J Ophthalmol. 1948;31:80-81

Sharma P et al. Strabismus fixus convergens secondary to amyloidosis. J Paediatr Ophthalmol Strabismus. 1991;28,4:236-237

Transactions 28th Meeting European Strabismological Association, de Faber (ed.)
© 2004 European Strabismological Association, ISBN 90 265 1965 6

Long-term results of augmented surgery for partially accommodative esotropia

Soochul Park*, MD, Donghyun Jee, MD, Mira Park, MD
Department of Ophthalmology, The Catholic University of Korea, Seoul, Korea

OBJECTIVE: To investigate the long-term stability of augmented surgery for partially accommodative esotropia and to define factors influencing success.

DESIGN: A retrospective medical record review of partially accommodative esotropes undergoing both medial recti augmented recession according to Wright 's formula.

METHODS: Postoperative observations from repeated measures were analyzed with polynomial re- gression analysis for long-term changes in alignment. To detect any contributing factors, the cha- racteristics of each group (success, under-corrected and over-corrected)were compared using ANOVA. A deviation of less than 10 PD was considered a successful outcome.

RESULTS: Of 79 patients with follow-up of 36 months or more, 53 (67. 1%)maintained the success- ful outcome at last follow-up and no significant change of alignment was observed with the time interval;the regression equation was Postoperative alignment (PD)=4. 59 – 0. 30 x Log Follow-up (month). No continuing exo-shift was not observed in both over-and under-corrected group as well. Of the potential contributing factors to the surgical outcome, target angle for augmented surgery was statistically different between groups.

CONCLUSIONS: Augmented surgery for partially accommodative esotropia maintains a stable posto- perative alignment even after long-term follow-up. To improve the surgical outcome, we recom- mend to increase the surgical number in case target angle is large than 45 PD and to decrease in case target angle is smaller than 25 PD.

REFERENCES

Wright KW, Bruce-Lyle L. Augmented surgery for esotropia associated with high hyper- metriopia. J Pediatr Ophthalmol Strabismus 1993;30:167-70.

Kushner BJ. Partially accommodative esotropia. Should you overcorrect and cut the plus?Arch Ophthalmol 1995;113:1530-4.

Transactions 28th Meeting European Strabismological Association, de Faber (ed.)
© 2004 European Strabismological Association, ISBN 90 265 1965 6

Clinical Risk Factors and Surgical Treatment of Convergence Insufficiency Pattern Consecutive Exotropia

Hyun Taek Lim, MD, Hyosook Ahn, MD
Department of Ophthalmology, Asan Medical Center, University of Ulsan College of Medicine, Seoul, South Korea

ABSTRACT: We studied the clinical risk factors of convergence insufficiency pattern consecutive exotropia (CICE) and the efficacy of our surgical treatment. Twelve consecutive patients who underwent surgeries to correct CICE following bimedial recessions were enrolled. Age of onset, amblyopia, refraction, and the detailed preop and postop characteristics were reviewed. Poor surgical outcome was associated with LR recession or MR advancement without slanted reattachment. All 6 patients who underwent MR advancement with slanted reattachment showed the successful alignment. The presence of a preoperative oblique dysfunction, A or V pattern, DVD, amblyopia, low hyperopia, excessive amounts of MR recession, and late timing of esotropia surgery seem to predispose to develop the CICE. Unilateral or bilateral medial rectus advancement and/or resection with slanted reattachment procedure may be a good surgical option for the treatment of CICE.

KEYWORDS: Consecutive exotropia, Convergence insufficiency, Slanted reattachment.

A consecutive exotropia is an outward deviation that develops immediately or for many years after surgery for esotropia. The overall incidence has been reported to range from 3% to 27% in various series. Factors usually mentioned as being responsible for the consecutive exotropia include excessive amount of surgery, amblyopia, high hyperopia, developmental delay, associated vertical deviations, A or V patterns, and nystagmus. Convergence insufficiency pattern, which is characterized by a greater exodeviation measured at near than at distance, also may be seen as a consecutive exotropia after esotropia surgery. Although consecutive exotropia itself has been well studied, convergence insufficiency pattern consecutive exotropia (CICE) has not been shed the proper light on. The aim of our study is to determine the clinical risk factors for the development of CICE and to evaluate the efficacy of our surgical treatment of CICE.

SUBJECTS AND METHODS

Twelve consecutive patients who were diagnosed as CICE at Asan Medical Center, pediatric ophthalmology and strabismus service, between 1998 and 2002 were studied. Data for 3 patients who underwent initial esotropia surgery at other eye clinics were retrieved from the old records provided by the surgeons who performed the surgery. Convergence insufficiency pattern consecutive exotropia was defined when the near exotropia exceeds the distance exotropia irrespective of the amount of the distance-near discrepancies.

To be included in this study, all patients must have undergone bimedial rectus recession to correct esotropia; must be treated surgically for CICE; and must be followed over 1 year after the correcting surgery for CICE. Patients were excluded if they had history of prematurity, neurologic abnormalities such as hydrocephalus, cerebral palsy, and any other ocular or systemic diseases.

The following data were collected; age of onset, amblyopia, refraction, and data for initial esotropia surgery and reoperations for exotropia including preoperative deviations, type of surgeries performed, and postoperative alignments at final visits. The amount of deviations were measured with prism and alternating cover tests while patients fixated on targets at 6 m and 1/3 m. Ductions and versions were examined before and after surgeries. We graded any limitation in horizontal ductions in the operative eye on a scale of 0 (full excursion) to -4 (inability to move into the field). Successful outcome was defined as both distance and near alignment less than 10 Δ of exotropia.

RESULTS

Initial esotropia surgery

Ten patients had congenital esotropia and 2 patients (No 11 and 12) had partially accommodative esotropia. The median age at surgery was 45 months with a range of 16 to 120 months. The mean preoperative esodeviation was 49.6 Δ with a range of 40 to 80 Δ. Mean surgical dosage of initial esotropia surgery (BMR recession) was 6.2 mm with a range from 5.0 to 7.0 mm. At postoperative 1 month, all patients had relatively good alignments with a range from orthophoria to 10 Δ of exotropia.

Reoperation for CICE

All patients showed the gradual increase of the amount of exodeviation during the follow-up period as compared to the alignment at the postoperative 1 month. At the time of reoperation, the mean exodeviation for distance was 17.6 Δ (range, 12 to 30 Δ) and at near, 23.4 Δ (range, 16 to 35 Δ). Only 3 patients exhibited a significant adduction deficiency of one or both eye, but on version testing, mild adduction deficiencies were suspected in more patients. Sixteen surgeries were performed in 12 patients. Two types of surgical procedures were performed: 8 for lateral rectus recession and the other 8 for medial rectus advancement with or without slanted reattachment technique.

Results of the reoperation

After the first reoperation, 7 out of 12 patients achieved the successful outcome (<10 Δ) and 4 patients needed further second reoperations. Poor surgical outcome after reoperation was associated with LR recession or MR advancement without slanted reattachment. All 6 patients who underwent MR advancement with slanted reattachment showed the successful alignment. Distance-near disparities were reduced after reoperations, in average, from 5.8 Δ to 2.4 Δ for overall group, from 4.5 Δ to 2.4 Δ for LR recession group, and from 6.8 Δ to 2.3 Δ for MR slanted advancement group, respectively.

Risk factors

In our series, the age at initial surgery was later than usual. Degree of hyperopia was lower than +1.5diopter as spherical equivalents in all patients. Amblyopia was identified in 4 (33%) patients. Large recessions of MR (in excess of 6mm) were performed in 10 (83.3%) patients, and furthermore, 8 of 10 were over 3 years of age at the times of initial surgery. Oblique dysfuntions, A and V pattern, or DVD were associated in 5 (42%) of total 12 patients.

DISCUSSION

Not infrequently consecutive exotropia with convergence insufficiency pattern occurred after successful esotropia surgery. The overcorrected strabismus with convergence insufficiency pattern is often difficult to handle and it is also difficult to predict the amount of surgery to correct a given deviation. Kushner (1992) stated that patients with consecutive exotropia and mild convergence insufficiency have a very high surgical undercorrection rate, even in the cases of no obvious underaction of the medial recti. The careful evaluation of the medial rectus function is highly essential in the management of consecutive exotropia. Convergence insufficiency pattern even in the absence of obvious underaction of the medial recti is probably a sign of subtle medial rectus underaction in consecutive exotropes. Medial rectus advancement and/or resection with slanted reattachment surgery could successfully reduce the exodeviations and collapse the distance-near disparities in our study. Nemet and Stolovitch (1990) reported good results using slanted medial rectus resection in three patients with convergence insufficiency. In addition, as the response to a given amount of surgery is usually smaller in the patients with consecutive exotropia, larger dosage of surgery than normally be indicated seem appropriate in the treatment of CICE.

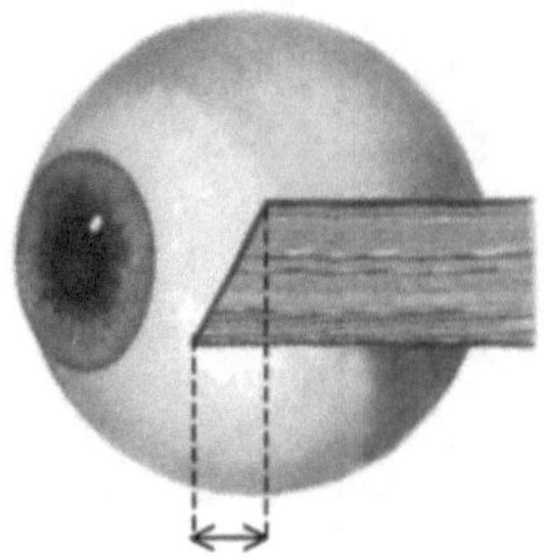

Figure 1. Diagram of a slanted medial rectus advancement surgery. 3mm anteriorly positioned lower horn of medial rectus

CONCLUSIONS

The presence of a preoperative oblique dysfunction, A or V pattern, DVD, amblyopia, low hyperopia, excessive amounts of MR recession, and late timing of esotropia surgery seem to predispose to develop the convergence insufficiency pattern consecutive exotropia. Unilateral or bilateral medial rectus advancement and/or resection with slanted reattachment procedure may be a good surgical option for the treatment of convergence insufficiency pattern consecutive exotropia.

REFERENCES

Biedner B. 1997. Treatment of convergence insufficiency by single medial rectus muscle slanting resection. Ophthalmic Surg Lasers 28(4):347-348.

Kushner B.J. 1992. Surgical pearls for the management of exotropia. Am Orthoptic J 42:65-71.

Mittelman D, & Folk E.R. 1979. The surgical treatment of overcorrected esotropia. J Pediatr Ophthalmol Strabismus 16(3):156-159.

Nemet P & Stolovitch C. 1990. Biased resection of the medial recti: a new surgical approach to convergence insufficiency. Binocul Vision Strabismus Q 5:213-216.

Table 1. Data for preoperative and postoperative characteristics of all patients studied.

Patient No.	Initial surgery: Age at BMR (yr)	Initial surgery: Preop Esotropia (PD)	Initial surgery: Surgical dosage (BMR,mm)	Initial surgery: 1 mo postop alignment (PD)	Reoperation: Age at reop (yr)	Reoperation: Preop exotropia (PD) D	Reoperation: Preop exotropia (PD) N	Reoperation: Type of surgery	Reoperation: Surgical dosage (mm)	Final status: Postop alignment D	Final status: Postop alignment N	Final status: Further reoperation	Final status: Deviation D	Final status: Deviation N	Final status: Associated findings
1	4	50	6.5	XT 5	5.5	12	16	LLR recession	7	XT 4	XT 4				BIOOA
2	6	45	11.0 limbus	XT 10	8	30	35	BMR adv	R5.0/L3.0	XT 16	XT 20	Re-adv 3.0 (L)	XT 10	XT 10	RIOOA 2+ Amblyopia
3	4	60	7	Ortho	5	12	18	LLR rec	5	XT 10	XT 12				BIOOA, DVD
4	10	30, 45(N)	5	XT 5	18	12	18	RMR slanted adv	5.0 (adj)	Ortho	XT 3				RSOOA, A pattern
5	3.5	80	7	XT 10	6	20	25	LLR rec	8	XT 12	XT 16	RLR rec 5.0	XT 5	XT 5	DVD(B) Amblyopia
6	2.5	45	6	Ortho	5	20	30	BMR slanted adv	5	Ortho	XT 3				
7	3	50	6	Ortho	21	25	35	BLR rec	5	XT 10	XT 18	LMR slanted res 3.0, adv (adj)	Ortho	XT 3	
8	4	50	6.5	Ortho	6	18	25	BMR slanted adv	4	ET 5	Ortho				BIOOA
9	1	45	11.0 limbus	XT 5	2.5	20	25	LLR rec	7.5	XT 15	XT 15	RLR rec 6.0	Ortho	Ortho	DVD(L) Amblyopia
10	3	45	6.5	Ortho	20	18	20	RLR rec	9	XT 5	XT 5				
11	5	30, 40(N)	5.5	XT 2	6	12	18	LMR slanted adv	4	Ortho	Ortho				
12	3	40	6	XT 10	5	12	16	RML slanted adv	4	XT 3	XT 3				Amblyopia

Transactions 28th Meeting European Strabismological Association, de Faber (ed.)

Vertical Retraction Syndrome

J. P. Mathews, A. Ansons
Manchester Royal Eye Hospital

ABSTRACT: Vertical retraction syndrome is considered much more rare than analogous syndrome of Duane's affecting the horizontal muscles. Most cases were the result of innervation abnormalitiest,[1,2] and the others were attributed to mechanical factors [3]. We report a case of unilateral vertical retraction syndrome in the right eye of a young male with normal ocular movements in the fellow eye.
KEYWORDS: Duanes retraction syndrome, vertical retraction

CASE REPORT

History

A 23-year-old male was seen in our clinic with diplopia on attempted up gaze of approximately 10-year duration. He was emmetropic with visual acuity of 6/6 in each eye.

OCULAR EXAMINATION

Globe examination and fundoscopy was normal in each eye. There was no ptosis and the function of levator palpebral superior (LPS) was normal. He was orthophoric in the primary position with no abnormal head posture (fig. 1).
There was restricted elevation of the right eye in all positions of upgaze with corresponding overaction in the left eye (fig.2).
The right globe showed retraction with narrowing of ipsilateral palpebral fissure on attempted elevation (fig.3a,b).

Bells phenomenon
Right eye - restriction -2.
Left eye - normal elevation.
Forced duction test
Right eye - +2 mechanical restriction in all elevated positions

DISCUSSION

Retraction of the globe on attempted elevation can be caused by

1. Mechanical factors
2. Aberrant regeneration
    - -congenital
    - -acquired

Mechanical factors were identified in our case, but it is uncertain whether this was the sole cause of the unilateral vertical retraction syndrome.

REFERENCES

Kommerell G, Bach M A new type of Duane's syndrome. Neuro-ophthalmology 1986;6:159-64.
Pruksacholwait K, Ishikawa S. Atypical vertical retraction syndrome. J Paed Ophthalmol 1976;13:215-20.
Khodadoust A, von Noorden G. Bilateral vertical retraction syndrome. Arch Ophthalmol 1967;78:606-12.

Transactions 28th Meeting European Strabismological Association, de Faber (ed.)
 ISBN 90 265 1965 6

Ocular motility disorders as a complication of Baerveldt implant

F.J. Noordhuizen, CO; W. Triemstra, CO; J.T.H.N. de Faber, MD
Orthoptic Department of the Rotterdam Eye Hospital, the Netherlands

ABSTRACT: Introduction: In one year 3 patients visited our department with diplopia after Baerveldt anti-glaucoma implant. Methods: Full ophthalmologic and orthoptic examination was performed. Results: Three patients have irreversible diplopia because of the incomitance. Conclusions: Diplopia following Baerveldt implantation is difficult to treat and patients should be warned for this complication before this glaucoma surgery.

KEYWORDS: Baerveldt, diplopia, strabismus

1. INTRODUCTION

Last year 3 adult patients visited our department with persistent diplopia after Baerveldt anti-glaucoma implant. These patients had mechanical ocular motility disorders due to the Baerveldt implant 350 mm^2. Baerveldt drainage is especially used in case of poor response to conventional surgical treatment. In our cases the Baerveldt implant was placed in the superotemporal quadrant. The lateral plate edges are directed under the superior and lateral rectus muscles. After implantation of the Baerveldt drainage a large filtering bleb will develop over the plate.

2. METHODS

Full ophthalmologic and orthoptic examination was performed. The patients had diplopia due to limitation of the ductions. Because of intractable glaucoma, removal of the Baerveldt implant was not an option. Strabismus surgery was not performed because this would interfere with the brittle regulation of the intra ocular pressure.

3. RESULTS

In primary position there is an exotropia of the right eye and a right-hypotropia (Fig. 1). The patient fixates with his left eye because it is his best eye. Most often the eye with the implant is the eye with the best vision. In right gaze there is a limitation of adduction, so the exotropia is increasing in rightgaze. In leftgaze the exotropia decreases. In downgaze there is a limitation of depression of the left eye. In upgaze there is a right-hypertropia because of a little reduced elevation of the left eye.

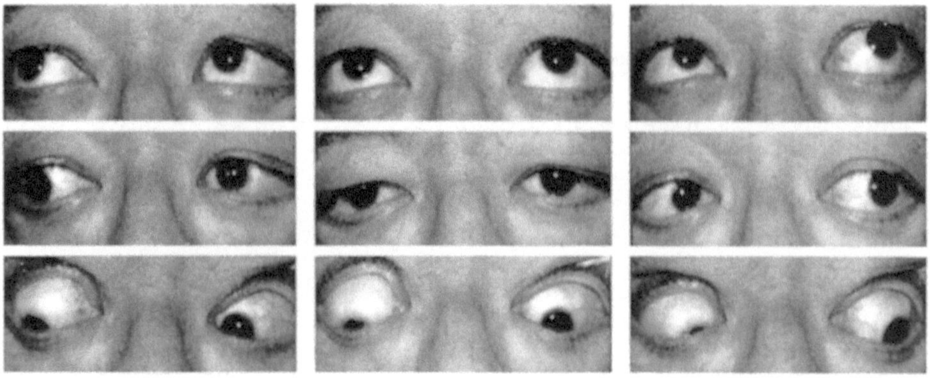

Figure 1.: Baerveldt implant OS

4. CONCLUSION

Diplopia following Baerveldt implantation is difficult to treat because of the incomitance of the strabismus and the poor fusional mechanisms caused by low vision and poor visual fields.
Prisms are not an option because the strabismus is very incomitant and the patients have poor fusional mechanisms. Our patients did not prefer prisms. Removal of the implant is also not an option because of the intractable glaucoma. Strabismus surgery of the involved eye (with the implant) caries the risk of disturbing the function of the implant and one has to realize that this is most often the eye with the best vision. Strabismus surgery of the fellow eye can be an option, but that will not resolve the mechanical restrictions of the involved eye. People should be warned for post-operative diplopia before Baerveldt implantation.

REFERENCES

Smith, M.F.,MD; Doyle, J.W.,MD,PhD; Sherwood, M.B.,MD. 1995. Comparison of the Baerveldt glaucoma implant with the double-plate Molteno drainage implant. Arch. Ophthalmol 1995 Apr; 113:444-447

Munoz, M., MD; Parrish II, R.K., MD. 1993. Strabismus following implantation of Baerveldt drainage devices. Arch. Ophthalmol. 1993 Aug; 111: 1096-1099

Krisha, R; Godfrey, DG; Budenz, DL; Escalona-Camaano, E; Gedde, SJ; Greenfield, DS; Feuer, W; Scott, IU. 2001. Intermediate-term outcomes of 350-mm^2 Baerveldt glaucoma implants. Opthalmology. 2001; Mar; 108(3): 621-6

Smith, SL; Starita, RJ; Fellman, RL; Lynn, JR. 1993. Early clinical experience with the Baerveldt 350-mm^2 glaucoma implant and associated extraocular muscle imbalance. Ophthalmology. 1993 Jun; 100(6): 914-8

Transactions 28th Meeting European Strabismological Association, de Faber (ed.)
© 2004 European Strabismological Association, ISBN 90 265 1965 6

About a case of acquired Brown's syndrome after insect bite

F. Ribaudeau-Saindelle
Le Mans, France

A. Péchereau
Service d'Ophtalmologie, Hôtel-Dieu, CHU Nantes, 44093 Nantes Cedex, France

ABSTRACT: We report a case of acquired Brown's syndrome presumed inflammatory. It concerns a 4 year old girl. After a walk in the forest (August 2001) the family noticed an obvious left hypotropia with a limitation elevation of the left eye. The investigations were normal. An excoriation in the internal part of the left superior eyelid was noticed. Three other cuts were on the nose, the superior lip and the chin. The syndrome was confirmed by a forced test duction. An MRI of the oculomotor muscles provided evidence of a very localized thickening at the level of the pulley. This limitation (April 2002) became occasional. The girl indicated the appearance of a click-syndrome. This syndrome of acquired Brown shows that a local inflammation can extend to the complex of the oblique superior pulley.

KEYWORDS: Acquired Brown's syndrome, insect bite, click-syndrome

1 INTRODUCTION

The Brown's syndrome is an oculomotor disorder characterized mainly by an elevation limitation of the eye in adduction with a forced positive duction test. It is one of the retraction's syndromes.

It results from a dysfunction of the complex trochlea - superior oblique tendon. This oculomotor disorder was described in association with numerous local and general inflammatory pathologies.

We report a case of acquired Brown's syndrome presumed inflammatory. It appeared as a consequence of an insect bite opposite to the trochlea. To our knowledge, this association has not been described before.

2 OBSERVATION

This observation concerns A R..., a 4 year old girl, without any previous medical history. As a standard check, an orthoptic examination was performed 9 months previously. It showed no abnormalities (a previous picture of June 23, 2001 showed a normal elevation of the left eye).

2.1 *August 2001*

Suddenly the day after a walk in the forest the family noticed that Alice began winking, then occluding with the left eyelids. These symptoms were initially interpreted as an irritation caused by the sun.

Some hours later, an obvious left hypotropia with the limitation of the left eye elevation appeared. This elevation limitation was dominant in adduction, it also existed on the median line and slightly in abduction (fig 1). The abduction and the depression were normal. The depression of the left eye was normal in adduction.

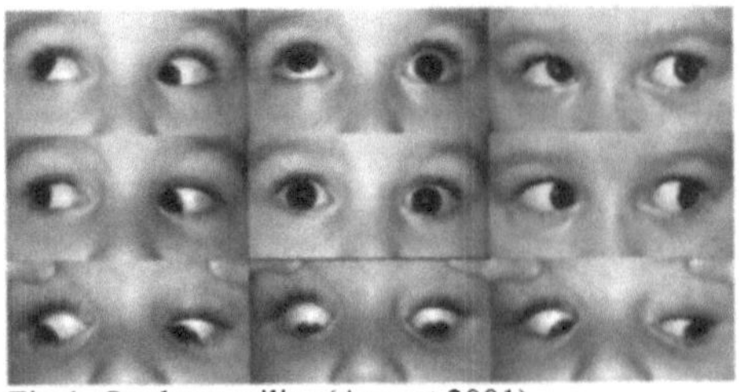
Fig 1. Ocular motility (August 2001).

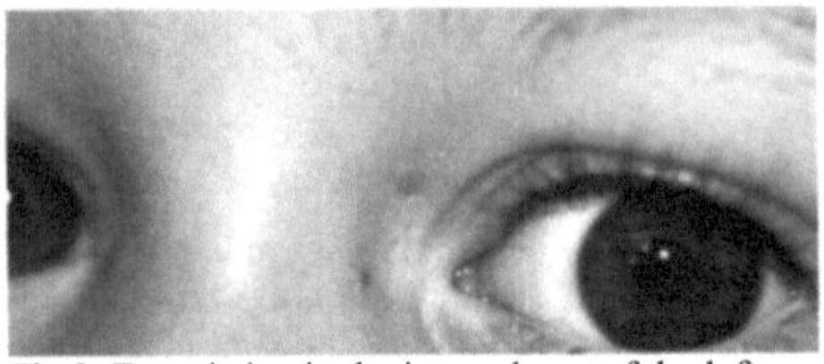
Fig 2. Excoriation in the internal part of the left superior eyelid.

This was in addition to a torticollis, a heightened chin, a head turned on the right-hand side, tilted on the left shoulder and an impression of the left exophtalmia.

The visual acuity was 10/10 to the two eyes. The investigations (ophtalmologic, neurological, pediatric, biologic (serology of Lyme) and MRI examinations) were normal.

The only noticed abnormality was an excoriation in the internal part of the left superior eyelid (fig 2). Three other cuts were identical on the nose, the superior lip and the chin. These cuts, having occurred after redness and then a crust, indicated insect bites.

An oral short cure of corticoids was prescribed.

One occlusion of the right eye enabled the diplopia to be relieved.

An orthoptic examination revealed the left hypotropia: 10 dioptres at far, 6 dioptres at near. There was a net degradation of stereopsia (Lang 1: 1 200 seconds of arc).

The Hess-Weiss's coordimetric examination found a left hypotropia, a disability of the left eye elevation in adduction, and also on the median line and in abduction. There is a compensatory hyperaction of the right superior rectus and of the right inferior oblique.

2.2 *September 2001*

The left Brown's syndrome was confirmed by a forced duction test under general anesthetic. The left eye was completely immobile, pointing downwards.

A second oral cure of corticoids was administered.

An MRI (fig 3) of the oculomotor muscles provided evidence of a very localized thickening at the level of the pulley of the left superior oblique.

Prisms were prescribed to treat the torticollis in the primary position.

The evolution is marked by an improvement of the sensory and motor capacities. The stereopsia (Lang 1) normalized. A marked limitation of the left eye elevation in adduction and on the median line was noted and also the normalisation of the depression in adduction.

2.3 *April 2002*

This limitation became occasional. Repeated elevation of the eye allowed a almost normal sudden excursion. The girl indicated the appearance of a click-syndrome (fig 4).

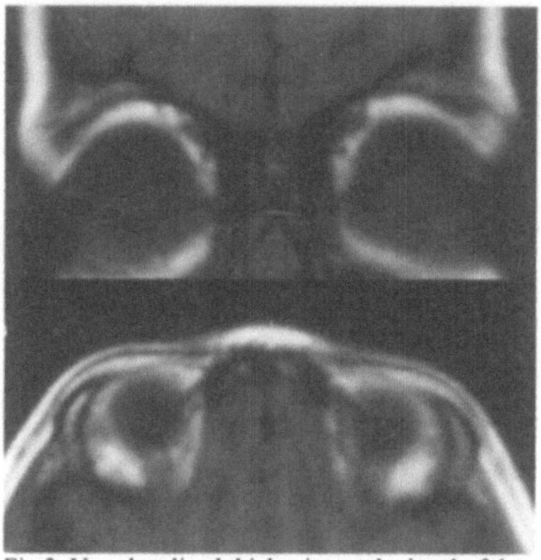
Fig 3. Very localized thickening at the level of the pulley of the left superior oblique (MRI).

3 DISCUSSION

The acquired characteristic of this Brown's syndrome is indisputable:
- Photos showing a normal oculomotor;
- Initial normal orthoptic examination;
- Sudden appearance of a diplopia associated with oculomotor troubles.

The origin of this Brown's syndrome should be connected with the cutaneous cuts, the most likely hypothesis being an insect bite. The progressive cure is a supplementary argument in favour of this hypothesis.

4 CONCLUSION

This syndrome of acquired Brown is exceptional because of its rarity (frequency of Brown's syndrome: 0,005%). It shows that a local inflammation can extend to the complex of the oblique superior pulley and expresses itself as the Brown's syndrome.

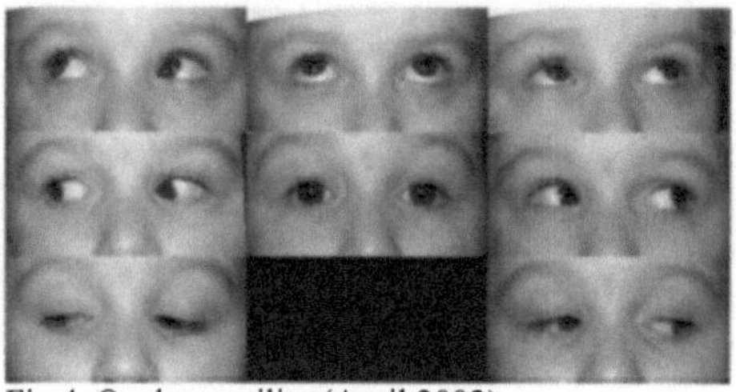
Fig 4. Ocular motility (April 2002).

Transactions 28th Meeting European Strabismological Association, de Faber (ed.)
© 2004 European Strabismological Association, ISBN 90 265 1965 6

Binocular vision after refractive surgery in hyperopic patients

R Gómez-de-Liaño, E. Piedrahita & A. Arias-Puente
Hospital Clínico San Carlos, Instituto Castroviejo, Universidad Complutense de Madrid, Spain

ABSTRACT: Objective: To evaluate if there are any Binocular Vision (BV) modifications after refractive surgery in patients with hyperopia or hyperopic astigmatism. Methods: Prospective study of patients with hyperopia or hyperopic astigmatism operated of refractive surgery between May 1999 and February 2002. There were 31 patients, aged between 18 and 59, who suffered a Refractive surgery with the Lasik technique. The preoperative study included: Best corrected visual acuity, cycloplegic refraction, motility evaluation, binocular vision examination, (Polarized Vectografic study, retinal correspondence and fusion amplitude with the synoptophore, TNO Estereopsis). We re-evaluate the patients with the same protocol at 3, 6 and 12 months of follow up after surgery. Results: 1. Postoperative BV was similar or better than the preoperative data in 76% of the cases. 2. The modifications were not homogeneous in all the tests 3. There is a tendency to the endoforia after surgery. 4. Patients without strabismus had a situation similar or better than the preoperative status in 71,42% of the cases but only one had esoforía with transitory asthenopia. 5. In the group of patients with strabismus there was a small progression towards endophoria in an important number of cases (10/14), 2 of them aggravated mildly their strabismus. 3 patients with accommodative strabismus were compensated after refractive surgery, although one need them for reading. Conclusions: After refractive surgery we have found modifications of BV or Ocular motility in an important number of cases (24%), but most of them are not symptomatic after 12 months of follow-up. We suggest to evaluate preoperatively Binocularity with a completely Orthoptic Protocol.

KEYWORDS: Refractive Surgery, Binocular Vision, Hyperopia, Strabismus

1 INTRODUCTION

Among complications of refractive surgery, may appear diplopia or strabismus[1-5]. In 1996 we studied retrospectively binocular outcome in myopic and myopic anisometropia patients after PRK[6].

The experience in surgery of the hyperopia so far has been smaller than that of the myopia, having a smaller predictability in their results[7,8]. Some hyperopic patients have lability in the BV and or strabismus. Their binocularity and degree of oculomotor compensation is frequently related to the correction of their refraction and the refractive surgery could decompensate them although there are encouraging results[9-11].

The objective of this study is, to evaluate prospectively, if there are any BV modifications after refractive surgery (Lasik technique) in patients with hyperopia or hyperopic astigmatism in normal as well as in strabismic patients.

2 METHODS

This is a prospective study of patients with hyperopia or hyperopic astigmatism, operated of refractive surgery between May 1999 and February 2002. All patients were operated by the same author (AAP). Refractive technique was Lasik with the MEL-70 G-Scan Laser (Asclepion-Meditec).

There were 31 patients, aged between 18 and 59 (mean 29,68 ± 8,77 years). We had three subgroups of patients. Group I, patients with no strabismus and normal binocular vision (N=14), Group II, patients with accommodative esotropia with Normal Retinal Correspondence (NRC) (N=3) and Group III, patients with strabismus and Anomalous Retinal Correspondence (ARC) (N=14).

Preoperative study included: 1. Best corrected visual acuity (EDTDS Test□). We classified Visual Acuity (VA) as the "best eye" and "worse eye". Best eye was considered as the dominant one, the one with better visual acuity, and if there was no difference the right eye. 2. Cycloplegic refraction. We considered the Spherical Equivalent (Sph.E). 3. Retinal correspondence evaluated with the synoptophore (Oculus□, foveolar charts). 4. Suppression with Polarized Vectografic test. 5. TNO Estereopsis. 6. Fusion amplitude (Synoptophore Oculus□, foveolar charts). 6. Motility evaluation (simple and dissociated cover-test, and Phoria under synoptophore.).

Table 1 Shoes preoperative and postoperative refractive data.

Table 1	No strabismus (N=14)		Accommodative ET + NRC (N=3)		Esotropia + ARC (N=14)	
	PRE LASIK	POST LASIK	PRE LASIK	POST LASIK	PRE LASIK	POST LASIK
VA dominant/better /RE	0.92 DS 0.15 (0.5 to 1.0)	0.93 DS 0.08 (0.7 to 1.0)	0.98 DS 0.03 (0.95 to 1.0)	0.97 DS 0.06 (0.90 to 1.0)	0.98 DS 0.03 (0.9 to 1.0)	0.83 DS 0.13 (0.6 to 1.0)
VA domined/worse / LE	0.89 DS 0.16 (0.5 to 1.0)	0.86 DS 0.12 (0.65 to 1.0)	0.80 DS 0.35 (0.40 to 1.0)	0.90 DS 0.10 (0.80 to 1.0)	0.79 DS 0.25 (0.3 to 1.0)	0.65 DS 0.23 (0.2 to 1.0)
Refr. better eye (Sph equivalent)	+2.96 DS 2.17 (-0.63 to +6.38)	+0.81 DS 1.16 (-0.38 to +3.25)	+4.46 DS 1.69 (+2.75 to +6.13)	+0.96 DS 1.16 (0 to +2.25)	+4.28 DS 1.31 (+2.16 to +7.00)	+0.51 DS 0.57 (-0.50 to +1.38)
Refr. worse eye	+3.34 DS 2.23 (-0.63 to +7.00)	+0.89 DS 0.96 (-0.50 to +2.75)	+4.75 DS 1.56 (+3.00 to +6.00)	+0.92 DS 0.88 (0 to +1.75)	+5.16 DS 1.44 (+3.16 to +7.75)	+1.00 DS 0.93 (0 to +2.50)
Anisoacuity	0.03 DS 0.09 (0 to 0.35)	0.07 DS 0.11 (-0.1 to 0.3)	0.18 DS 0.32 (0 to 0.55)	0.07 DS 0.12 (0 to 0.2)	0.19 DS 0.24 (0 to 0.65)	0.18 DS 0.21 (0 to 0.65)
Anisometropia	0.48 DS 0.37 (0 to 1.00)	0.38 DS 0.26 (0 to 0.75)	0.38 DS 0.33 (0.13 to 0.75)	+0.29 DS 0.26 (0 to 0.5)	0.88 DS 0.79 (0 to 3.25)	0.53 DS 0.56 (0 to 1.75)

Although there is no difference in the mean pre- and postoperative visual status there are interindividual changes in the visual acuity (Graph 1 and 2).

We re-evaluated patients with the same protocol at 3, 6 and 12 months of follow up after surgery. The follow-up since surgery was 11.10 ±7,64 months (4-31 months.)

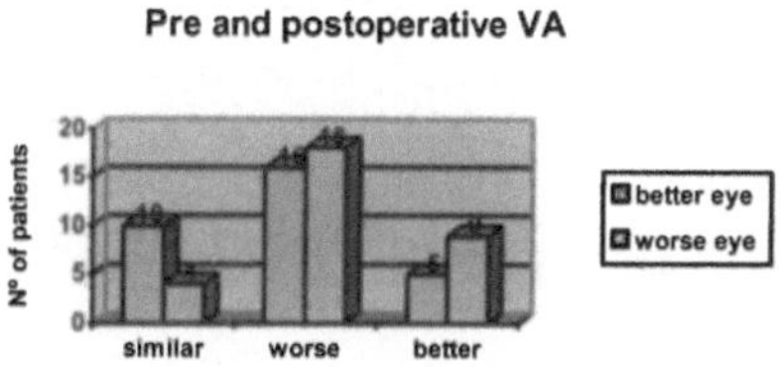

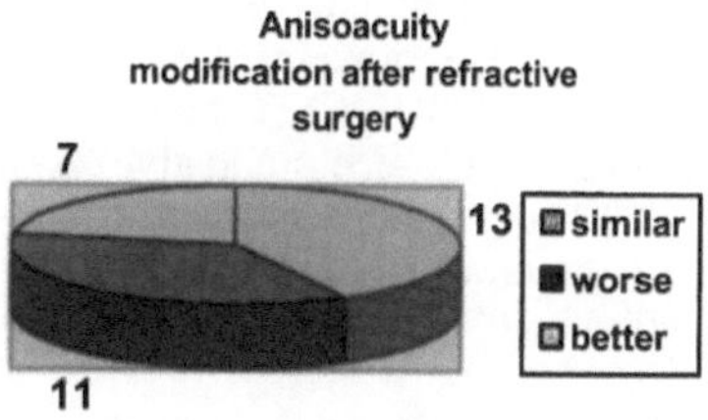

Graph 1(left): Graph 2 (right): Difference in Visual Acuity between both eyes (anisoacuity) pre and post refractive surgery

We analysed our results with the T Student test for independent series and paired series, Fisher exact test to analyse expected frequency below 5 and Pearson Correlation. We studied also bifactorialy with interactive graphs. We considered statistically significant a p below 0.05.

3 RESULTS

The comparative study of BV and ocular motility pre- and postoperative showed that Postoperative BV was similar or better than the preoperative data in 76,47- 77,42% of the cases. The modifications were not homogeneous with all the tests, some patients failed in one test and others did it in another test.

In the comparative study of the pre- and postoperative binocular vision we observed the following data:

1.*Distance Fusion or dominance* with vectographic tests: The situation was similar or better

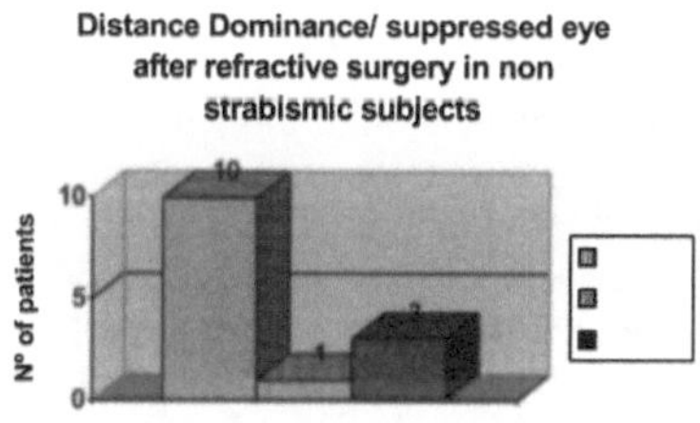

Graph 3

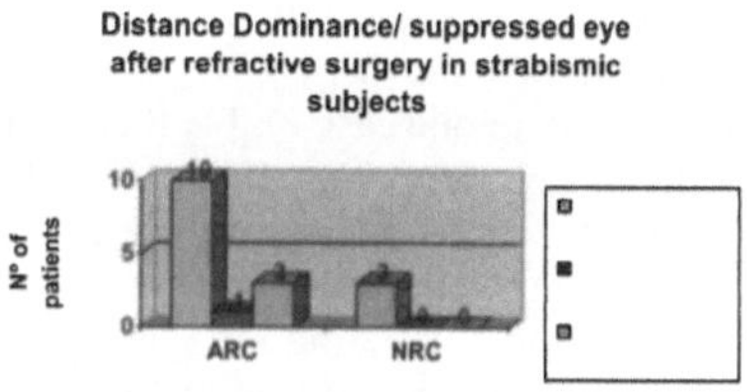

Graph 4

to the preoperative situation in 24 patients (77.42%), they deteriorate or there was as dominant change in 7 (22.58%). The situation was similar in the previous normal binocular patients and in the strabismus group. (Graph 3 and 4).

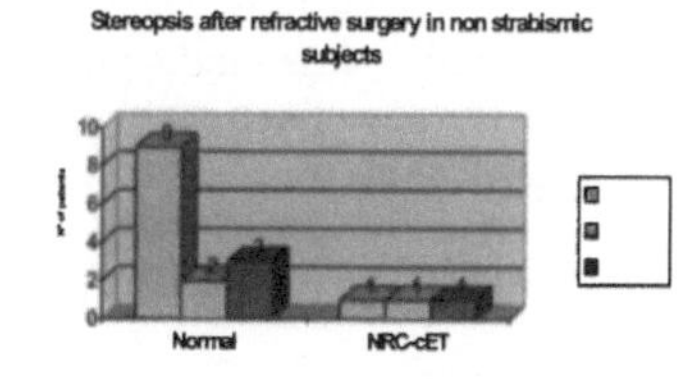

Graph 5

2. *Estereopsis*: (Out of 17 patients with CRN) (Graph 5) The situation was similar or better than in the preoperative 13 patients (76.47%). 4 patients had a deterioration (23.53%). 6/7 patients that their Estereopsis improved registered an improvement of the VA.

3. *Fusion amplitude:* We found a similar situation of the fusion amplitude as in the preoperative 13 (76.47%), and improvement in 3/14 patients and a deterioration 3 (23.53%). (Graph 6) Among the 3 patients with NRC-Accommodative esotropia (NRC-AccET) 1 had a small improvement and one a regression. Evolution of fusion amplitude was related with VA evolution (C=0,562, p=0.019).

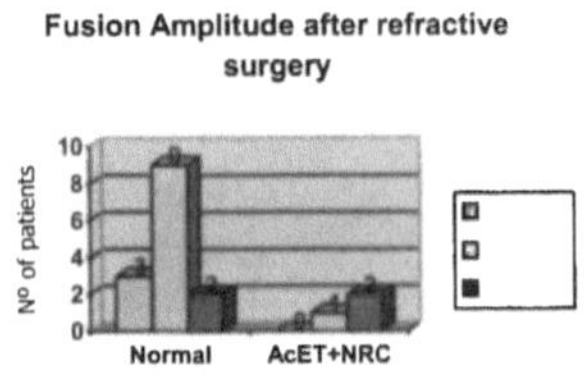

Graph 6

4. *Ocular Motility:* It is more frequent with a tendency of progression towards endophoria (17/31 patients (54.83%), overalls in the ARC patients. (Graph 7). 3 patients with Accommodative esotropia were ortotropic after the refractive surgery although 2 need residual hyperopic glasses for reading.

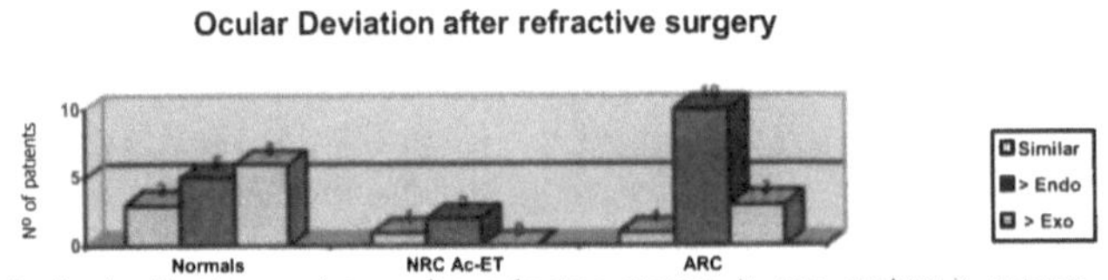

Graph 7: Ocular Motility evolution after refractive surgery in non strabismic patients. Accommodative esotropia with NRC and ARC Esotropia

5. *Symptomatology:* 5 patients (16.13%) mentioned binocular disconfort, being all patients with ARC strabismus (35,71%) (Fisher=0.012).

Patients without strabismus had similar BV as the preoperative situation with the three tests in 71,42% of the cases. (Graph 3, 5 and 6). 3 patients suppressed partially. 3 patients deteriorated their estereopsis and 2 their fusional amplitude. 2 Patients ameliorate their estereopsis and 9 their fusional amplitude. Improvement of BV was related with VA improvement (C=0,562, p=0.019). At the ocular motility examination patients without previous strabismus were stable after refractive surgery with small changes in a similar trend towards esophoria or Exophoria. (Graph 7). They were not symptomatic, but in one case referring to transitory asthenopia in the first postoperative months.

Patients with ARC partially accommodative esotropia, had a similar binocular situation as the postoperative one in 10/14 cases (71,43%), 3 that were alternators transformed into one-eye dominants, and in one case (1/14) there was a change in the dominant eye. (Graph 4) Changes in de dominance pattern were related with the residual refraction. We found more modifications at the oculomotor deviation than in normal subjects. There was a small progression towards endophoria in an important number of cases (10/14), 2 of them aggravated mildly. (Graph 7). They were more symptomatic than the normal patient group (5/14 = 35.71%) 3 of them needed further refractive surgery and 2 of them glasses, but none of them had any intractable diplopia.

We have operated 3 Patients with NRC Accommodative esotropia, all 3 maintained their fusion at distance but 2/3 had a slight deterioration in the estereopsis and fusion amplitude (Graphs 4, 5 and 6). At the ocular motility examination in 2/3 cases we found a residual esophoria (1 case small, 1 case moderate) (Graph 7). They could compensate deviation without glasses although one needed them for reading. This situation was related with the hyperopia regression after refractive surgery.

4. CONCLUSIONS

1. We registered a similar or better situation of binocular vision than the preoperative one in 76% of the cases.

2. Each patient's answers were not homogeneous with all the tests.
3. There is a tendency of evolution towards endophoria that affects in higher degree ARC patients.
4. Patients without strabismus had slight modifications but had no functional repercussion.
5. In the group of patients with ARC strabismus we registered a similar or better situation than in the initial examination in 7/14 patients, they had a greater tendency to progression towards esophoria and were more symptomatic.
6. 3/3 patients with NRC accommodative Esotropia were ortotropic after the refractive surgery, but 1 had a moderate residual esophoria and needed glasses for reading.

5. BIBLIOGRAPHY

Duling K, Wick B. Binocular vision complications alter radial keratotomy. Am J. Optom & Physiol Optics, 1988: 65(3): 215-223.

John ME, Howard C. Esotropia following radial keratotomy. J. Cataract Refract Surg 1991; 17:246-247.

Zwaan J. Strabismus induced by radial keratotomy. Mil Med 1996 Oct;161(10):630-1.

Mandava N, Donnenfeld ED, Owens PL, Kelly SE, Haight DH. Ocular deviation following excimer laser photorefractive keratectomy. J Cataract Refract Surg 1996 May;22(4):504-5.

Kowal, L. Refractive surgery and diplopia. Clin Experiment Ophthal 2000; 28:344-346.

Gómez de Liaño R, Arias A, Ragai N et al. Visión binocular tras la cirugía fotorrefractiva. Acta Estrabológica 1996; 25: 185-188.

Dausch D, Klein R, Schroeder E. Excimer laser photorefractive keratectomy for hyperopia. J. Refract Corneal Surg 1993; 9: 20-28.

Nagy Z, Krueger R, Hamberg-Nyström H et al. Photorefractive Keratectomy for hyperopia in 800 eyes with the Meditec Mel 60 Laser. Journal Refractive Surg 2001 17: 525-533.

Hoyos J, Cigales M, Hoyos-Chacón J et al. Hyperopic laser in situ keratomileusis for refractive accommodative esotropia. J. Cataract Refract Surg 2002; 28:1530-1538.

Nemet P, Levenger S, Nemet A. Refractive surgery for refractive errors which cause strabismus. A report of 8 cases. Binocular Vision Strabismus Quarterly. 2002 Fall; 17(3): 187-90; discussion 191.

Stidham DB, Borissova O, Borissov V et al. Effect of hyperopic laser in situ keratomileusis on ocular alignment and stereopsis in patients with accommodative esotropia. Ophthalmology 2002; 109(6): 1148-53.

Rosario Gomez de Liaño. Prof. Dr
Fortuny 51
28010 Madrid, Spain
rgomezdeliano@med.ucm.es

Transactions 28th Meeting European Strabismological Association, de Faber (ed.)

The results of the systemic treatment of binocular vision and of amblyopia in children with eccentric fixation

Teresa Baranowska-George,Lidia Puchalska-Niedbal
I Klinika Okulistyczna Pomeranian Medical Academy,Szczecin.Poland

Occlusion of the normal eye with an eye patch and the localization treatment are the standard treat- ment for amblyopia with squint in childhood.
We present the behaviour of visual acuity in a squinting eye with initial excentric fixation by mean of long-term systematic treatment with the localization method. The material for studies included 20 children with initial poor visual acuity of the squinting eye (0.02 Snellen test).The subjects were systematic treatment with an eye patch and localization method during 6 years period received.They also had tests of binocular function carried out and a test of their capacity to perceive binocular rivalry using slides in a synoptophore. We pay attention to the improvement of visual acuity depends on the consolidation of the normal binocular vision.

Transactions 28th Meeting European Strabismological Association, de Faber (ed.)
© 2004 European Strabismological Association, ISBN 90 265 1965 6

Refraction over cycloplegia: 2 versus 3 eyedrops use of cyclopentolate.

Sellami L,Le Lez ML,Denoyer A,Santallier M,Pisella PJ,Arsène S.
Department of ophthalpmology,Tours,France.

Introduction: Children refraction is usually made under cycloplegia using a three eyedrops cyclopentolate (5 mg/ml)protocol. Instillations are given using a 5 minutes interval of time. Standard protocol is based on a two drops of cyclopentolate administration,at 10 minutes interval. The objective refraction is realised 45 minutes after the first eyedrop in both cases. The aim of the study is to compare results of refraction in these two protocols of cycloplegia.

Methods: 30 healthy volunteers aged of 16 to 29 years,without any oculomotors troubles were included in this study. Both protocols were conducted simultaneously on each patient at one week interval. Objective refraction was evaluated using an autorefractometer before and every 15 minu- tes after instillation until 90 minutes.

Results: Analysis confirmed that cycloplegia was maximal 45 minutes after the first instillation. Moreover there was no statistical difference for sphere and cylinder values,at this time,between the two protocols.

Conclusion: Cycloplegia could be realised using the two eyedrops protocol with less toxicity than the three one and with the same efficiency.

Transactions 28th Meeting European Strabismological Association, de Faber (ed.)
© 2004 European Strabismological Association, ISBN 90 265 1965 6

Congenital third nerve palsy in septo-optic dysplasia

A. Langmann, S. Lindner
Department of Ophthalmology, University Graz, Austria

ABSTRACT: The most likely cited mechanism for congenital third nerve palsy is perinatal injury. However associated brain stem signs and neurologic anomalies can occure. We present three cases of congenital third nerve palsy in septo-optic dysplasia (de Morsier syndrome). All children had bilateral optic nerve hypoplasia, mid brain malformations and hypothalmohypophseal dysfunction. One child died during febril illness despite intensive medical care. Conclusion: In children with congenital third nerve palsy we have to pay attention to optic nerve hypoplasia for early diagnosis (brain ultasound, MRI, endocrinologic workup) and treatment of de Morsier syndrome. KEYWORDS: optic nerve hypoplasia, congenital third nerve palsy, septo-optic dysplasia

1. INTRODUCTION

Pediatric oculomotor nerve palsies are rare lesions. The most frequently cited mechanism is perinatal injury to the peripheral third nerve (4), although they may be due to congenital absence of the nerve and/ or nucleus and be accompanied by neurological deficits (1) as well. Septo-optic dysplasia, described by De Morsier in 1956 consists of optic hypoplasia, mid brain malformations and hypothalamohypophyseal dysfunction. For pathogenesis intrauterine or perinatal injury, genetic defects and toxic agents are discussed. These children are at risk of sudden death during febril illness by dehydration, hypoglycemia and thermorgulatory distress. Early diagnosis and adequate treatment of endocrinological deficits is necessary. We present three children with congenital third nerve palsy and septo-optic dysplasia. To the best of our knowledge there are only two cases reported in literature with the same malformations.

2. PATIENTS

We report on three children, 3 girls out of 20 patients with de Morsier syndrome and congenital third nerve palsy. All of them had bilateral optic nerve hypoplasia, small pale discs, with visual function from light projection to 0,05 and manifest nystagmus. MRI revealed absent septum pellucidum, thinning of corpus callosum and posterior pituitary ectopia with anterior pituitary hormone deficiency - growth hormone, adrenocorticotrophic hormone and hypothyroidism-in case one and two, and infundibular hypoplasia predicting anterior and posterior pituitary hormone deficiency, with additional diabetes insipidus in the third case. There were no other associated brain or ocular anomalies. These children had no positive history in terms of trauma, drugs or toxic agents. Parents were not related.
Orthoptic examination:
Case 1 (fig.1) had unilateral, leftsided, pupil sparing third nerve palsy, with a fixed exodeviation of 45 ° and extreme hypotropia of 30°, no aberrant regeneration, no ptosis.

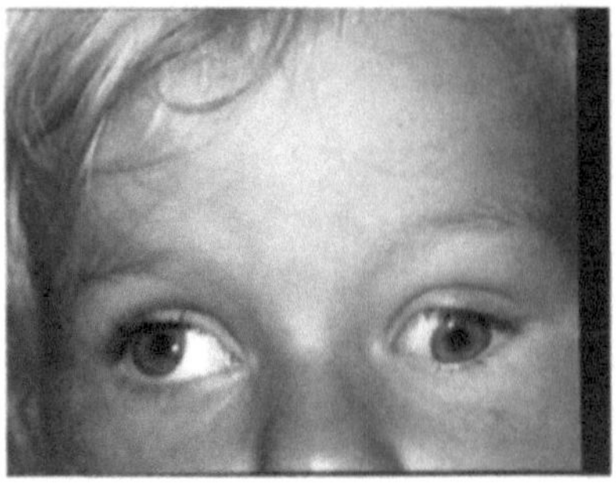

Fig1. Third nerve palsy left side, right gaze, elevation and adduction deficit, some depression

Case 2 (fig.2), fixing with the paretic left eye, demonstrated an elevation deficit of –3, adduction deficit of –2 on this side but good depression. There was no ptosis, nor anisocoria, or aberrant regeneration of the oculomotor nerve.

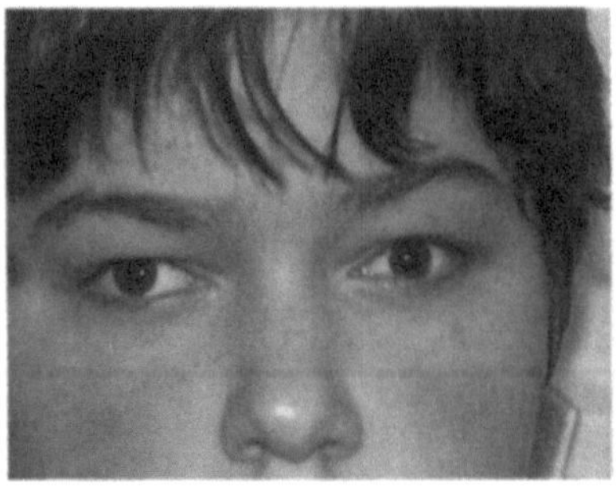

Fig2. Third nerve palsy left side, fixing with paretic eye

The third case was brought to our attention immediately after birth with bilateral third nerve palsy and pupil involvement on the left side (Fig3, 4). The diameter of this pupil was 6 mm and it was non reactive to light. Orthoptic examination revealed defective medial gaze and elevation on both sides (left side worth than right side) and defective depression on left side. In course of the first year of life pupillary reaction recovered without aberrant regeneration. At the age of 12 years the child died during febril illness, despite intensive medical care with increased dosage of
steroids.

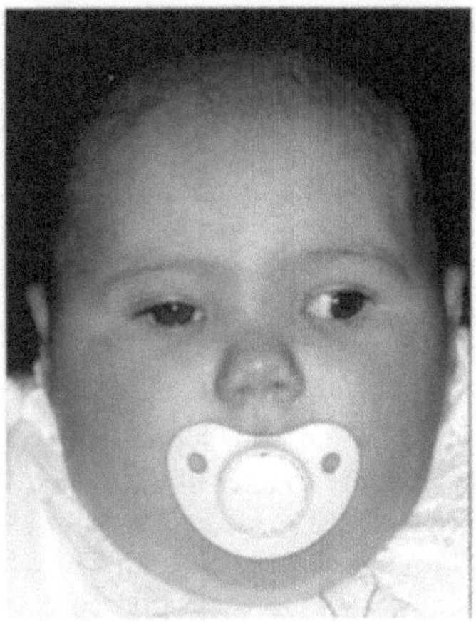

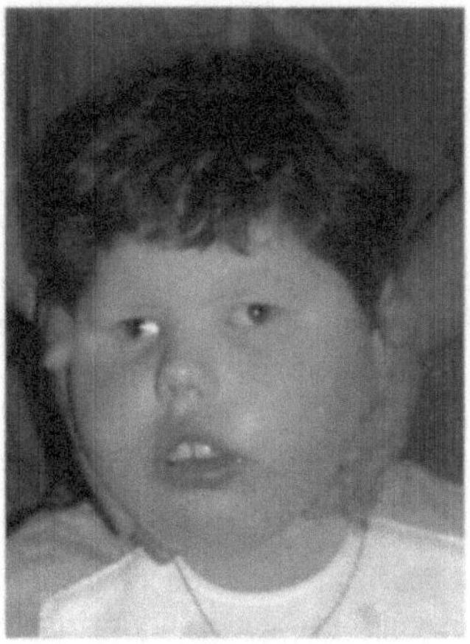

Fig3. Bilateral third nerve palsy with pupillary involvement left side
Fig4. Bilateral third nerve palsy, age 10 years

3. DISCUSSION

Third nerve paresis or palsy occurs uncommonly in children and is often (45%, 9) congenital caused by adverse intrauterine events or traumatic delivery. The presumed mechanism is compression of the nerve crossing the tentorial edge or a diffusely increased intracranial pressure. Direct injury to the nerve during amniocentesis is discussed as well. Although congenital third nerve palsy is mostly an isolated defect accompanied neurological deficit are known (1, 2). We present three children with congenital third nerve paresis/palsy in septo-optic dysplasia, de Morsier syndrome. These children had unilateral palsy in two cases and bilateral palsy in one case. There was no ptosis and no involvement of the contralateral rectus superior in the two patients with unilateral nerve disturbance, indicative perhaps for peripheral nerve defect, although there was no evidence of perinatal trauma and no aberrant regeneration. A possible explanation for the lack of aberrant regeneration may be due to extreme atrophy or even absence of the third nerve (10). The child with bilateral third nerve palsy (case 3) had postnatal pupillary involvement in one eye, with regeneration within one year. Thus underlining the hypothesis that fibrotic changes in eye muscles found in strabismus surgery in the patient with third nerve palsy of Schulz (8) who had an additional miotic pupil on the involved eye after regeneration of pupillary involvement were secondary abnomalities rather than developmental muscle deficiencies. Peripheral nerve damage as well as nuclear defects may have been responsible. Previous reports in the literature showed that several kinds of brain damage could result in congenital oculomotor palsies, such as brainstem infarction, cerebellar and midbrain hypoplasia, absence of basal ganglia etc (3, 6). Two theories have been proposed regarding the pathogenesis of septo-optic dysplasia, a variable combination of absent septum pellucidum, optic nerve hypoplasia and pituitary abnormalities. As all components arise from different tissues and processes at different times developmental anomaly or dysplasia makes little embryologic sense. Genetic causes are exceptional (11). A vascular disruptive sequence similar to porencephaly, possibly involving the proximal trunk of the anterior cerebral artery is discussed by Lubinsky (5). Our findings of congenital third nerve palsy in de Morsier syndrome do not support this hypothesis, as the third cranial nerve and its nuclei are not within the territorial distribution of the anterior cerebral artery and there were no additional defects in the median and paramedian areas of the frontal lobes. The partial palsy in case two, with some amount of adduction, elevation and depression and the recovery of the pupillary involvement in case three implicate probably

prenatal traumatic, infectious or toxic insults, thus supporting the second theory of secondary degeneration, although prenatal and perinatal history was unremarkable in our cases.
Case 2 prefered fixation with the paretic eye. We think for nystagmus dampening as no additional ocular anomalies were found in our patient, that could explain the phenomenon. No occlusion therapy was necessary for the visual function in this patient was only light projection.
Children with corticotropin deficiency in de Morsier syndrome are at risk of sudden death (2) during febril illness. During infection with release of circulating pyrogens hypothalamic thermoregulatory dysfunction may predipose to life threatening hyperthermia. A second thermoregulatory disturbance occurs in children who become hypothermic during episodes of hypoglycemia. All of our three cases with congenital third nerve palsy had growth problems, and hypocortisolism. Case 3 suffered from additional diabetes insipidus, another risk factor for dehydration and thermoregulatory disturbance and died despite intensive medical care and increased dosage of cortisol. Even subclinical hypopituitarism can manifest as acute adrenal insufficiency following for instance surgery under general anesthesia (7). Because children with third nerve palsy may require strabismus surgery ophthalmologists must be attuned to careful preoperative mangement. None of our children was operated.
Conclusion: Ophthalmologists may be the first to recognize the features of septo-optic dysplasia and its neuroendocrinologic disturbances. Our case reports illustrate the necessity of careful optic nerve examination in congenital third nerve palsy for early diagnosis and treatment of de Morsier syndrome

REFERENCES

BalkanR, Hoyt CS.1984.Associated neurological abnormalities in congenital third nerve palsies.*A J ophthalmol* 97:315-319

Brodsky M., Contc F., Taylor D.ct.al. 1997.Suddcn death in septo-optic dysplasia..*Arch ophthalmol 115: 66-7*

Flanders M., Watters G., Draper J., O`Gorman A. 1989. Bilateral congeital cranial nerve palsy.*Can J ophthalmol; 24:28-300*

Hamed LM.1991.Associated neurologic and ophthalmologic findings in congenital oculomotor nervepalsy.*Ophthalmology* 98:708-714

Lubinsky M.1997. Hypothesis: Septo-optic dysplasia is a vascular disruption sequence.*Am J Med Genet 69:235-236*

Norman MG.Unilateral encephalomalacia in cranialnerve nuclei in neonates: report of two cases. 1974. *Neurology; 24:424*

Scherlock DA., McNicol LR. 1987. Anaesthesia and septo-optic dysplasia:implications of missed diagnosis in perioperative period.*Anaesthesia;42:1302-130*

SchulzE., Jung H. 2001.Unilateral congenital oculomotor nerve palsy, optic nerve hypoplasia and pituitary malformation. A preliminary report. *Strabismus 9(1): 33-5*

Schumacher-Feero LA, Yoo KW,.Solari FM., Biglan AW. 1999. Third cranial nerve palsy in children. *Am J Ophthalmol*128: 2: 216-221

Sun Ch.Ch.,.Kao L-Y 2000.Unilateral congenital third nerve palsy.*Chan Gung Med J* 23:12; 776-780

Tajima T., Hattorri T., Nakajima T., et al. 2003. Sporadic heterozygous frameshift mutation of HESX1 causing pituitary and optic nerve hypoplasia and combined hormone deficiency in a Japanese patient. *J-Clin-Endocrinol_Metab 8: 88(1): 45-5*

Transactions 28th Meeting European Strabismological Association, de Faber (ed.)

Orbital fracture referrals: outcome results

M. L. Pedersen
Orthoptic Department, Royal Victoria Infirmary, Newcastle-upon-Tyne, United Kingdom

ABSTRACT: A retrospective study investigated management outcome of patients referred to the Orthoptic Department with ocular motility abnormalities following orbital injury. 73 patients were identified. 7% had spontaneous resolution within four months. 81% were unresolved. 63% of the unresolved cases had orbital surgery while the rest did not. 40% of patients who underwent orbital repair recovered while 43% had unresolved symptoms. Strabismus surgery only occurred in 4/73 of cases (3 following orbital repair). Long term resolution (4-12 months) occurred in 10/73 of cases. 10% (7/73) were discharged with untreated unresolved symptoms. 29% failed to attend or was lost to follow-up. This study has led to an improved liaison between Orthoptics and the Maxillary-Facial Department.

KEYWORDS: Orbital fracture, blow out fracture, orbital repair.

1 AIM

The aim of this study was to investigate the following in patients referred to the Newcastle Royal Victoria Infirmary Orthoptic Department:

- Incidence of patients requiring orbital repair and/or strabismus surgery.
- Outcome of patients undergoing orbital repair.
- Outcome of patients not undergoing orbital repair.

2 METHODS

A respective review of computer held record of patients referred to the Orthoptic Department over the period 2000 – 2002. Data was collected on the incidence of:

- Time span for resolution of diplopia or ocular motility problems,
- Patients requiring intervention for resolution of diplopia or ocular motility problems,
- Patients with persistent diplopia or ocular motility problem.

3 FINDINGS

73 patients were identified with confirmed ocular motility abnormality caused by orbital injury, shown in Table 1. Resolution was defined as complete recovery of diplopia or the presence of minimal residual non-symptomatic diplopia. Outcome of patients undergoing orbital repair is shown in Table 2 and outcome of patients not undergoing orbital repair is shown in Table 3.

Table 1. Results of confirmed ocular motility abnormalities (n=73).

Outcome	Number	(%)
Spontaneous resolution (< 4 months)	7	(10)
Unresolved (>4 months)	59	(81)
Orbital repair	37	(63)
No orbital repair	22	(37)
Failed to attend or lost to follow-up	7	(10)

Table 2. Outcome of patients undergoing orbital repair (n=37).

Outcome	Number	(%)
Resolution	15	(40)
Unresolved symptoms	16	(43)
Strabismus surgery	3	(63)
Under review for ?strabismus surgery	1	(6)
Long term resolution (> 4 months)	6	(38)
Prism management	2	(12)
Patients managing with diplopia	4	(25)
Unknown outcome	6	(17)
Failed to attend	1	(16)
No feedback from Max-Fax	5	(84)

Table 3. Outcome of patients who had no orbital repair (n=22).

Outcome	Number	(%)
Strabismus surgery	7	(10)
Under review for possible strabismus surgery	1	(5)
Prism management	4	(19)
Awaiting follow-up	1	(5)
Long term resolution (<4 – 12 months)	4	(19)
Patient managing with diplopia	3	(14)
Unknown – failed to attend/lost to follow-up	3	(14)
Unknown – no feedback from Max-Fax	5	(24)

4 CONCLUSION

15/37 (40%) patients resolved following orbital repair. This amount increased to 73% if including patients with long-term resolution and if assuming resolution occurred in patients not seen again. Overall, only 4/73 (5%) patients, with a confirmed ocular motility abnormality due to orbital injury, had strabismus surgery. 7/30 (23%) patients were discharged with unresolved symptoms. Patients adopted compensatory strategies to cope. Prisms or strabismus surgery were not appropriate or necessary in these cases. Long term resolution occurred in 10/59 (17%). The longest period of resolution in this study was 12 months at time of completion. A total of 21/73 (29%) either failed to attend or was lost to follow-up. In many of these cases there was no feedback from the Maxillary-Facial Department.

5 OUTCOME

An improved liaison has now been established between the Orthoptic and the Maxillary-Facial Department. In order to assess the actual benefit of Orthoptic assessment of suspected/confirmed orbital fracture cases all patients have a review appointment with Orthoptics.

The Maxillary-Facial Department now refers directly to Orthoptics via fax and completed Orthoptic reports are being faxed back.

Transactions 28th Meeting European Strabismological Association, de Faber (ed.)
© 2004 European Strabismological Association, ISBN 90 265 1965 6

The early natural history of acquired non-accommodative esotropia

Brian G. Mohney, MD. 1 , Anna S. Kitzmann, B. A. 2 , Nancy Diehl, B. S. 3
Department of Ophthalmology 1 , Mayo Medical School 2 , and the Division of Biostatistics 3 Mayo Clinic and Mayo Foundation, Rochester, Minnesota

Purpose: Although the angle of deviation in patients with congenital esotropia has been shown to increase during the early preoperative period, little data exists with regards to other forms of child- hood esotropia. The primary objective of this study was to investigate whether the angle of deviati- on increases with time in patients with acquired nonaccommodative esotropia (ANAET).

Methods: The medical records of all children diagnosed with ANAET at East Tennessee State University College of Medicine from August 1, 1995, through July 31, 2001, were retrospectively reviewed. All patients were assessed for any change in the amount of their strabismic angle and as- sociated risk factors.

Results: Eighty-two patients with ANAET were identified, and all except 3 children had more than one examination. Of the 79 children with more than one examination, 26 (32. 9%)displayed an in- crease of 10 or more prism diopters (PD)during a median follow-up period of 2. 9 months. Those patients who increased by 10 or more PD were diagnosed (28. 4 months vs. 45. 5 months, p=0. 003) and underwent surgery (35. 9 months vs. 56. 8 months, p=0. 003)at a significantly younger median age than those whose angle progressed less than 10 PD.

Conclusions: Approximately one third of patients with ANAET in this study had a progressive in- crease in their angle of deviation of at least 10 prism diopters during the early preoperative period. This increase is more likely in younger patients and underscores the importance of performing serial measurements of the deviating angle prior to surgical intervention.

Transactions 28th Meeting European Strabismological Association, de Faber (ed.)
© 2004 European Strabismological Association, ISBN 90 265 1965 6

Visual conversive syndrome disorder: a case report

E.Lala 1 , ML Le Lez 1 , J.Malvy 2 , F Madern 1 , PJ.Pisella 1 , S.Arsène 1
1 Department of Ophthalmology, Tours, France 2 Department of Psychiatry, Tours, France

Introduction:Ophthalmologists are often solicited in first intention in case of somatopsychic disturbances affecting visual system.They have to keep in mind these disorders without misdiagnosing organic dysfunction.

Case report:Marion, a 16 years old girl, has consulted in emergency for an isolated right eye 's positive scotoma, which appeared five days ago.Visual acuity was conserved, clinical ophthalmological examination was normal, without any abnormality of fundus neither pupillary reflex.The scotoma was found in the inferio-temporal visual field, non-systematised, in two successive exami- nations.Neither the angiofluorography, neither the cerebral CTscan, neither visual evoked potential showed any organic damage.Ultimately, the scotoma disappeared spontaneously following a nightmare and the psychiatrist diagnosed a visual conversive disorder following upon a conflict.

Discussion/conclusion:Somatopsychic disturbances exist in ophthalmology, in the form of disorders of eye motricity and of visual perception ranging from a slight amblyopia, often associated with limitation of the field of vision, to complete amaurosis.In the lid region, nictation tics and tri- chotillomania of the eyebrows and eyelashes occur;dyslexia or dysorthography often occur as se- condary phenomena. Ophthalmologists have to confirm the suspicion of non-organic visual dysfunction by demonstra- ting the functional integrity of the visual system and the non-physiologic nature of the visual com- plaints. Clinical investigation between ophthalmologists and psychiatrists will provide the most appropriate patient management.

Transactions 28th Meeting European Strabismological Association, de Faber (ed.)
© 2004 European Strabismological Association, ISBN 90 265 1965 6

E.M.A.N. (Eye Movement and Accommodation Analyzer) device for vergence accommodation synkinesis recording and analysis

M. Dostálek
Department of Ophthalmology (Ortoptic Section), City Hospital, Litomyšl, Czech Republic

J. Dušek
Department of Radioelectronic, Faculty of Electrical Engineering, Czech Technical University, Prague, Czech Republic

ABSTRACT: The non-invasive and safe simultaneous recording of the dynamic changes of horizontal eye position (i.e. horizontal duction) and refractive status (i.e. accommodation) is necessary for the study of reactions to standardised stimulus (step change of the fixation target distance) in children. Some methodological aspect of our Eye Movement and Accommodation Analyzer are discussed.

KEYWORDS: Hirschberg principle, excentric photorefraction, simultaneous recorging, accommodation, duction, image analysis.

1 INTRODUCTION

E.M.A.N. (Eye Movement and Accommodation Analyzer) is a videometric device consisting of three video circuits (Fig. 1) and a controlling PC located in three rooms (two of them are dim). The videometric unit is the main component of the device. It is based on a digital monochromatic area scan camera DALSA CA-D1-0256A. Image sensor DALSA IA-D1 offers peak spectral responsivity at near infrared (NIR) wavelength band (825 nm) and 100 % fill factor thanks to the frame transfer technology. The spacial resolution of the sensor is low (256 x 256 pixels), pixels are large (16 x 16 µm). The time resolution of the camera, i.e. the number of captured frames per second is high (203 fps). The excentric photorefraction shield with the measuring NIR light source (LCD array) (Fig. 4) is attached to the custom camera lens. Controlling PC co-ordinates (1) grabbing (transformation and recording) frame sequences from videometric unit, (2) emmiting of measuring NIR light, and (3) switching the fixation target (colour live video of mother's face) from distant (3.12 m) to near (0.37 m) (or *vice versa*) fixation monitor of stimulational video-circuit. Both monitors are located at the common cyclopean visual axis of the proband and are of identical angular subtense and of approximately similar luminance. The observational video-circuit offers a mother visual feed-back contact with her child fixating her face on the fixation monitor.

The off-line processing of all frames follows the on-line grabbing of the videometric frame sequence. The image analysis of particular image frames from the frame sequence represents particular measurements of actual refractive power and angle of eye rotation at the time of frame capture.

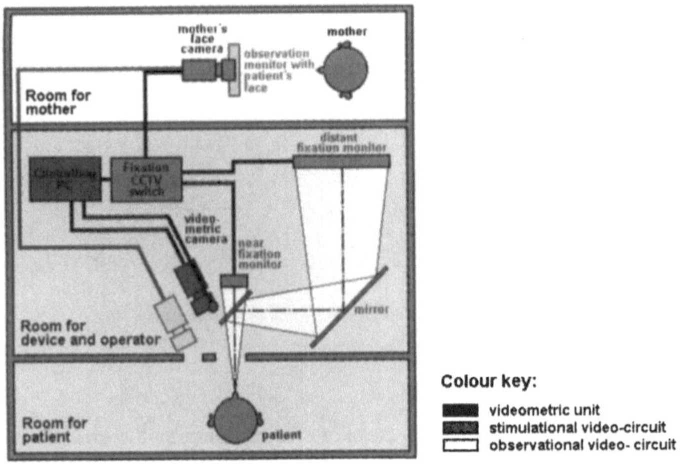

Figure 1. Eye Movement and Accommodation Analyzer hardware diagram (dash-and-dot line = cyclopean eye visual axis, view from above)

There are three consequent procedures during the off-line processing: (1) image analysis of each frame to obtain the set of primary measurements (Fig. 2), (2) transformation and individual calibration of this primary data set and graphical reconstruction of duction and accommodation responses´ (qualitative) morphology, and finally, (3) extraction of parameters quantifying some characteristics of pulse controller dynamics (latency, average initial speed, time constant, etc.), step controller stability (parameter of undulation), and saccadic replacement of version during initial segments of duction reactions (saccadic contribution).

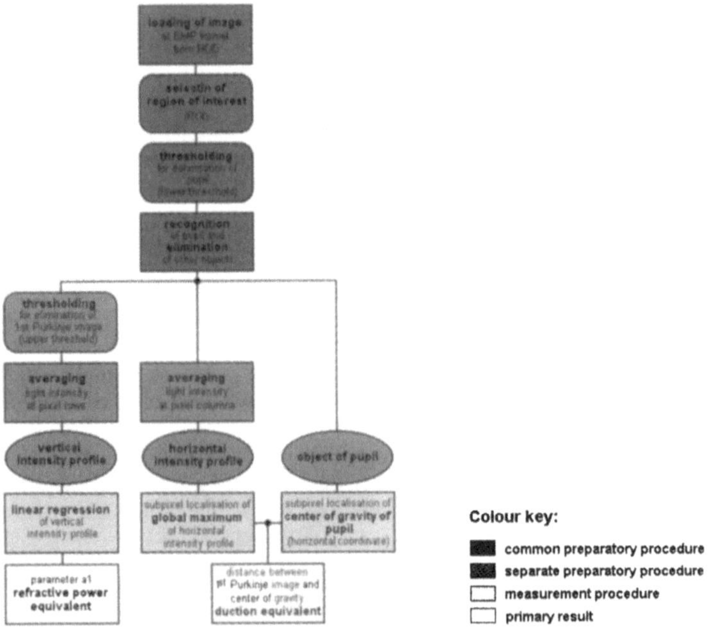

Figure 2. Algorithm of image analysis procedures applied to all particular images fromvideometric frame sequences (rectangle = automatic processing, rectangle with rounded corners = manually controlled processing, oval = result of preparatory processing)

2 SOME METHODOLOGICAL PROBLEMS RELATED TO PROCESSING OF RECORDED VIDEOMETRIC FRAME SEQUENCES

2.1 Problem 1: How to sufficiently balance the time and spatial resolution of the videometric device and cope with IR light hygienic standards?

The optimal balance of the time and spatial resolution of measurements is one of the prerequisites for the reliability of results. Our approach to this problem is based on harvesting the maximal time resolution through hardware setting. Resulting reduction in spatial resolution is compensated by software concept.

The application of 2 x 2 pixel binning to the image sensor enlarges the pixel area four times (32 x 32 □m) and reduces the light energy necessary for creating a quality image even during reduced shutter opening time. This setting enables us to obtain average of 325 frames (measurements) per second. Software philosophy is based on an effort to extract information from all relevant image pixels and on the wide usage of subpixel calculations. The separation of the image object of pupilla by thresholding and consequent averaging of sets of bearing pixels precedes mathematical processing of primary results on subpixel accuracy (Dušek et al. 2003).

Extra large pixels, 100 % fill factor and peak spectral responsivity at NIR wavelength band of used image sensor enable to usage of safe intensity of infrared measuring light for videorefraction. Maximum possible exposure of NIR light energy used in the device $RE_{max.}$= $1.531\ 10^2\ J/m^2$ is eleven times less than maximum permitted exposure MPE = $1.727\ 10^3\ J/m^2$. The device cope with standard ČSN-EN 60825-1.

2.2 Problem 2: How to obtain two parameters (refractive power and eye position) from one frame ?

The videometrics of the horizontal ductions is based on the Hirschberg principle: measurement of the horizontal distance between the center of gravity of the pupil and the center of the 1st Purkinje image (i.e. corneal reflex) of measuring NIR light source (Hirschberg 1885, Du Bois-Reymond 1886). The refractive status is measured by using excentric, slope-based (Schaeffel et al. 1987, Roorda et al. 1997) photorefraction principle (Howland 1980). The measurement of 1st Purkinje image´s displacement from the center of pupil must be performed at the plane of measured eye rotation whereas the measurement of refractive power changes is independent on the orientation of the measuring plane, thanks to the presumed rotational symetry of crystalline lens change during accommodation. We have experimented with rectangular orientation of the measuring planes. Our crossed intensity profiles principle of image analysis of measuring frames is presented in Figure 3.

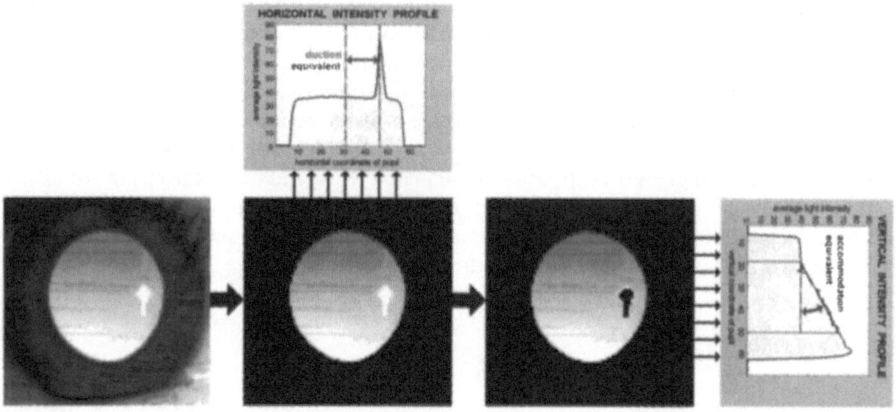

Figure 3. Crossed intensity profiles principle of image analysis (bold arrow = tresholding, thin arrows = averaging)

The NIR LED array located at the semilunar shield in aperture of the front-end optics of the videometric unit (Fig. 4) primarilly serves as a source of measuring light for excentric photorefraction. The array simultaneously serves as a source of light generating 1st Purkinje image. Point source offers optimal accuracy for the Hirschberg principle application, whereas array of point sources with different excentricity are beneficial for the excentric, slope-based, photorefraction measurement (Roorda et al. 1997). The array of four LEDs aligned to the row parallel to the pixel columns at which we perform an averaging of light intensity to create the horizontal intensity profile is an effective compromise.

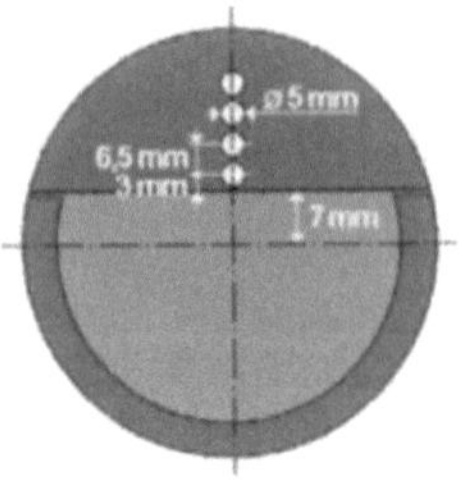

Figure 4. Photorefractive shield on front-end optics of the videometric unit (deep gray =shield, grey = camera lens, white = NIR LED, view from the position of patient)

2.3 Problem 3: Are measurements of accommodation and duction by E.M.A.N. device independent ?

The absence of an interrelationship between the measurements of accommodation and duction is an important condition of the reliability of results. The rapid change of the habitually slow course of accommodation at the close time relation to the saccadic eye movement we consider a sensitive indicator of coupling between measurements of both reactions.

The majority (62.2 %) of 280 reviewed vergence-accommodation records showed no signs of remarkable interrelationship of both measured processes (Fig. 5a).

In the rest of the reviewed records, the interindividually different degree of interrelationship were found and measurements of left eyes were more coupled (49.9 %) than measurements of right eyes (29.8 %). Two forms of coupling could be denoted. The difference lay in whether the accommodation measurements artificial changes are of same (Fig. 5b) or opposite (Fig. 5c) direction as the change of duction angle

The fact that 83.7 % of interferences reviewed of right eye records were of the opposite direction and that 78.7 % of interferences of left eye records were of the same direction could be explained by the changes at off-axis refraction (Schaeffel et al. 1999). Horizontal refraction profile (Fig. 8) represents the change of refraction if measured against excentric points of retinal surface different from ideal spheroid (without change at accomodation).

Rotation of eye relatively to the stationary videometric camera (on left side of fixating monitors) cause the change of excentricity of illuminated retina and hence the change of off-axis refraction independent on the accommodation. During inward rotation, illuminated retinal spot moves centrally at right eye and periferally at the left eye (Fig. 9). The opposite artificial change at measured refractive power results probably from this antagonism

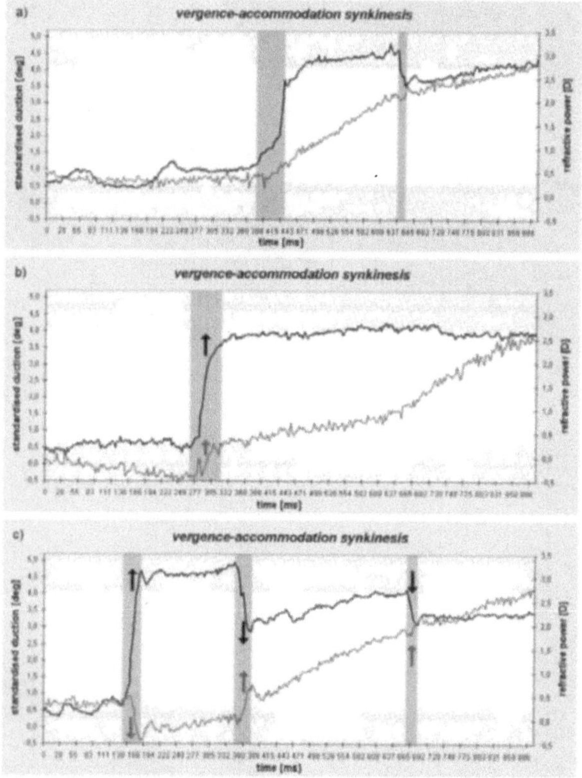

Figure 5. Vergence-accommodation synkinesis record: a) no significant interference between both processes, b) parallel direction of interference between both processes, c) opposite direction of interference between both processes (black curve = duction, grey curve = accommodation, grey strip = saccadic fragment of duction movement)

3 CONCLUSION

The methodological approach applied at E.M.A.N. shows the potential of the device to provide relevant measurement results and promises the possibility of further development and elaboration.

REFERENCES

Du Bois-Reymond, C. 1886. Ueber Schielmessung. *Centralbl prakt Augenh* 9: 1-5.

Dušek, J., Dostálek, M., Hozman, J., Hromádka, Z. 2003, Automatic detection of Purkinje images′ horizontal coordinates. *Physician and Technology* 34: 47-59.

Hirschberg, J. 1885. Ueber Messung des Schielgrades und Dosirung der Schieloperation. *Centralbl prakt Augenh* 8: 325-327.

Howland, H.C. 1980. The optics of static photographic skiaskopy (comments on paper by K. Kaakinen: A simple method for screening of children with strabismus, anisometropia or ametropia by simultaneous photography of the corneal and the fundus reflexes). *Acta Ophthalmol (Kbl.)* 58: 221-225.

Roorda, A., Campbell, C.W. & Bobier, W.R. 1997. Slope-based eccentric photorefraction: theoretical analysis of different light source configurations and effects of ocular aberrations. *J Opt Soc Am A* 14: 2547-2556.

Schaeffel, F., Farkas, L. & Howland, H.C. 1987. Infrared photoretinoscope. *Appl Opt* 26: 1505-1509.

Schaeffel, F., Weiss, S. & Seidl, J. 1999. How good is the match between the plane of the text and the plane of focus during reading? *Ophthal Physiol Opt* 19: 180-192.

 ISBN 90 265 1965 6

Clinical features of isolated inferior rectus paralysis

A. Yaman
Fellow, Department of Ophthalmology, Dokuz Eylül University, İzmir,Turkey

AT. Berk
Professor, Department of Ophthalmology, Dokuz Eylül University, İzmir,Turkey

Aim: Our aim was to evaluate diagnosis and treatment of isolated inferior rectus paralysis
Method: Medical records of 4 patients who were diagnosed as isolated inferior rectus paralysis were reviewed.
Results: The mean age of patients was 30.2 years (min:6 max: 64 years) the aetiology was congenital in 3 patients and vascular in one patient. Three of 4 patients were female. The ophthalmologic examination and ocular motility were performed. Hypertropia was presenting symptom in all patients. Severe limitation in down-ward gaze, head posture, secondary deviation were revealed in examination. An associated exotropia (range 10-90 prism diopters) was present in three patients. Forced duction test was positive in three congenital patients who underwent surgical procedure. One patient required one operation, 2 had two. As surgical approach, superior rectus recession and inferior rectus resection was performed in two eyes, but in one of them, combined lateral rectus recession was also performed for associated exotropia. In one patient, lateral rectus recession-medial rectus resection with infraplasman and superior rectus recession and contralateral inferior rectus recession was performed. The mean postoperative deviation of hypertropia was 4 prism diopters (0 to 12) The patient who developded sudden onset of vertical diplopia especially down-ward gaze had myastenia gravis and diabetes mellitus.
Conclusion: This study shows that isolated paralysis of the inferior rectus muscle responds to surgical correction with significant improvement. Surgery consist of recession of the tight superior rectus combined with or without resection of the paralysed inferior rectus seemed to be effective.

Key word: Isolated inferior rectus paralysis, hypertropia

Clinical features of isolated inferior rectus paralysis
An isolated inferior rectus paralysis without involvement of other muscles supplied by the oculomotor nerve is rare and often congenital(1). It may occur following orbital trauma vascular disease, intracranial metastasis or primary lesion, and in conjuction with myastenia(2-3). Our aim was to evaluate diagnosis and treatment of isolated inferior rectus paralysis.
Method: Medical records of 4 patients who were diagnosed as isolated inferior rectus paralysis were retrospectively reviewed.

Case 1: 6-year-old girl had a history of deviation in right eye since birth. Visual acuity was 20/30 in RE, 20/20 in LE without correction. She had mild amblyopia in right eye. Pupillary examination was normal. The patient preferred to fixate with the left eye. She had a right hypertropia of 25 prism diopters and exotropia of 10 prism diopters by cover test(figure 1). Ocular version testing demonstrated a severe reduction of depression in right eye, particularly in abduction. Fundus examination with dilated pupils was normal. Forced duction test was positive. As a surgical approach, 4.5 mm. superior rectus recession and 5 mm. inferior rectus resection was performed. Postoperatively, there was no deviation in right eye in primary gaze and ductions of right eye improwed. Postoperative eye motility of patient is shown in figure 2.
Case 2: 22-year-old woman with hypertropia in her right eye underwent ophthalmic examination. Visual acuity was 20/20 bilaterally. She had hypertropia and exotropia in right eye and prefered to fixate with left eye. In primary gaze, there were 20 prism diopters of right hypertropia and 20 prism diopters of right exotropia. Ductions of the left eye were normal. The right eye had moderate limitation of depression when the eye was abducted . Compensatuar head posture consist of head tilt and face turn towards nonparalyzed eye was observed. Pupils were equal, round and reactive to light. Fundus examination was normal. Forced duction test was positive. In first operation 7 mm. lateral rectus recession and 4.5 mm superior rectus recession were performed. After first operation, there were 14 prism diopters of hypertropia and 6 prism diopters exotropia in right eye (figure 3). As a second operation, 4.5mm. inferior rectus resection was performed for residual hypertropia. Postoperatively she had 4 prism diopters of right hypertropia in primary gaze. Ocular motility and head posture slightly improved. Her ocular motility in last examination is shown in figure 4.
Case 3: 33-year-old woman with history of strabismus from birth presented with right hypertropia and exotropia. Ophthalmologic examination disclosed a best corrected visual acuity of right eye 20/30 (-2.00 x 165) and left eye 20/20. She had mild ambliopia in right eye. Pupillary examination was normal. The patient preferred to fixate with the left eye. With the left eye fixing, she had a right hypertropia of 25 prism diopters and exotropia of 90 prism diopters by cover test (figure 5). Ocular version testing demonstrated a severe reduction of depression and mild limitation of adduction in right eye. Fundus examination with dilated pupils was normal. Forced duction test was positive. 9 mm. lateral rectus recession and 6 mm. medial rectus resection with one full tendon width infraplacement were performed in first operation. After this operation, she had 25 prism diopter of right hypertropia and 20 prism diopters of right exotropia in primary gaze. After 8 months, 5 mm. right superior rectus recession and 4 mm left inferior rectus recession were performed. In last follow-up examination, there were hypertropia of 12 prism diopters and exotropia 30 prism diopters in right eye in primary position. Downward gaze slightly improved in right eye. Ocular versions after surgery is shown in figure 6.
Case 4: 64-year-old man was refered to our department for evaluation of binocular vertical diplopia. He noted diplopia in primary and inferior gaze that he was able to eliminate with a face turn to left and chin-down head posture . He had been diagnosed as having diabetes mellitus. His neurological history was unremarkable. His visual acuity was 20/30 without correction. In slit-lamb examination, grade 1 nuclear sclerosis was detected in two eyes. Pupils were equal, round and reactive to light, with no relative afferent pupillary defect. Ductions of left eye were normal. The right eye had moderate limitation of depression particularly in abduction. In primary gaze, there were 8 prism diopters hypertropia and 4 prism diopters exotropia in right eye (figure 7). There was no blepharoptosis. Other cranial nerve testing were unremarkable. Ophthalmoscopic findings were normal bilaterally. Right isole inferior rectus paralysis was diagnosed. Single fiber electromyelography revealed myastania gravis. We could not treat this patient because of social insurancy problem. He was unavalible for follow-up. We learned that systemic corticosteroid treatment was planed but he did not receive the medication. He died because of systemic respiratuar complication of myastenia gravis.

RESULTS

The mean age of patients was 30.2 years (min:6 max: 64 years) the aetiology was congenital in 3 patients and myastenia gravis in one patient. Three of 4 patients were female. The ophthalmologic examination and motility analysis were performed. Hypertropia was presenting symptom. Mean deviation of hypertropia was 18 prism diopters (range 8-25 prism diopters).Severe limitation in down-ward gaze, head posture, secondary deviation was revealed in examination. No other manifestation of partial third nerve involvement such as pupillary anomalies, ptosis were present. An associated exotropia (range 4-90 prism diopters) was present in all patients. Forced duction test was positive in three congenital patients who underwent surgical procedure. One patient required one operation, 2 had two. As an surgical approach, superior rectus recession and inferior rectus resection was performed in two eyes, but in one of them, combined lateral rectus recession was also performed for associated exotropia. In one patient, lateral rectus recession-medial rectus resection with infraplasman and superior rectus recession and contralateral inferior rectus recession was performed. The mean postoperative deviation of hypertropia was 5 prism diopters (0 to 12). Postoperatively, ductions of affected eye were improved in three patients The patient who developed sudden onset of vertical diplopia especially in downward gaze had diabetes mellitus and myastenia gravis. The ocular finding of patients was shown in table 1.

CONCLUSİON

The diagnosis of inferior rectus paralysis must rely on testing the ductions and versions and measuring the deviation in the diagnostic position with the either eye fixating. Associated clinical signs such as compensatuar head posture, secondary deviation may be helpfull in diagnosis of this condititon. Exotropia was associated findings in our patient. von Noorden had noted that there were exotropia in 5 of 14 patients and esotropia in 3 of them.

This study shows that isolated paralysis of the inferior rectus muscle responds to surgical correction with significant improvement. Three patients who were treated surgically improved signifigantly. Compensatuar head porture was eliminated. Surgery consist of recession of the tight superior rectus combined with or without resection of the paralysed inferior rectus seemed to be effective.

von Noorden(2) have recommended to performed combined recession-resection operation in larger deviation and only resection of paralised muscle in smaller deviations.

Burke and Keech (4) had performed the procedure consist of full transposition of the horizontal recti in affected eye of 5 patients with paralysis of the inferior rectus muscle. Single binocular vision in primary position of gaze had been achieved without use of the prisms in these patients. He had underlined that additional surgery may be required to correct residual vertical diplopia.

As a conclusion, isolated inferior retus paralysis respond to surgical correction with improvement in ocular deviation and single binocular vision in primary position.

REFERENCES

von Noorden GK , Campos EC.Binocular vision and motility. Theory and management of strabismus. Sixth ed. İn ed: Lambert R. Mosby comp. Chapter 20. paralytic strabismus. P:414-458.

von Noorden GK, Hansell R. 1991. Clinical characteristic and treatment of isolated inferior rectus paralysis. Ophthalmolgy. 98: 253-57.

Harrison AR, Wirtschafter JD. 1999. Isolated inferior rectus paresis secondary to a mesencephalic cavernous angioma. Am J Ophthalmolgy. 127:617-9.

Burke JP, Keech RV. 1995. Effectiveness of inferior transposition of the horşzonta lrectus muscle for acquired inferior rectus paresis.

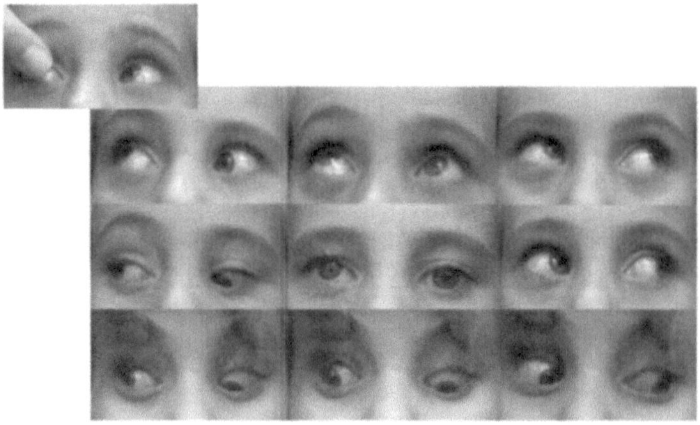

Figure 1: Ocular motility of case 1 preoperatively

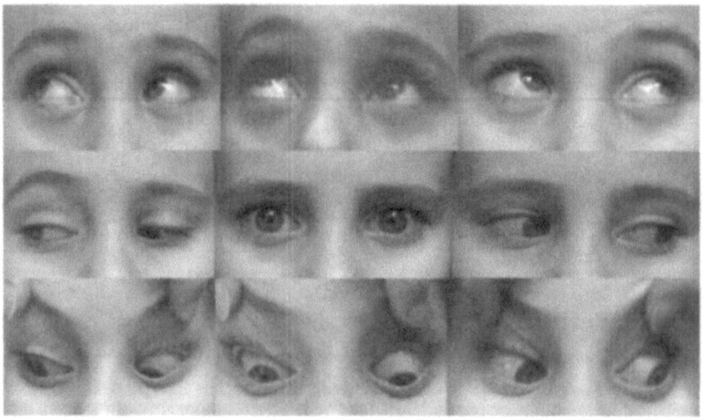

Figure 2: Ocular motility of case 1 postperatively

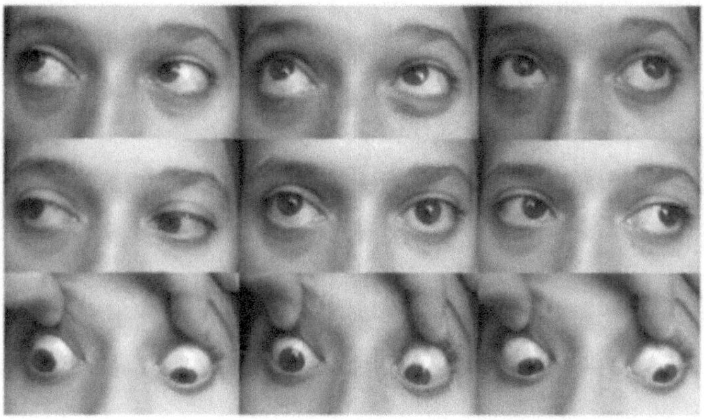

Figure 3: Ocular motility of case 2 just before undergoing second surgery

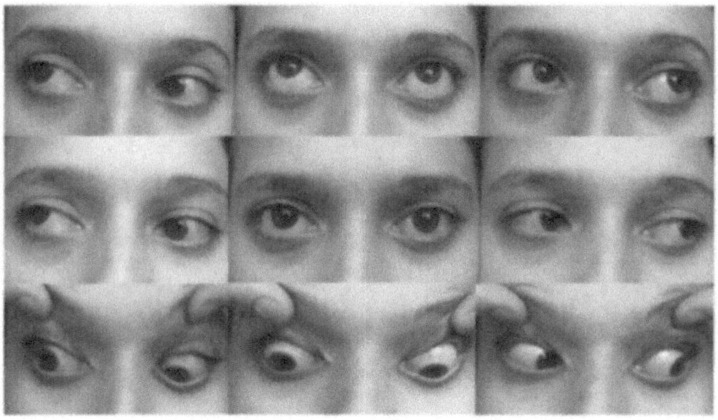

Figure 4: Ocular motility of case 2 postperatively

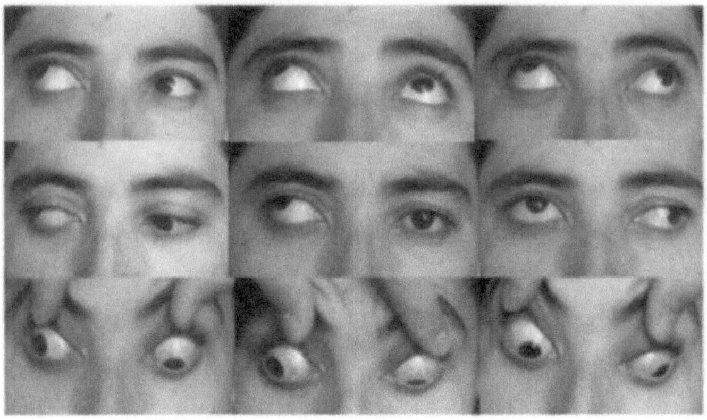

Figure 5 Ocular motility of case 3 preoperatively

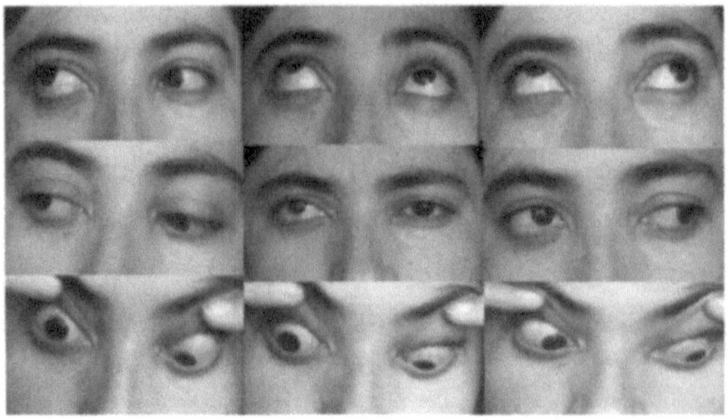

Figure 6 Ocular motility of case 3 postperatively

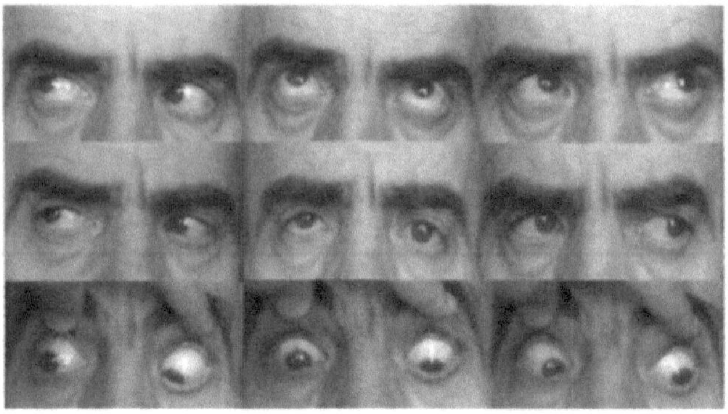

Figure 7 Ocular motility of case 4

Case	Age Sex	Eye	VA R/L	Cause	Angel of Deviation (pd)	Ductions	Surgery	Second surgery	Residual deviation
1	6 F	R	20/30 OD 20/20 OS	Congenital	25 ΔHT 10 ΔXT	Limitation of DWG in abduction	4.5 mm SR recession 5 mm IR resection	-	Ortho
2	22 F	R	20/20 OU	Congenital	20 ΔHT 20 ΔXT	Limitation of DWG in abduction	7 mm LR recession 4.5 mm SR recession	4.5 mm IR resection	4 ΔHT
3	33 F	R	20/30 –2.00D X 165 OD 20/20 OS	Congenital	25 ΔHT 90 ΔXT	Limitation of DWG and adduction	9 mm LR recession 6 mm MR resection with 1 tendon width infraplacement	5 mm SR recession contralateral 4.5 mm IR recession	12ΔHT 30ΔXT
4	64 M	R	20/30 OU	Myastenia Gravis	8 ΔHT 4 ΔXT	Limitation in DWG	-	-	-

Table 1: Ocular findings of patients

Δ: indicates prism diopters, HT: hypertropia of affected eye, XT: exotropia of affected eye, DWG: downward gaze Ortho: Orthophoric

Transactions 28th Meeting European Strabismological Association, de Faber (ed.)
© 2004 European Strabismological Association, ISBN 90 265 1965 6

Infantile Orofacial Hemangioma with Ipsilateral Peripapillary Excavation in Girls-A Variant of PHACE Syndrome

C. Kniestedt & K. Landau
University of Zürich, Switzerland

M. Brodsky, P. North & M.Waner
University of Arkansas for Medical Sciences, Little Rock, Arkansas, U.S.A.

ABSTRACT

Objective: To describe two girls with large infantile orofacial hemangiomas and ipsilateral excavated optic disc anomalies.

Methods: Description of clinical and neuroimaging findings in these two cases.

Results: Two girls with resolved orofacial hemangiomas were found to have decreased vision in the ipsilateral eye. Ophthalmologic evaluation disclosed an ipsilateral morning glory optic disc anomaly in one patient and an ipsilateral peripapillary staphyloma in the other patient. Magnetic resonance angiography disclosed ipsilateral intracranial vascular anomalies in both cases.

Conclusion: The findings in these two cases suggest that the association of infantile orofacial hemangioma and excavated optic disc in girls falls within the spectrum of PHACE syndrome.

References:

1. Holmstrom G, Taylor D: Capillary haemangiomas in association with morning glory disc anomaly. Acta Ophthalmol Scand 1998;76:613-616.

2. Metry DW, Dowd CF, Barkovich AJ, and Frieden IJ: The many faces of PHACE syndrome. J Pediatr 2001;139:117-123.

Transactions 28th Meeting European Strabismological Association, de Faber (ed.)
© 2004 European Strabismological Association, ISBN 90 265 1965 6

The outcome of strabismus surgery in patients with Graves' Ophthalmopathy without prior orbital decompression.

D.L.T. Donker, J.T.H.N. de Faber & J.A.M. van Everdingen
The Rotterdam Eye Hospital, the Netherlands

ABSTRACT

The purpose of this study was to review the results of strabismus surgery in patients with strabismus secondary to Graves' Ophthalmopathy without prior orbital decompression and to identify the factors which can possibly influence the outcome of surgery. In all cases, binocular Single Vision (BSV) in primary- and reading position was restored. 76.9% had an excellent outcome. Additional prisms were needed in 23.1% of the cases. 15.4% needed more than one surgical procedure to restore BSV. Preoperative factors like age, sex, duration of Graves' Ophthalmopathy, orbital irradiation, number of muscles operated on, number of operations, deviation and intra-individual asymmetry in duction limitation between both eyes, had no significant influence on the final outcome in our study.
However, two preoperative factors appeared to have an influence on the outcome of surgery. Patients who still needed prism correction to regain BSV had significantly more limitation of abduction preoperatively (p=0.024). In cases of more than one surgical procedures, significantly more different muscles were recessed (p=0.001).

KEYWORDS: Graves' Ophthalmopathy, strabismus surgery, diplopia

1. OBJECTIVE

The objective was to identify factors which can possibly influence the outcome of surgery by reviewing the results of strabismus surgery on patients with strabismus secondary to Graves' Ophthalmopathy without prior orbital decompression.

2. MATERIAL AND METHODS

A population, existing of the records of 72 patients with Graves' Ophthalmopathy who underwent strabismus surgery between 1996 and 2002 was retrospectively reviewed, from which we analysed the results of strabismus surgery in the 43 cases that had not undergone prior orbital decompression. 4 Patients were excluded of this study for reasons of respectively having strabismus surgery elsewhere, intracranial hypertension, an existing 4th nerve palsy and a Herpes Simplex keratitis with corneal scars apart from Graves' Ophthalmopathy. For analysis, a stable eye disease was required in all 39 patients, which means three similar orthoptic measurements within six months. All but two patients were operated by one surgeon at the Rotterdam Eye Hospital, the Netherlands. From 39 patients, 11 were male and 28 were female, with their age ranging from 34 to 85 years. The rectus inferior muscle has been operated most frequently.

Binocular Single Vision (BSV) in primary- and reading position without the use of prisms was used as criterion for excellent result. BSV in both positions with the use of prisms was used as criterion for good result. Diplopia in primary- or reading position despite the use of prisms was used as criterion for fair result and diplopia in both positions with the use of prisms was used as criterion for poor result (Ruttum, 2000).

RESULTS

BSV in primary- and reading position was restored in all cases. 76.9% had an excellent outcome. Additional prisms were needed in 23.1% of the cases. For the fact that all 39 patients had a good or excellent result, we compared these two groups to analyse whether some of the patients still needed a prism postoperatively to restore BSV (table 1).

Table 1.

	BSV without prism N=30	BSV with prism N=9	P-value
Male/Female	7/23	4/5	0.238
Mean age yrs (range)	57 (34-78)	60 (36-85)	
Duration of Thyroid disease (yrs) ± SD	Median=1.91 ± 2.8	Median=1.87 ± 2.4	1.000
Orbital irradiation (%)	9 (30.0)	6 (66.7)	0.063
Mean number of muscles ± SD	2.1 ± 0.8	2.1 ± 0.8	0.840
Mean number of operations ± SD	1.2 ± 0.6	1.22 ± 0.4	1.000
Mean preop deviation (PD) ± SD Horizontal	9.3 ± 12.8	4.9 ± 6.1	0.588
Vertical	11.9 ± 8.1	23.3 ± 16.9	0.059
Mean preop ductions ODS (Degree) ± SD			
Adduction	39.7 ± 3.4	39.8 ± 2.4	0.668
Abduction	39.2 ± 2.9	36.6 ± 3.4	0.024
Elevation	26.7 ± 5.0	21.8 ± 6.5	0.054
Depression	30.7 ± 1.2	31.0 ± 0.0	0.425
No of patients with asymmetric ductions > 5 □			
Adduction (%)	3 (10.0)	0 (0.0)	1.000
Abduction	2 (6.7)	3 (33.3)	0.070
Elevation	7 (23.3)	7 (77.8)	0.005
Depression	1 (3.4)	0 (0.0)	1.000

N= number of patients

No significant differences between both groups in duration of thyroid disease, irradiation, mean number of muscles, mean number of operations and mean preoperative deviation were observed. However, patients who postoperatively still needed prisms to restore BSV had preoperatively significant more abduction limitation than patients with BSV without prisms. Another outcome of the review of patient records was that having asymmetric ductions between both eyes did not lead to a significant increase of requiring prisms postoperatively.

Of the population, 15.4% needed more than one surgical procedure to restore BSV. Surgery of more than one muscle in the first operation did not increase the chance of requiring prisms or a reoperation. However, in cases where patients had more than one operation, statistically more muscles where operated on.

3. CONCLUSION

BSV in primary- and reading position was restored in all 39 cases. 76.9% had an excellent outcome. Additional prisms were needed in 23.1% of the cases.
Preoperative factors like age, sex, duration of Graves' Ophthalmopathy, orbital irradiation, number of muscles operated on, number of operations, deviation and intra-individual asymmetry in duction limitation between both eyes, had no significant influence on the final outcome in our study. However, two preoperative factors appeared to have an influence on the outcome of surgery. Patients who still needed prism correction to regain BSV had significantly more limitation of abduction preoperatively (p=0.024). In cases of more than one surgical procedures, significantly more different muscles were recessed (p=0.001).

REFERENCES

Ruttum, MS. 2000. Effect of prior orbital decompression on outcome of strabismus surgery in patients with thyroid ophthalmopathy. *J AAPOS* 4:102-5.

Transactions 28th Meeting European Strabismological Association, de Faber (ed.)
 ISBN 90 265 1965 6

A Model for the Prediction of Outcomes of Recession / Resection Surgery for Primary Constant Esotropias

A. Kailasanathan, S. Mirza & R.D. Brown
University Hospital Of North Staffordshire, Stoke-On-Trent, United Kingdom

ABSTRACT: No strict guidelines exist for strabismus surgery because of the large degree of variation in outcome between surgeons. Trainees may only be able to predict outcome after experience is gained. We looked at the results of recession/ resection repairs for primary constant esotropias performed by one surgeon and his trainees. The results were calculated in prism dioptres of change per millimetre of surgery for both lateral rectus and medial rectus muscles. Regression analysis was performed to separate the relative effects of each muscle. This showed that the two muscles provided different amounts of correction per millimeter of surgery. We suggest that strabismus surgeons create individualized graphs/curves to serve as a model for predicting their outcome from surgery. This is useful when planning surgery and may also serve as a teaching aid.

KEYWORDS: primary constant esotropia, esotropia, surgery, recession, resection,

1 INTRODUCTION

No strict guidelines exist for strabismus surgery because of the variation in outcome between surgeons. Junior surgeons will only be able to predict outcomes after experience is gained. We propose that strabismus surgeons develop a dose response curve/graph/table to evaluate the results of their surgery. This would provide a framework for planning future surgery as well as for teaching juniors.

2 METHODS

We looked retrospectively at the results of uniocular recession/resection repairs for 88 patients with primary constant esotropias with and without an accommodative element performed by one surgeon and his trainees. We included patients who had childhood esotropia with onset of esotropia after 6 months of age. The management of amblyopia was independent of surgery. Patients were excluded if they had neurological disease, paralytic squints, previous strabismus surgery or had strabismus syndromes and pattern deviations. None of the patients underwent prism adaptation therapy. All patients had preoperative esotropia measurements the day before surgery and all measurements were taken with full refractive correction .Postoperative measurements were taken 2 – 6 weeks after surgery and once more all measurements were taken with full refractive correction.

The results were calculated as prism dioptres of change against millimetres of surgery performed. The variables of age at surgery, refractive error, medial rectus surgery, lateral rectus surgery and surgeon grade were subjected to regression analysis testing. The results were analysed to separate the relative effects of lateral rectus and medial rectus muscles.

3 RESULTS

The data followed a normal distribution pattern. Our results show that the lateral rectus and medial rectus muscles provide different amounts of correction per millimetre of surgery. The lateral rectus had more effect for distance angle than the medial rectus. The opposite was the case for the angle for near.

Table 1. Change in prism dioptres for distance

Lateral rectus resection (mm)		0	1	2	3	4	5	6	7	8	9
Medial rectus recession (mm)	0	-9	-5	-1	4	8	12	17	21	26	30
	1	-7	-3	2	6	10	15	19	23	28	32
	2	-5	-1	4	8	12	17	21	26	30	34
	3	-3	2	6	10	15	19	23	28	32	26
	4	-1	4	8	13	17	21	26	30	34	39
	5	2	6	10	15	19	23	28	32	36	41
	6	4	8	13	17	21	26	30	34	39	43
	7	6	10	15	19	23	28	32	36	41	45
	8	8	13	17	21	26	30	34	39	43	47
	9	10	15	19	23	28	32	36	41	45	50

Formula = -9.259 + (4.346 x lateral rectus resection) + (2.183 x medial rectus recession)

Residual SD = 6.45

68% of patients had an outcome within ±6.5 PD (1 standard deviation) of the predicted value

95% of patients had an outcome within ±13PD (2 standard deviations) of the predicted value

Table 2. Effects on distance angle in prism dioptres

Surgery (mm)	2	3	4	5	6	7	8	9	10
Lateral rectus resection	4.1	8.4	12.8	17.1	21.4	25.8	30.1	34.5	38.8
Medial rectus recession	-0.3	1.9	4.1	6.3	8.5	10.7	12.8	15.0	17.2

Table 3.Change in prism dioptres for near

Lateral rectus resection (mm)		0	1	2	3	4	5	6	7	8	9
Medial rectus recession (mm)	0	-12	-8	-5	-2	1	4	8	11	14	17
	1	-7	-4	-1	2	5	9	12	15	18	21
	2	-3	0	3	6	10	13	16	19	22	26
	3	1	4	7	11	14	17	20	23	27	30
	4	5	8	11	15	18	21	24	28	31	34
	5	9	12	16	19	22	25	28	32	35	38
	6	13	17	20	23	26	29	33	36	39	42
	7	18	21	24	27	30	34	37	40	43	46
	8	22	25	28	31	35	38	41	44	47	51
	9	26	29	32	36	39	42	45	48	52	55

Formula = -11.592 + (3.202 x lateral rectus resection) + (4.171 x medial rectus recession)

Residual SD = 8.5

68% of patients had an outcome within ±8.5 PD (1 standard deviation) of the predicted value

95% of patients had an outcome within ±17PD (2 standard deviations) of the predicted value

Table 4. Effects on near angle in prism dioptres

Surgery (mm)	2	3	4	5	6	7	8	9	10
Lateral rectus resection	0.6	3.8	7.0	10.2	13.4	16.6	19.8	23.0	26.2
Medial rectus recession	2.5	6.7	10.9	15.1	19.2	23.4	27.6	31.7	35.9

The effects of age at surgery, refractive error, surgeon grade and need for further surgery was insignificant.13.3% of patients needed further surgery.

4 DISCUSSION

We are only reporting the results of surgery by one surgeon and his trainees and not a new surgical formula.These results may not apply to other surgeons as there is a large variability in results based on technique. However, any one individual surgeons results may be predictable and our current system for predicting the results of strabismus surgery have evolved from those used in this study. Dose response curves have been created for bilateral medial rectus recession procedures by Mims (1986), Kushner (1987) and more recently by Tran (2002). However, as far as we are aware no such data have been produced for monocular recession/resection procedures although various recommendations have been published such as those of the American Academy of Ophthalmology (2002-2003).

A linear relationship was noted between the amount of surgery and the diopteric change in angle of esotropia. We note that Tran (2002) found an exponential relationship for bilateral medial recession repairs and we also note that Infeld (1993) did not find a significant change in results when varying the amount of lateral rectus resection. However, our findings may in part be as a result of the lack of data for large angle esotropias Large angle esotropias were recorded as >45 dioptres on many occasions because of difficulties measuring large angles in young children. Our data are therefore inadequate for these large angles as these patients were omitted from the study. Furthermore, the data for the esotropia angles below 12 dioptres and above 45 dioptres provided on the above tables were extrapolated by the computer based on the linear relationship found for surgery for esotropia with angles between 12 and 45 dioptres in size. Therefore, the lower and upper end of the figures provided above are probably inaccurate and we do not use them in planning our surgery.

The trainer and his trainees had comparable outcomes. This suggests that surgical results are related to similarities in technique. For distance angle, standard deviation was 6.5 while for near angle, standard deviation was 8.5 and these results are comparable to results published by Keenan (1993).

There are conflicting opinions on the factors that influence the results of surgery. .Like Kushner (1993), we found that refractive error did not influence our outcome. Age at surgery may be important for predicting outcomes for surgery for congenital esotropias (Bateman 1983) however, no such relationship was shown for primary constant esotropias.

5 CONCLUSION

It would be nice to think that multicentre studies would be able to provide an ideal graph or with an ideal 'normal range' for expected results from surgery which could be used for planning surgery. While individual results may vary, it is unlikely that the overall shape of the graph would vary widely between individual surgeons.

We suggest that trainers create similar personalised graphs and tables which may be used as teaching aids. We are looking at ways of evaluating our large angle esotropias more accurately. We would then like to continue this study prospectively.

REFERENCES

American Academy of Ophthalmology, 2002-2003. *Paediatric Ophthalmology and Strabismus* :166-167

Bateman, J.B., Parks, M.M. & Wheeler, N. 1983.Discriminant Analysis of Congenital Esotropia Surgery.*Ophthalmology* 1983;90:1146-1153

Infeld,D., Prior, C., Ryan, H. & O'Day, J.1993.The long term results of surgical correction Of childhood esotropia.*Australia and New Zealand Journal of Ophthalmology.* 1993;21(1):23-28

Keenan, J.M. & Willshaw, H.E. 1993.The Outcome of Strabismus Surgery in Childhood Esotropia. *Eye* 1993;7:341-345

Kushner, B.J. & Morton, G.V. 1986. The Effect of Surgical technique and Amount, Patient Age, Abduction Quality and Deviation, Magnitude on Surgical success rates in Infantile Esotropia. *Binocular Vision* 1987;2(1):25-40

Kushner, B.J., Fisher, M.R., Lucchese, N.J. & Morton, G.V. 1993. Factors *Influencing* Response to Strabismus Surgery. *Arch Ophthalmol.*1993;111:75-79

Mims, J.L., Treff, G. & Wood, R.C. 1986. Variability of *Strabismus* Surgery for Acquired Esotropia. *Arch. Ophthalmol.*1986;104:1780-1782

Tran, H.M., Mims, J.L. & Wood, R.C. 2002. A New Dose-Response curve for Bilateral Medial Rectus Recessions for Infantile Esotropia. *JAAPOS* 2002;6:112-9

Transactions 28th Meeting European Strabismological Association, de Faber (ed.)
© 2004 European Strabismological Association, ISBN 90 265 1965 6

Globe preserving treatment of an unilateral retinoblastoma by brachychemoradiotherapy

G.Langmann , A.Langmann , * P.Sovinz & * C. Urban
Department of Ophthalmology, University Graz, Austria, Department of Pediatric Haematology/ Oncology, Unviversity Graz, Austria*

ABSTRACT: A 2 years old female was admitted for possible globe preserving treatment of an unilateral retinoblastoma (12 x 19 x 13 mm), after the mother had noticed leucocoria in some gazing position of the eye. The child received 2 cylces of Cyclophosphamid, Carboplatin and Etoposid. Between the first and second course a Ruthenium 106 plaque with a duration of 14 days and a low dose rate was sutured at the base of the tumor. After a follow up of 13 months tumor regression could be observed to a tumor prominence of 3,4 mm and a base of 9 x 4 mm with a typical cottage cheese regression pattern. After 5 months of occlusion therapy visual acuity is now 20/32. Conclusion: Even in a large unilateral retinoblastoma with localized vitreous seeding the globe and some useful central vision may be preserved with new treatment modalities like combined chemotherapy and Ruthenium 106 plaque brachytherapy (chemoirradiation or brachychemoradiotherapy) thus avoiding enucleation or external beam irradiation. KEYWORDS:Unilateral retinoblastoma, primary chemotherapy, Ruthenium 106 brachytherapy, brachychemoradiotherapy.

1 INTRODUCTION

A decreasing trend in enucleation has been found in retinoblastoma over the past decades (96-75% (9). In medium sized tumors thermochemotherapy or thermoradiotherapy (6) have replaced external beam irradiation to a wide extend since second cancers in the field of irradiation have been found (1). Limitation to primary brachytherapy with Ruthenium 106 is a prominence of 5 mm (5) , in case of Jodine 125 eight millimeters tumor thickness (10) .
We report a case of successful treatment of a 12 mm prominent stage 4 b retinoblastoma treated by a low dose rate Ruthenium 106 plaque and simultaneous intravenous chemotherapy thus preserving reading vision.

1. CASE REPORT

A 2 years old female was referred to our hospital with a 12 x 19 x 13 mm exophytic unilateral retinoblastoma (figure.1), after the mother had noticed leucocoria in some gazing position.
Treatment: In a first step intravenous chemotherapy at the Department of Pediatric Haematology / Oncology was initiated according to a regimen proposed by Bornfeld and Havers (2) (table 1). The patient received the first course of Vincristin 0,05 mg /kg, Cyclophosphamid 40 mg/ kg and Carboplatin 10 mg / kg. 4 days later a Ruthenium 106 CCB plaque (diameter 20 mm, dose rate 2,47 Gy/ h) was sutured at the base of the tumor, surrounding 1 mm tumor-free healthy retina (duration 15 days, total dose (base) 888 Gy, dose (apex) 18 Gy, 50 Gy at 7,6 mm). Plaque therapy was uneventful. 22 days after the first course chemotherapy was continued with the second course consisting of Vincristion 0,05 mg/ kg, Cyclophosphamid 40 mg/kg and Etoposid 15 mg/kg. The whole regimen was repeated once, starting with course 1 at day 64, amounting in a total of 6 courses of chemotherapy (table 1).

During the following 13 months tumor height regressed to a prominence of 3,4 mm and a base of 9 x 4 mm. Initially a type II regression pattern was seen, followed by a type I (cottage cheese regression pattern - figure. 2) . After 5 months of occlusion therapy visual acuity is now 20/ 32.

2. COMMENT

Successful tumor regression in spite of the fact, that the tumor in our child exceeded the maximum prominence for brachytherapy (5,10) was due to 3 possible mechanism of the treatment:

1. Breakdown of the retinal blood barrier and the vessels of the retinoblastoma by radiotherapy with a better penetration of the chemotherapeutic agent into the tumor. Wilson (13) found a significantly higher level of carboplatin in the vitreous cavity 24 hours after cryotherapy of the retina.
2. Combined cytotoxic effect of the beta irradiation and chemotherapeutic drug.
3. Preservation of the central vision due to the low dose rate and long duration of the beta source Ruthenium 106.

1. CONCLUSION

Combinded low dose rate Ruthenium 106 brachytherapy with chemotherapy may be another treatment option for large retinoblastomas as an alternative to percutaneous teletherapy or enucleation.

REFERENCES

Abramson, D.H & Frank, C.M. 1998. Second nonocular tumors in survivors of bilateral retinoblastoma: a possible age effect on radiation- related risk. *Ophthalmology* 105: 573- 579, discussion 579-580

Bornhfeld, N. & Lommatzsch, P.K., Havers, W., Schüler, A. Retinoblastoma. In: Lommatzsch PK(ed).*Ophthalmologische Onkologie. Stuttgart 1999; 329- 361. Enke Verlag*

Bornfeld, N., & Schüler, A. Bechrakis, Henze, N., Havers, W .1997. Preliminary Results of Primary Chemotherapy in Retinoblastoma. *Klin.Pädiatr*. 209216- 221.

Gombos,D. & Kelly, A., Coen,P., Kinston, J., Hungerford,J. 2002 Retinoblastoma treated with primary chemotherapy alone: the significance of tumor size, location and age. *Br J Ophthalmol* 86 (1): 80 - 83

Lommatzsch, P.K. 1977 . Beta irradiation of retinoblastoma with 106 Ru/Rh applicators.. *Mod. Probl. Ophthalmol.* 18: 128 - 136

Murphree AL & Villablanca J.G., Deegan III, W.F. et al. 1996. Chemotherapy plus local treatment in the management of intraocular retinoblastoma. *Arch.Ophthalmol* 114: 1348- 1356

Murray, T.G.& Cicciarelli, C.M. ,McCabe, et al. 1997. In vitro efficacy of carboplatin and hyperthermia in a murine retinoblastoma cell line. *Invest Ophthalmo Vis sci* 38: 2516-2522

Shields,C.L. & Santos, M.C., Diniz, W., Gündüz, K., Mercady, G., Cater, J.R., Shields, J.A. 1999. Thermotherapy for Retinoblastoma. *Arch Ophthalmol* 117: 885- 893

Shields, J.A., Shields, C.L., Sicalingam;V., 1989 Decreasing frquenzy of enuclation in patients with retinoblastom. *Am J Ophthalmol*; 108: 185- 188

Shields, C.L., Shields, J.A. Minell, S.1993. Plaque radiotherapy in the management of retinoblastoma. *Am J Ophthalmol* 100: 185-188

11.Shields, C.L., Shields, J.A., 1999. Recent Developments in the Management of Retinoblastoma. J *Pediatr. Ophthalmol Stabismus* 36: 8-18

12 White, L. 1991. Chemotherapy for retinoblastoma. Where do we go from here ?: A review of published literature and meeting abstracts, including discussions during the Vth Internatinal Symposium on Retinoblastoma. October 1990. *Ophthalmic Pediatr.Genet.* 12 :115- 130.
13 Wilson, T.W. & Chan, H.S., Moselhy, .G. et al. 1996 Penetration of chemotherapy into vitreous is increased by cryotherapy and cylosporin in rabbits. *Arch Opthalmol* 114 : 1390- 1395.

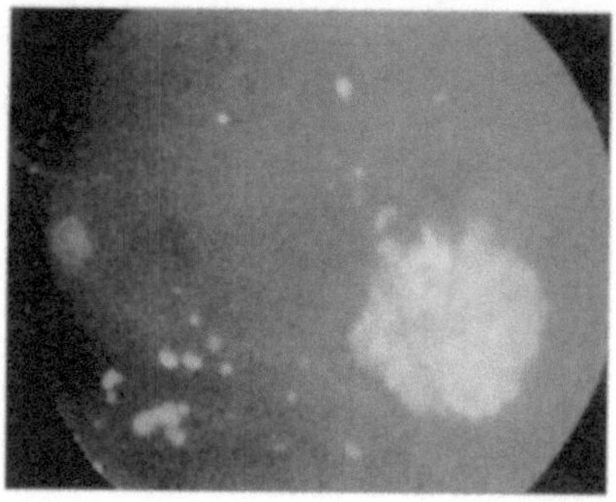

Figure 1. 12 mm prominent exophytic retinoblastoma with adjacent subretinal fluid at the posterior pole prior therapy.

Figure 2. 16 months after brachychemoradiotherapy: cottage cheese regression pattern, prominence (A - scan echography: 3,8 mm, visual acuity: 20/ 32)

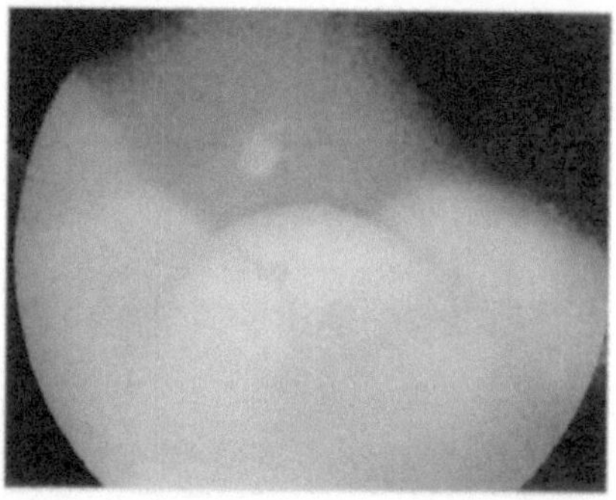

TABLE 1
Chemotherapy regimen as proposed by Bornfeld and Havers (2)

Course 1 (day1+64)	Vincristine 0,05 mg/ kg	Cyclophoshamid 40 mg/ kg	Carboplatin 10 mg/ kg
Course 2 (day 22+86)	Vincristine 0,05 mg/ kg	Cyclophoshamid 40 mg/ kg	Etoposid 15 mg/ kg
Course 3 (day43+107)	Vincristine 0,05 mg/ kg	Etoposid 15 mg/ kg	Carboplatin 10 mg/ kg

Transactions 28th Meeting European Strabismological Association, de Faber (ed.)
© 2004 European Strabismological Association, ISBN 90 265 1965 6

The dragged-Fovea Diplopia Syndrome

David L. Guyton, MD, M. Elaine De Pool, MD, Sheena O. Broome, OC(C), COMT
The Zanvyl Krieger Children 's Eye Center at the Wilmer Institute The Johns Hopkins University School of Medicine, Baltimore, Maryland, U. S. A.

Objectives:To identify the clinical characteristics of the "dragged-fovea diplopia (DFD)syndrome, " to introduce a simple diagnostic test to identify this syndrome, and to provide a simple treatment option to provide relief from the diplopia in some of these cases.

Methods:We reviewed the records of our patients with a diagnosis of maculopathy, internal limiting membrane contracture, or "dragged fovea, "and complaint of diplopia.

Results:Fifty-two affected eyes in 47 patients met the criteria for inclusion in the study. In 32 patients the small-field central fusion test (viewing a single white letter on the black background of a distance visual acuity display)showed central fusion with the room lights off and peripheral fusion with central diplopia with the room lights on. Diplopia recurred despite prism trial, as the patient adapted to the prism power in seconds to minutes. In 15 eyes, a pars plana vitrectomy with membrane peeling had been performed. In 6 of these patients, the diplopia was noticed only after the pars plana vitrectomy with membrane peeling. In 17 of the 32 patients, diplopia was effectively reli- eved using a piece of Scotch TM "Satin TM"tape.

Conclusions:The dragged-fovea diplopia syndrome consists of central diplopia in the presence of peripheral fusion that does not respond to prism therapy or eye muscle surgery. The small-field central fusion test ("lights on/off test")can be used to confirm the diagnosis in patients with clinical characteristics compatible with the DFD syndrome. A strip of Scotch "Satin"tape, applied vertically on the rear surface of the spectacle lens of the non-preferred eye, provides an aesthetic form of monocular occlusion. Epiretinal membrane peeling surgery can unmask or precipitate the develop- ment of the DFD syndrome.

References: 1. Burgess C, Roper-Hall G, Burde R. Binocular diplopia associated with subretinal neovascular membranes. Arch Ophthalmol 1980;98:311-317. 2. Bixenman WW, Joffe L. Binocular diplopia associated with retinal wrinkling. J Pediatr Ophthalmol Strabismus 1984;21:215-219. 3. Steffen H, Holz FG, Lolling GH. Macular dystrophy as a retinal model of fixation disparity. Strabismus 1996;4(4):179-184.

Transactions 28th Meeting European Strabismological Association, de Faber (ed.)
© 2004 European Strabismological Association, ISBN 90 265 1965 6

Binocular outcome of EOM-surgery for esotropia with onset later than one year of age

Elisabeth Schulz, MD, PhD;Beate Schmal, CO;Alexander Fell, MD;Kristin Rettig, CO
Orthoptic Department, University Eye Clinic, D-20246 Hamburg, Martinistrasse 52

Background:Esotropia of sudden onset below the age of 3 years is rarely reported to show normal binocular vision before or even after surgery. High resolution stereopsis was demonstrated in normal infants in the first year of life.

Purpose:To investigate the quality of binocular vision after EOMsurgery in infants and children with onset of strabismus after their first year of life.

Patients and methods:We evaluated the files of 83 patients, in whom the reported/observed onset of esotropia was later than 1 year of age and who were referred for EOM surgery to our Clinic. Onset of strabismus was minimum 1 year 1month, maximum 8 years 7 months, mean 3 years 4 months. Patients older than 5 years at onset of squint were neglected in the further study. Patients with alternate day squint and with DVD were rejected. Binocular vision was classified as:Lang I pos, Titmus Ring 6 pos (minimum), Titmus animals/fly pos, Bagolini striated glasses pos, no bino- cular vision.

Results:62 patients were remaining. They were emmetropic to hyperopic (minimum 0, maximum +7, 0 D, mean+2. 6D, SD 1, 58). High cylindric refractive errors were rare. (minimum 0, maximum -4, 5 D, mean -0. 4 D, SD 0, 7D).
There was no correlation of refractive error to onset of strabismus. Surgery was done minimum 0. 8 month, maximum 353 months , mean 44 months after onset of strabismus. The surgical outcome showed
Orthotropia in 19 patients (27. 4%)
Microtropia in 17 patients (30. 6%)
Exodeviation*in 7 patients (11. 3%)*all kinds
Esotropia in 19 patients (30. 6%)
Binocular vision in the first days after surgery was demonstrated to be
Lang pos 12 (19. 7%)patients
Titmus Ring 6 --
Titmus fly/animals 7 (11. 4%)
Bagolini striated glasses24 (39. 0%)
29 patients could be seen by us or reported on by the ophthalmologist 's office months later. 8 additional patients had improved to Lang pos, 5 to Titmus pos. This adds to confirmed 32, 8 % Lang pos. and 19, 7%Titmus pos. out of 61 patients. Good binocular qualitiy was more frequent in later onset strabismus (3 years), but positive Lang-test could be achieved in individual cases (3 out of 22)with earlier onset (1. 5 years).

Discussion:Good or fair binocular vision can be achieved after EOMsurgery in patients with relatively later onset esotropia (suspected normosensory esotropia in a less strict sense). These patients seem to be more frequent than reported normosensory esotropics in a strict sense (deDecker: 18%in ET starting above 3 years of age). Referral for surgery is very late in general. This may account for less favorite binocular outcome in most of the relatively early onset cases (below 3 years).

Transactions 28th Meeting European Strabismological Association, de Faber (ed.)

Correlation between asthenopic symptoms and different measurements of convergence and reading ability

Yair Morad, MD, (1)Ori Segal, MD, (1)Robert Lederman, FCOVD, (2)Daniela Atzmon, CO, (1)Emmanuelle Azoulay, CO, (1)Isaac Avni, MD
(1) Department of Ophthalmology, Assaf Harofeh Medical Center (1)and Vision Center, Efrat (2)

Purpose:To find correlations between asthenopic symptoms, reading skills and convergence amplitude, as assessed in various methods.

Methods:66 children aged 8-10 years were examined. Convergence was evaluated using 1)Non-accommodative target at near and distance;2)A near computerized stereogram and 3) Measurement of the near point of convergence (NPC). Reading ability was examined by:1)A reading comprehension test in which children had to answer questions regarding a paragraph they read and 2)The Developmental Eye Movement Test (DEM), which evaluates saccadic speed and accuracy. Asthenopic symptoms were scored by an Asthenopic Symptoms Questionnaire.

Results:Asthenopic symptoms score was correlated with the near point of convergence (r=-0. 4, p=0. 003), convergence on a near stereogram (r=0. 38, p=0. 01)and distant light (r=0. 27, p=0. 04)but not with convergence on a near non-accommodative target (r=0. 07, p=0. 6). The DEM score was correlated with the asthenopic symptoms score (r=-0. 32, p=0. 01), but the reading comprehension test score was not (r=0. 12, p=0. 4). There was correlation, however, between the time for completi- on of the reading comprehension test and the asthenopic symptoms score (r=-0. 39, p=0. 006).

Conclusion:Asthenopic symptoms score was correlated with convergence amplitude as measured while accommodation is controlled and with automatic reading skills as measured by the DEM. Further study on a larger cohort of children is needed to evaluate the usefulness of the Asthenopic Symptoms Questionnaire as a screening tool for children with convergence insufficiency.

Transactions 28th Meeting European Strabismological Association, de Faber (ed.)
© 2004 European Strabismological Association, ISBN 90 265 1965 6

Duane retraction syndrome –case report

Susanna Pelle, Agnes Sallai, Katalin Virágos Kis
Department of Ophthalmology of Pándy Kálmán County Hospital, Gyula, Hungary.

Introduction: The Duane retraction syndrome (DRS)is an autosomal dominant hereditary disea-se, with a sporadical manifestation. The cause of pathological innervation of muscles of the bulbus is due to the congenital defect of intracranial centers. Instead of sixth cranial nerve, the lateral rec- tus muscles are innervated by the third cranial nerve. Main symptoms are: decreased abduction and adduction of the affected eye, narrowing of palpebral fissure and retraction of the bulbus oculi. There are three types by Huber according the clinical symptoms. We present a girl of 6 years suffering a bilateral form of DRS.

Methods: Urgent ophthalmological examination of the patient was carried out according to the pe- diatric departement, where the girl had been hospitalised because of prompt by symptomes of gid- diness, trembling, numbness of limbs and palpitation, accompaniing recurrent infection of the up- per part of respiratory tract. Bilateral paresis of abducent nerves was detected and cerebral pro- cess was suggested. The ophthalmolagical examination detected DRS. Detailed anamnestical data from the mother conserning to other symptoms and previous fine signs, data of the members of the family were asked. Visual acuity, refraction, eye movements, Lang test, refraction of the eyes, audiometry, repeated neurological examination, cardiological and MRI and routine laboratory test showed normal results.

Results: Very fine facial asymmetry, mild amblyopie of the left eye, minimal hyperopia of both eyes with astigmatismus on the left side. Normal fundus and optic nerve, positiv Lang stereotest were detected. Eye movements: parallell state in primary position, totally paretic abducent muscles, di- minished adduction and retraction on both side with narrowing of the palpebral fissure.

Conclusion: The possibility of DRS in cases of paretic abducent nerves in childhood is worthwile to be more commonly known, mainly in other, sometimes exciting symptoms, which may show se- rious intracranial processes. The relative rarity of the bilateral DRS emphasizes the interesting ma-nifestation of our case.

References: Duane A. : Congenital deficiency of abduction, associated with impairment of adducti- on retraciton movements contraction of the palpebral fissure and oblique movements, of the eye. 1905 /classical article/. Arch Ophthalmol 114, 1255-1256 /1996/. Kanski J. J. : Clinical Ophthalmolgy. Butterworth-Heinemann Linacre Hause Jordan Hill, Oxford, p. 448. /1994/.

Transactions 28th Meeting European Strabismological Association, de Faber (ed.)

Acute-onset adult esotropia: Bielschowsky type

Pérez, Inés MD, Fernández, Marta MD.
Centro Médico POVISA. Vigo, Spain.

Introduction:We report a case of acute-onset esotropia with intermittent deviation and diplopia associated with diminished visual acuity secondary to an accommodative spasm.

Methods:A 26-year-old woman, in her 29 weeks of pregnancy, was referred with diplopia. Motility examination revealed intermittent esotropia of 45 PD. There was a minimal limitation of abduction in her right eye. No other ocular or neurologic disturbances were found. The patient returns to the office in six months. The motility examination did not change but her visu- al acuity have diminished to 0, 1 in both eyes and accommodative spasm was diagnosed.

Results:The study was negative for neurologic disorders, Myastenia Gravis/Eaton-Lambert and congenital myopathy. Chemodenervation (BOTOX ®)was performed without success. The intermittent esotropia and diplopia remain two years later but she does not complain and refuse surgery.

Conclusion:Acute-onset adult esotropia may be secondary to a sixth cranial nerve palsy or another neurologic disease presenting as comitant esotropia. The case we report did not show a significant incomitance and deviation and diplopia remained intermittent. The diagnostic was uncertain but the motility exploration and the presence of an ac- commodative spasm make us consider a Bielschowsky type esotropia.

References: Hoyt CS, Fredrick DR. Serious neurologic disease presenting as comitant esotropia. In: Rosenbaum, Santiago, editor. Clinical Strabismus Management. Principles and surgical techniques. Philadelphia:W. B. Saunders Company;1999. p. 152-158.

AUTHOR INDEX